SOLVING PATIENT PROBLEMS:

Ambulatory
Care

SOLVING PATIENT PROBLEMS:

Ambulatory Care

Editor
Marjorie A. Bowman, M.D., M.P.A.

Professor and Chair
Department of Family Practice and
Community Medicine
University of Pennsylvania
Philadelphia, Pennsylvania

Associate Editor
Judith A. Fisher, M.D.

Assistant Professor
Department of Family Practice and
Community Medicine
University of Pennsylvania
Philadelphia, Pennsylvania

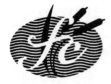

Typesetter: Pagesetters, Brattleboro, VT
Printer: Port City Press, Baltimore, MD

Distributors:

United States and Canada
  Blackwell Science, Inc.
  Commerce Place
  350 Main Street
  Malden, MA 02148
  Telephone orders: 800-215-1000 or 781-388-8250
  Fax orders: 781-388-8270

Australia
  Blackwell Science, PTY LTD.
  54 University Street
  Carlton, Victoria 3053
  Telephone orders: 61-39-347-0300
  Fax orders: 61-39-347-5001

Outside North America and Australia
  Blackwell Science, LTD.
  c/o Marston Book Service, LTD.
  P.O. Box 269
  Abingdon Oxon, OX 14 4XN England
  Telephone orders: 44-1-235-465500
  Fax orders: 44-1-235-465555

2 3 4 5 6 7 8 9 10

Contents

Contents

Contributors

Mark D. Andrews, M.D.
Assistant Professor
Department of Family and Community Medicine
Wake Forest University School of Medicine
Winston-Salem, North Carolina

Lisa M. Bellini, M.D.
Assistant Professor
Program Director
Department of Medicine
University of Pennsylvania School of Medicine
Philadelphia, Pennsylvania

Amy J. Behrman, M.D.
Assistant Professor
Division of Occupational Medicine
University of Pennsylvania School of Medicine
Philadelphia, Pennsylvania

Marjorie A. Bowman, M.D., M.P.A.
Professor and Chair
Department of Family Practice and Community Medicine
University of Pennsylvania School of Medicine
Philadelphia, Pennsylvania

Kent D. W. Bream, M.D.
Clinical Instructor
Department of Family Practice and Community Medicine
University of Pennsylvania School of Medicine
Philadelphia, Pennsylvania

Russell S. Breish, M.D.
Clinical Assistant Professor
Family Practice Center
Chestnut Hill Hospital
Philadelphia, Pennsylvania

Victor Caraballo, M.D.
Assistant Professor
Department of Emergency Medicine
University of Pennsylvania School of Medicine
Philadelphia, Pennsylvania

Robert K. Cato, M.D.
Assistant Professor
Department of Medicine
University of Pennsylvania School of Medicine
Philadelphia, Pennsylvania

Jason D. Christie, M.D.
Assistant Instructor
Department of Medicine
University of Pennsylvania School of Medicine
Philadelphia, Pennsylvania

Robin M. Clemons, M.D., M.P.H.
Assistant Professor
Department of Family Medicine
University of Medicine and Dentistry of New Jersey
Stratford, New Jersey

Elizabeth M. Datner, M.D.
Assistant Professor
Department of Emergency Medicine
University of Pennsylvania School of Medicine
Philadelphia, Pennsylvania

Peter DeLong, M.D.
Assistant Instructor
Department of Medicine
University of Pennsylvania School of Medicine
Philadelphia, Pennsylvania

Kevin S. Ferentz, M.D.
Associate Professor
Department of Family Medicine
University of Maryland School of Medicine
Baltimore, Maryland

Judith A. Fisher, M.D.
Assistant Professor
Department of Family Practice and Community Medicine
University of Pennsylvania School of Medicine
Philadelphia, Pennsylvania

Kevin M. Fosnocht, M.D.
Assistant Professor
Division of General Internal Medicine
University of Pennsylvania School of Medicine
Philadelphia, Pennsylvania

Marilyn V. Howarth, M.D.
Assistant Professor
Division of Occupational Medicine
University of Pennsylvania School of Medicine
Philadelphia, Pennsylvania

William H. Hubbard, M.D.
Assistant Professor
Department of Family and Community Medicine
Wake Forest University School of Medicine
Winston-Salem, North Carolina

Julienne K. Kirk, Pharm.D.
Assistant Professor
Department of Family and Community Medicine
Wake Forest University School of Medicine
Winston-Salem, North Carolina

Mark P. Knudson, M.D., M.S.P.H.
Associate Professor
Department of Family and Community Medicine
Wake Forest University School of Medicine
Winston-Salem, North Carolina

Katherine C. Krause, M.D.
Department of Family Practice and Community Medicine
University of Pennsylvania School of Medicine
Philadelphia, Pennsylvania

Steven C. Larson, M.D.
Assistant Professor
Department of Emergency Medicine
University of Pennsylvania School of Medicine
Philadelphia, Pennsylvania

Judith A. Long, M.D.
Robert Wood Johnson Clinical Scholar
Yale University School of Medicine
New Haven, Connecticut

Marc W. McKenna, M.D.
Clinical Associate Professor
Family Practice Center
Chestnut Hill Hospital
Philadelphia, Pennsylvania

Gaetano P. Monteleone, Jr., M.D.
Assistant Professor
Department of Family and Community Medicine
Wake Forest University School of Medicine
Winston-Salem, North Carolina

Richard A. Neill, M.D.
Assistant Professor
Department of Family Practice and Community Medicine
University of Pennsylvania School of Medicine
Philadelphia, Pennsylvania

James A. Nicholson, M.D.
Clinical Instructor
Department of Family Practice and Community Medicine
University of Pennsylvania School of Medicine
Philadelphia, Pennsylvania

David E. Nicklin, M.D.
Assistant Professor
Department of Family Practice and Community Medicine
University of Pennsylvania School of Medicine
Philadelphia, Pennsylvania

Kevin A. Pearce, M.D., M.P.H.
Associate Professor
Department of Family and Community Medicine
Wake Forest University School of Medicine
Winston-Salem, North Carolina

Valerie P. Pendley, M.D.
Clinical Assistant Professor
Family Practice Center
Chestnut Hill Hospital
Philadelphia, Pennsylvania

Eileen E. Reynolds, M.D.
Assistant Professor
Division of General Internal Medicine
University of Pennsylvania School of Medicine
Philadelphia, Pennsylvania

Iris M. Reyes, M.D.
Assistant Professor
Department of Emergency Medicine
University of Pennsylvania School of Medicine
Philadelphia, Pennsylvania

Ilene M. Rosen, M.D.
Assistant Instructor
Department of Medicine
University of Pennsylvania School of Medicine
Philadelphia, Pennsylvania

Matthew H. Rusk, M.D.
Assistant Professor
Division of General Internal Medicine
University of Pennsylvania School of Medicine
Philadelphia, Pennsylvania

David A. Simpson, M.D.
Assistant Director
Family Medicine Residency Program
Christiana Care Health Services
Wilmington, Delaware

Robert V. Smith, M.D.
Medical Director
Cathedral Village
Philadelphia, Pennsylvania

Sarah A. Stahmer, M.D.
Staff Physician
Emergency Department
Cooper Medical Center
Camden, New Jersey

Marcia B. Szewczyk, M.D.
Assistant Professor
Department of Family and Community Medicine
Wake Forest University School of Medicine
Winston-Salem, North Carolina

Laure L. Veet, M.D.
Assistant Professor
Division of Medicine
Veterans Affairs Medical Center
Philadelphia, Pennsylvania

R. Parker Ward, M.D.
Assistant Instructor
Department of Medicine
University of Pennsylvania School of Medicine
Philadelphia, Pennsylvania

James T. Whitfill, M.D.
Assistant Instructor
Department of Medicine
University of Pennsylvania School of Medicine
Philadelphia, Pennsylvania

Preface

The goal of this text is to help third- and fourth-year medical students diagnose and treat common medical problems in adults in ambulatory settings. It is one of a series of books that emphasizes clinical reasoning through *key symptom and sign differentiation* among categories of illnesses and *pattern recognition*. The other books in the series concern internal medicine, obstetrics and gynecology, pediatrics, surgery, and psychiatry.

Key symptoms and signs help to differentiate among categories of illnesses (and among individual illnesses). For example, fever, often a key symptom or sign, is associated mostly with infection and inflammation (categories of illnesses). Expert diagnosticians often use these key symptoms first to categorize illness broadly and then to differentiate individual diseases within the broad category. For example, back pain that is worse with specific movements suggests a musculoskeletal origin rather than infection; the diagnostician then attempts to differentiate important causes of musculoskeletal pain, such as rib fracture or strain. A key sign to differentiate rib fracture is localized tenderness over a small area of rib.

Pattern recognition is defined as identifying the combination of symptoms, signs, and patient characteristics that are commonly associated with an illness. Pattern recognition is frequently used by experienced physicians and often distinguishes the decision-making process of the expert from that of the novice physician. For example, an overweight middle-aged woman complaining of lethargy, dry skin, and constipation who has an enlarged thyroid is often quickly recognized by an expert physician as having hypothyroidism, but the student may get lost in the long differential diagnoses of each of the individual complaints. It is the recognition of patterns that helps the physician quickly determine that thyroid tests would confirm the diagnosis.

Of course, patterns are rarely absolutely specific. The recognition of the patterns can lead to more specific testing or trials of appropriate medication, but the physician needs to keep in mind that patients may not have the disease suggested by the pattern.

This text is divided into three sections. Section I presents common patient complaints, discusses key associated signs and symptoms, provides tables of common patterns of symptoms and signs associated with illnesses, and presents several patient cases. Section II provides specifics on the diagnosis of common medical illnesses of adults seen in the ambulatory care setting and gives succinct summaries of treatment options. Section III consists of a table of commonly used drugs and their uses. Because drug information books often only cite the approved uses as specified by the Food and Drug Administration, this table provides a quick reference that considers the potential patient problems for which a given drug is used.

MARJORIE A. BOWMAN, M.D., M.P.A.

Introduction

One of the major problems in medical education is that the traditional approach (memory-based approach) to educating future physicians inadequately prepares them for clinical problem-solving. Thus, problem-based learning was designed to place the teaching of content (and memorization) and problem-solving skills on an equal footing. Surveys of both traditional and problem-based educational programs have determined the following: most students in traditional programs feel that more than 50% of what they learn is memorized without understanding; however, most students in problem-based programs feel that less than 20% of what they learn is memorized without understanding. Unfortunately, because of the deficiencies in the traditional (memory-based) approach to medicine, students are handicapped by their memorization of large amounts of information that they are unable to apply to clinical problems.

These books are designed to help the reader develop an approach to clinical problem-solving. While traditional medical education demands that students memorize vast amounts of information without understanding, problem-based learning is based on the concept of practicing the process of problem-solving while acquiring the knowledge (content) used in the process. George Bordage, M.D.[1] states in his article "Elaborated Knowledge" that "less is better for beginning students when introducing new material"; that is, in order for the student to be able to organize information for later recall, less information, preferably using prototypical case presentations, must be provided so that students are able to understand, incorporate, and then use what they learn. Students who have the most trouble with clinical reasoning seem to have a poorly organized knowledge base, making rational approaches to patient problems almost impossible.

There is no question that knowledge is important in problem-solving. The more the student knows, the better he or she can test the hypotheses that are entertained. It is the quality of the hypotheses and the skill in testing them that distinguish the expert from the novice. Failure to consider more than one hypotheses is one of

[1] Bordage G: Elaborated knowledge: a key to successful diagnostic thinking. *Acad Med* 69:883–885, 1994. George Bordage, M.D., is Professor and Director of Graduate Studies in the Department of Medical Education at the College of Medicine, University of Illinois at Chicago, Chicago, Illinois.

the basic deficiences of inexperience. One of the goals of this text is to help the student move from novice to expert in this critical area of medical diagnosis.

The purpose of the *Solving Patient Problems Series* is to assist students at all levels in developing their clinical problem-solving or reasoning skills by leading them through the clinical reasoning process around common presenting complaints in the various clinical rotations. The most common diseases that students are likely to encounter given the chief complaints are presented. These prototypical diseases are the foundation upon which the student may then begin to build a more extensive differential. Only by comparing and contrasting the diagnostic features of two or more common diseases can students build a knowledge base that will allow the inclusion of other possible causes of the same complaint, thereby moving from the prototypical problems to more complex problems and then to life-threatening problems that must not be overlooked.

In no way is this text meant to be inclusive but rather a supplement, guide, and aid to the success of students as diagnosticians. It is deliberately pocket-sized to be carried on clinical rotations. More extensive reading about patients is necessary. However, facts learned about diseases in the context of patient presentations are bound to be easier to retain and retrieve. What seems to be "intuition" and part of the "art" of medicine is actually a combination of experience and a very highly organized knowledge base, which allows physicians to differentiate quickly between differential diagnoses—a necessary skill that this text has been designed to help students develop.

S. Scott Obenshain, M.D.[2]

[2]S. Scott Obenshain, M.D., is the Associate Dean for Undergraduate Medical Education and Professor of Pediatrics and Family and Community Medicine at the University of New Mexico School of Medicine, Albuquerque, New Mexico.

SECTION I
Pattern Recognition of Symptoms

CHAPTER 1
Chief Complaint: Headache

David E. Nicklin, M.D.

CASE 1-1

INITIAL PRESENTATION

M. White, a 30-year-old man, has had a fronto-occipital headache several days each week for the past month. He has had similar headaches occasionally in the past. He is under increased stress at work, and the headaches come on during the day. He recently had a severe one after arguing with his wife. There is no history of aura before onset, nausea, vomiting, or fever. Physical examination is normal.

What is the first task that a physician should do when presented with a patient complaining of a headache?

Discussion

There are several essential tasks in evaluating the patient with a headache. The first is to evaluate for life-threatening causes and start emergent care if they are found. If none are found, the next task is to determine the likely cause of the headache and begin treatment for symptomatic relief. Also, it is important in all visits to ask patients about their fears. Many patients with headaches worry about brain tumors. If evaluation shows other causes, the patients should be reassured that their headache symptoms are inconsistent with a brain tumor.

Headache diagnoses requiring emergency treatment include meningitis, encephalitis, subarachnoid hemorrhage, hypertensive encephalopathy, temporal arteritis, and intracranial neoplasm

> Headaches requiring emergency treatment: meningitis, intracranial hemorrhage, temporal arteritis, increased intracranial pressure

with increased intracranial pressure. A brief history and survey for fever, neck stiffness, depressed level of consciousness, temporal tenderness in the elderly, severely elevated blood pressure, and papilledema will exclude these causes in most patients.

Most Common Causes of Headache Tension Migraine	A thorough history and physical examination usually reveals the cause of the headache. Common causes of chronic, recurrent headache include tension and migraine—typical and atypical. Common causes of acute, nonemergent headache are sinusitis and viral illnesses.

KEY SYMPTOMS, SIGNS, AND OTHER FACTORS

The *historical pattern* and *location* of a headache may indicate its cause. Headaches occurring over a period of months are usually caused by tension or migraine. Migraine headaches often first appear in adolescence. If there is a history of trauma, chronic headaches also can be postconcussion or caused by a subdural hematoma. Having had similar headaches in the remote past strongly suggests a benign source of headache, such as tension or migraine. New, acute headache suggests urgent diagnoses as discussed above.

Tension headaches tend to be frontal, occipital, or in both locations. The classic migraine headache is unilateral, as are cluster headaches. Sinus headaches are often located over the maxillary or frontal areas. A very focal headache may signify a neoplasm.

Increased emotional stress often causes tension headache. Migraine headaches may be triggered by particular foods or stress and may be related to the menstrual cycle.

Headaches that occur yearly in the same season suggest that a cluster headache or *seasonal allergies* may be the cause.

Many patients with migraine headaches have first-degree relatives with migraine headaches, suggesting that there is a *family history* involved.

Headaches may be a presenting symptom of *depression*. Migraine headaches are common in depressed patients.

Upper respiratory tract infection and sinus congestion also may cause headache. A history of head trauma and alcohol use with blackouts suggests a *subdural hematoma*.

An *aura*, a sensation that a headache is about to occur before the actual pain begins, is highly suggestive of migraine. The most common aura is a flickering in part of the visual field. A transient focal neurologic deficit followed by severe headache suggests a migraine headache. Eighty percent of migraine headaches are not preceded by aura.

Nausea and vomiting are nonspecific findings but suggest that the headache is severe. They commonly occur in typical migraine headaches and are frequently seen with benign viral illnesses.

A *stiff neck* or nuchal rigidity suggests meningitis or subarachnoid hemorrhage. Mild stiffness can be seen in tension headaches with spasm of paracervical spine muscles.

Fever suggests infection such as acute sinusitis, meningitis, or Rocky Mountain spotted fever. However, any high fever can cause headache.

Blood pressure is often modestly elevated due to pain. Moderate blood pressure elevation will not cause headache. Blood pressures above 180/110 mm Hg may cause headache.

Blurring of disk margin suggests *increased intracranial pressure* as a result of a brain tumor, other space-occupying lesions, or a pseudo-tumor. Retinal hemorrhages and exudates are generally seen in hypertensive encephalopathy.

Fixed *neurologic deficits* are not seen with common benign causes of headache and suggest a brain tumor. Acute stroke, while usually pain free, can cause headache and new, fixed deficits. Transient neurologic deficits can occur with migraine headaches. Lyme disease and cranial nerve palsies, particularly peripheral seventh nerve palsy (Bell's palsy), can cause headache.

COMMON DIAGNOSTIC PATTERNS

Symptoms	Signs	Diagnosis
Acute Headache Syndromes (Days to Weeks)		
Nasal congestion; pain over frontal, maxillary, or ethmoid areas	Sinus tenderness and fever	Sinusitis
Fever, stiff neck; more common in children and the elderly	Fever, stiff neck, and lethargy	Meningitis
"Worst headache of my life"; generally acute onset	Stiff neck, lethargy, and confusion	Subarachnoid hemorrhage
Bilateral pain; pounding	Severely increased blood pressure, confusion, and retinal changes	Hypertensive encephalopathy
Subacute Headache Syndromes (Weeks to Months)		
History of head trauma or alcohol abuse and chronic headaches	Often normal examination; may have focal neurologic deficits	Subdural hematoma
Patient over 60 years old, fatigue, and weight loss	Tender temporal arteries and high sedimentation rate	Giant cell arteritis
Pain progressive over weeks; generally obese younger adult patient; may have decreased vision	Funduscopic examination shows bilateral papilledema; may have optic atrophy	Pseudotumor cerebri

COMMON DIAGNOSTIC PATTERNS (CONTINUED)

Symptoms	Signs	Diagnosis
Persistent, progressive, worse in mornings; may be very localized; often with vomiting that relieves headache; may have petit or grand mal seizures	May have papilledema or focal neurologic loss	Primary or metastatic intracranial neoplasm (brain tumor)

Chronic Headache Syndromes (Months to Years, Recurrent)

Chronic frontal or occipital pain; associated with increased life stress	Normal neurologic examination; spasm in trapezius muscles	Tension headache
Unilateral pain; photophobia; preceded by aura; nausea and vomiting; lasts a few hours	Normal examination; may have transient, brief neurologic deficits	Migraine headache with aura (classic migraine)
Unilateral or bilateral pain, no aura	Normal examination	Migraine without aura (common migraine)
Severe unilateral headache; occurs every year at same time of year	Normal examination	Cluster headache

DIAGNOSIS: TENSION HEADACHE

Discussion

Early diagnosis of intracranial neoplasms is a challenge even to experienced physicians. The disease is relatively rare but must be considered when evaluating headache patients. While many cases present with neurologic signs, including seizures or focal neurologic deficits, the presentation can be subtle without dramatic abnormalities. Changes in intellectual function or personality are suggestive of this disease, as is a highly localized headache that is not over a sinus. Any new headache persisting over weeks that does not seem to fit into other diagnostic categories raises the concern of tumor, and obtaining a computed tomography scan or magnetic resonance imaging should be considered.

CASE 1-2

INITIAL PRESENTATION

A 24-year-old woman comes into the office and complains of unilateral severe headaches, which she says have been occurring over the past year. The headaches occur several times each month, sometimes on the right side of her head and sometimes on the left side. When the pain is severe, she vomits. Sometimes she experiences a few minutes of a "flickering" area in vision prior to the headache.

DIAGNOSIS: MIGRAINE HEADACHE WITH AURA (CLASSIC MIGRAINE HEADACHE)

CASE 1-3

INITIAL PRESENTATION

A 30-year-old man with no history of headache comes into the office with a sudden onset of "the worst headache of my life." The headache is bilateral. He is afebrile, and his blood pressure and funduscopic examination are normal. He is sleepy but arousable, and his neck resists flexing and turning on examination.

DIAGNOSIS: SUBARACHNOID HEMORRHAGE

SUGGESTED READING

Akpek S, Arac M, Atilla S, et al: Cost-effectiveness of computed tomography in the evaluation of patients with headache. *Headache* 35(4):228–230, 1995.

Couch JR: Headache to worry about. *Med Clin North Am* 77(1):141–167, 1993.

Coutin IB, Glass SF: Recognizing uncommon headache syndromes. *Am Fam Phys* 54(7):2247–2252, 1996.

Kumar KL, Cooney TG: Headaches. *Med Clin North Am* 79(2):261–286, 1995.

Perkins AT, Ondo W: When to worry about headache. Head pain as a clue to intracranial disease. *Postgrad Med* 98(2):197–201, 204–208, 1995.

Saper JR: Diagnosis and symptomatic treatment of migraine. *Headache* 37 (Suppl 1):S1–14, 1997.

Smith R: Chronic headaches in family practice. *J Am Board Fam Pract* 5(6):589–599, 1992.

Spence J: Migraine and other causes of headache. *Ann Emerg Med* 27(4):448–450, 1996.

CHAPTER 2
Chief Complaint: Earache

Judith A. Fisher, M.D.

CASE 2-1

INITIAL PRESENTATION

S. Fox, a 55-year-old attorney, comes into the office complaining of a right earache. He recently began to swim at the local YMCA on his lunch hour. The physician looks into his ear and sees a red, swollen ear canal. The tympanic membrane is visible and clear with a good light reflex.

What is the most likely cause of this acute earache?

Discussion

Earaches are common in children and adults alike. Earaches can be acute or chronic, unilateral or bilateral. An earache may be due to referred pain from many areas of the head, neck, esophagus, or heart. Acute ear pain (1–2 days) is usually due to an infection somewhere in the ear, throat, or neck. Chronic earaches (more than 2 weeks) are usually due to problems with the temporomandibular joint (TMJ), teeth (particularly the wisdom teeth), or enlargement of the lymph nodes. Any of the causes of ear pain could be unilateral or bilateral.

> The most common cause of acute ear pain is an infection somewhere in the head, ear, throat, or neck region.

KEY SYMPTOMS, SIGNS, AND OTHER FEATURES

Fever is the sign of an acute infection, bacterial or viral. Acute otitis media (AOM) is perhaps the most common diagnosis when ear pain is associated with fever. Less commonly, a low-grade temperature of less than 100°F, which may wax and wane or be associated with *lymphadenopathy* and night *sweats*, may lead to a diagnosis of lymphoma; other cancers; chronic infections such as tuberculosis, cytomegalovirus, toxoplasmosis, or Epstein-Barr virus; cat scratch fever; or sarcoidosis.

Upper respiratory tract congestion with ear pain is most commonly secondary to an upper respiratory tract infection (URI) or environmental allergies. The cause of the ear pain may be due to eustachian tube dysfunction, AOM, serous otitis media (SOM), or mastoiditis.

Chest pain with ear pain may be due to gastroesophageal reflux disease (GERD). GERD symptoms may include a sour taste in the back of the mouth ("brackwash") after a meal, when lying down, or when bending over. Chest pain associated with ear pain can also be an angina equivalent. Chest pain and ear pain with a positive medical history or a family history of cardiovascular disease, diabetes mellitus, high cholesterol, sedentary life style, male gender, or being postmenopausal would make one consider angina.

> Many areas of the body refer pain to the ears. These include the mastoids; temporomandibular joints; lymph nodes of neck, teeth, oropharynx, esophagus, and heart.

Location is an important consideration. Pain in the central ear is more common for otitis externa, otitis media, angina, and GERD. Pain in front of the ear is common in problems with TMJ, teeth, or lymph nodes. Pain behind the ear is more common in mastoid and skin disease. Acute or chronic *decreased hearing* occurs with most middle and inner ear problems.

Eczema and psoriasis are *skin conditions* associated with ear pain, especially if these conditions cause cracking and infection of the skin around the ear or in the external ear canal.

Dental problems such as cavities, an abscess, impacted wisdom teeth, and teeth grinding (bruxism) may cause ear pain.

A history of recurrent pharyngitis or cryptic tonsils with food trapping or an abscess can be important in the diagnosis of earache.

COMMON DIAGNOSTIC PATTERNS

Symptoms	Signs	Diagnosis
Acute Ear Pain		
Outside ear hurts, +/− low-grade fever, ear pierced, eczema, or psoriasis	Red, tender auricle or pinna	Infection of the outer ear
Ear pain, no fever, +/− recent swimming or ear irrigation, and +/− discharge	External ear canal red, swollen, +/− exudate, and pain on pulling the auricle or with pressure on the pinna	Otitis externa

COMMON DIAGNOSTIC PATTERNS (CONTINUED)

Symptoms	Signs	Diagnosis
Ear pain, decreased hearing, fever, and upper respiratory tract congestion	Red or injected TM, which may be bulging	AOM
Ear fullness or pain, decreased hearing, no fever, and upper respiratory tract congestion	Fluid behind the TM, a dull looking TM, or no movement of the TM with pneumatoscopy	SOM
Pain behind or in the ear, +/− fever, and upper respiratory tract congestion	Normal ear with tenderness behind ear (area behind ear can be red, swollen, and warm)	Mastoiditis
Pain in or below the ear, +/− fever, and body aches	Tenderness below the ear at the jaw angle, +/− redness, swelling, warm to touch, and may palpate a lymph node	Infected or enlarged lymph node
Ear pain, +/− mouth or face pain, and +/− bad breath (halitosis)	Normal ear, teeth tender with palpation in posterior jaw area, tenderness to pressure on or underneath the teeth, +/− redness, swelling, and warm to touch	Dental abscess or dental cavities
Fever, +/− sore throat, and +/− difficulty swallowing (dysphagia)	Red or injected, swollen oropharynx or tonsils with or without exudate	Pharyngitis or tonsillitis
History of a blow to the head or ear	Black and blue (ecchymosis) around or behind the ear, on the auricle, or in the canal; may have a perforated TM and blood in the external or middle ear	Trauma

	Chronic Ear Pain	
Pain may be intermittent, history of skin condition or environmental allergies, and itching	Skin around or behind ear or in ear canal has fissures, rash, or redness	Eczema, psoriasis, or seborrheic dermatitis with secondary skin infection

COMMON DIAGNOSTIC PATTERNS (CONTINUED)

Symptoms	Signs	Diagnosis
Ear pain in front of or in the ear, increased pain after eating or in early morning, history of grinding teeth while sleeping, dentist might say teeth are rubbing down or malaligned, or history of arthritis	Tender in front of ear or in anterior canal as patient opens and closes jaw and molar teeth can be flat (without usual groves)	TMJ syndrome
Decreased hearing with or without dizziness	Wax (cerumen) plug in canal	Cerumen plug
Concurrent and intermittent vertigo, may have decreased hearing, ringing of the ear (tinnitus), nausea, fluctuating symptoms, and ear pain is more of a pressure	Nystagmus	Meniere's disease
+/− Decreased hearing, dizzy, complains of a feeling of spinning (vertigo), and tinnitus	Normal ear examination, increased bone conduction of sound to ear with pain, decreased whisper appreciation to same ear, and +/− nystagmus or ataxia	Acoustic neuroma or other space-occupying lesion
Pain in or below ear, low-grade fevers, +/− night sweats, and fatigue	Increased size of lymph node, tender below ear, +/− abnormal chest examination, +/− abnormal chest x-ray, +/− other palpable lymph nodes, and +/− hepatosplenomegaly	Lymphoma, sarcoidosis, cytomegaloviral infection, infectious mononucleosis, toxoplasmosis, tuberculosis of the lymph node (scrofula), or cat scratch fever
Ear pain, mouth or face pain, and presence of wisdom teeth	Normal examination, wisdom teeth partially visible, jaw can be tender with palpation, +/− gum redness, swelling, and tender to touch around teeth	Wisdom teeth impaction

COMMON DIAGNOSTIC PATTERNS (CONTINUED)

Symptoms	Signs	Diagnosis
Ear pain, mouth or face pain, and +/− fever	+/− Redness, swelling, area around a molar may be tender to palpate, and dental x-ray shows a root abscess	Infected root canal
History of large tonsils, history of frequent tonsillitis, fever, and can have change in voice	Tonsils with crypts, +/− exudate, redness, swelling, and tonsils may cross midline of throat	Tonsillar abscess
History of large tonsils and frequent tonsillitis	Tonsils with crypts, +/− exudate, and no redness or swelling	Food trapping in tonsillar crypts
Ear pain, +/− throat pain, intermittent pain after patient has eaten or when bending over or lying down (brackwash), +/− halitosis, and +/− chest pain	+/− Red oropharynx and epigastric area may be tender with palpation	GERD
+/− Chest pain, +/− history of angina, intermittent chest pain, +/− jaw pain, and +/− pain on exertion	Normal HEENT examination, +/− S_3 or S_4, +/− cardiac murmur, and +/− ECG changes	Ischemic heart disease: acute myocardial infarction or angina

Note. TM = tympanic membrane; AOM = acute otitis media; SOM = serous otitis media; TMJ = temporomandibular joint; GERD = gastroesophageal reflux disease; S_3 = third heart sound; S_4 = fourth heart sound; ECG = electrocardiogram; HEENT = head, ears, eyes, nose, and throat.

DIAGNOSIS: ACUTE OTITIS EXTERNA

CASE 2-2

INITIAL PRESENTATION

A 35-year-old woman visits the office complaining of right ear pain. On further questioning the physician finds out that this has been going on for 6 months. At a recent dental visit she was asked if she grinds her teeth at night. Her dentist found a flat-tening of all tooth surfaces. The patient is going through a divorce.

Stress often exacerbates TMJ syndrome.

DIAGNOSIS: TEMPOROMANDIBULAR JOINT SYNDROME

CASE 2-3

INITIAL PRESENTATION

A 70-year-old man complains of decreased hearing associated with low-grade right ear pain over the past month. He is somewhat dizzy. The physician looks into his ear and sees a large wax plug. After gentle ear irrigation with warm water, the patient is relieved of his symptoms.

DIAGNOSIS: CERUMEN IMPACTION

CHAPTER 3
Chief Complaint: Chest Pain

Judith A. Fisher, M.D.

CASE 3-1

INITIAL PRESENTATION

M. Davis, a 50-year-old workaholic, comes to the office complaining of intermittent dull substernal chest pain that occurs only when he runs 2 miles. The patient is overweight and leads a sedentary life style. His chest pain began 2 weeks ago when he began his own running program to lose weight. The chest pain is associated with some shortness of breath and sweating. The patient wants to understand why his left shoulder also hurts. The patient attributes these symptoms to "I'm just out of shape." The electrocardiogram in the office is normal.

What is the most likely cause of this chest pain?

Discussion

Chest pain is a common complaint. The most common etiologies depend on the age and gender of the patient. Chest pain can be episodic or persistent.

KEY SYMPTOMS, SIGNS, AND OTHER FACTORS

Age and gender can be risk factors for cardiac chest pain. Individuals less than 50 years old are more likely to have noncardiac chest pain. This statement excludes individuals with a positive family history of ischemic cardiac disease in family members less than 50 years of age or other standard risk factors. Men greater than 50 years of age and postmenopausal women are at greater risk for ischemic cardiac chest pain.

The standard independent *risk factors* for ischemic heart disease are: a positive family history, male sex, diabetes mellitus, hypertension, hyperlipidemia, or cigarette smoking. Some physicians feel that being postmenopausal and female and having a sedentary life style should be included in any list of risk factors.

Anxiety associated with *panic disorder* is the most common cause of chest pain in younger women. Many other types of chest pain are associated with concurrent anxiety.

Barlow's syndrome, or *mitral valve prolapse*, is a frequent cause of chest pain in younger women. Mitral valve prolapse may cause chest pain, palpitations (usually a supraventricular tachycardia), and anxiety symptoms. In a young woman with any of these symptoms, the physician should auscultate for a click and murmur in the area of the mitral valve.

The risk factors for *pulmonary embolus* are: the use of birth control pills or estrogen replacement therapy; surgery; cancer; a personal history or family history of pulmonary emboli, deep venous thrombosis, or a hypercoagulable state; confinement to bed or wheelchair; and a long car ride or air flight.

Shortness of breath is associated with chest pain from cardiac and pulmonary causes as well as anxiety. *Gastrointestinal complaints* of nausea and vomiting are associated with pneumonias located near the diaphragm, inferior wall myocardial infarctions, and many of the gastrointestinal diseases. *Fever*, which is a sign of inflammation or infection, is associated with pericarditis, pneumonia, bronchitis, pancreatitis, and acute gallbladder disease.

Pinpoint tenderness is associated with pleurisy, pulmonary embolus, and rib fractures. *Pain with movement* is characteristic of pneumonia, pleurisy, thoracic disk disease, rib fracture, and musculoskeletal strains.

COMMON DIAGNOSTIC PATTERNS

Symptoms	Signs	Diagnosis
Episodic Chest Pain		
Dull ache or squeezing pain often on exertion, which may radiate to the left arm, shoulder, neck, jaw, or ear; may be associated with SOB, DOE, sweating (diaphoresis), and nausea	At the time of the chest pain: pale, scared, sweating, SOB, tachycardia, S_4, a diastolic murmur in the axilla, and ECG with nonspecific ST–T-wave changes or T-wave inversions	Angina
Burning or spasm central chest, occurs after eating when lying down or bending over, and +/− associated with bad breath in mouth	+/− Epigastric tenderness	GERD

COMMON DIAGNOSTIC PATTERNS (CONTINUED)

Symptoms	Signs	Diagnosis
Acute or severe SOB, lightheadedness, and diaphoresis associated with global chest heaviness or point tenderness, which is exacerbated with inspiration	Tachypnea, tachycardia, and low blood oxygen (hypoxemia)	Pulmonary embolus
Acute or severe SOB, lightheadedness, and diaphoresis associated with chest heaviness	Tachypnea, tachycardia, and normal blood oxygen	Anxiety
Dull pain with or without palpitations and feelings of anxiety	Midsystolic click with or without a diastolic murmur in the mitral area	Prolapsed mitral valve
Persistent Chest Pain		
Dull ache or squeezing pain, which may radiate to the left arm, shoulder, neck, jaw, or ear; may be associated with SOB, DOE, diaphoresis, and nausea or vomiting	At the time of pain: pale, scared, sweating, SOB, tachycardia, S_4, a diastolic murmur in the axilla, and ECG may have ST–T-wave changes	Acute myocardial infarction
Dull or sharp, knife-like pain, which changes with changing position; may occur with a URI, after a myocardial infarction, or with a collagen–vascular disease	Cardiac rub	Pericarditis
Fever, cough, SOB, and localized pain	Rales or rhonchi, wheezes, and increased WBCs	Pneumonia
Localized pain with inspiration, +/− cough, and +/− SOB	Pleural rub and normal blood oxygen	Pleurisy
Sharp pain just lateral to the sternum, and pain increases with inspiration or movement of the arms	Point tenderness reproducible over the costochondral junction of one or more ribs	Costochondritis (Tietze's syndrome)
History of sudden onset of pain precipitated by cough or trauma and increased pain with inspiration	Point tenderness over one or more ribs and pain at fracture site or sites with pressure over the sternum	Fractured rib or ribs
Pain in the distribution of a thoracic dermatome, +/− pain over the same thoracic vertebrae, history of cough or trauma, and no rash	+/− Tenderness of the thoracic vertebrae, parathoracic muscle spasm, and range of motion increases pain	Thoracic disk disease

COMMON DIAGNOSTIC PATTERNS (CONTINUED)

Symptoms	Signs	Diagnosis
Pain along the distribution of a thoracic dermatome, often prior to rash in same area, and history of chicken pox	+/− Red base with blisters (vesicles) in one or more dermatomal distributions	Herpes zoster

Note. SOB = shortness of breath; DOE = dyspnea on exertion; S_4 = fourth heart sound; ECG = electrocardiogram; GERD = gastroesophageal reflux disease; URI = upper respiratory tract infection; WBCs = white blood cells.

DIAGNOSIS: NEW ONSET ANGINA

CASE 3-2

INITIAL PRESENTATION

An 18-year-old college student gives a 7-day history of a low-grade fever, upper respiratory tract congestion, and sore throat. In the past 24 hours, she developed a cough productive of yellow sputum and chest pain on the left side. On physical examination, she has a temperature of 102°F and rhonchi in her left axillary area. Her chest x-ray shows a left lingular infiltrate. A complete blood count shows 20,000 white blood cells with a left shift.

DIAGNOSIS: LEFT LINGULAR PNEUMONIA

CASE 3-3

INITIAL PRESENTATION

A 20-year-old college student began to smoke cigarettes in the past 2 weeks. He has had upper respiratory tract congestion and a marked dry cough. Last night while coughing, he had sudden onset of left chest pain. The pain continued today and is increased with coughing, inspiration, or movement. The patient is able to point to the exact spot where his chest hurts. On physical examination the physician is also able to reproduce his pain by palpating over the left seventh rib at the anterior axillary line.

DIAGNOSIS: FRACTURED LEFT SEVENTH RIB

CHAPTER 4
Chief Complaint: Back Pain

Judith A. Fisher, M.D.

CASE 4-1

INITIAL PRESENTATION

T. Chang, a 24-year-old laborer, complains of acute onset of lower back pain while shoveling a load of dirt. He has no pain down his legs and no urinary or bowel complaints. On physical examination, he has full range of motion of his lower back but tightness in the paravertebral muscles of the lumbosacral area. Neurologic, vascular, motor, and reflex examinations are within normal limits.

What is the most likely cause of back pain?

Discussion

Back pain is a very common complaint. Lower back pain is the leading cause of long-term disability in the United States. While back pain is often musculoskeletal, there are many other causes of back pain which must be explored. It is probably easiest to evaluate back pain as upper back pain (above the diaphragm) and lower back pain (below the diaphragm). A few conditions, such as muscle strain or sprain, dislocated disk, aortic dissection, and herpes zoster, can occur in either area of the back.

KEY SYMPTOMS, SIGNS, AND OTHER FACTORS

If *movement* affects the pain, musculoskeletal causes and pleurisy in the upper back are likely causes; in the lower back musculoskeletal causes are most likely.

Unilateral *neurologic* symptoms or signs such as numbness, urinary retention, motor weakness, sensory changes, or asymmetry of the reflexes point to disk disease.

If the pain follows a *dermatome*, intervertebral disk disease and herpes zoster are common causes.

A patient complaining of upper back pain and *fever* should be examined for signs of infection or inflammation in the heart and lung areas. Fever and lower back pain suggest infection or inflammation in the gastrointestinal (GI) and genitourinary systems. Bony or joint infections in the back are rare.

Weight loss points to cancer or a chronic problem that has been associated with loss of appetite (anorexia).

Common causes of back pain associated with GI complaints are pancreatitis, gallbladder disease, and peptic ulcer disease. Diverticulitis is a common cause of these symptoms in the elderly.

Pain in the costovertebral angle in the lower back associated with *hematuria* and *dysuria* is usually due to a problem in the urinary tract.

Pelvic pain and *dyspareunia* (painful sexual intercourse) point to uterine and ovarian diseases.

A patient presenting with upper back pain and several *cardiac risk factors* may be having an acute myocardial infarction or a thoracic aortic dissection, which the physician needs to exclude immediately. When several cardiac risk factors and lower back pain are present, dissection of an abdominal aortic aneurysm is a possibility. In dissecting aortic aneurysm, the pulses on either side of the body may have different qualities.

Medical history is always helpful since many causes of back pain are recurrent or preceded by an inciting event.

COMMON DIAGNOSTIC PATTERNS

Symptoms	Signs	Diagnosis
Upper or Lower Back		
Pain or ache, may feel spasmodic; a history of exercise or trauma is common	Tight paravertebral muscles, increased pain with range of motion of spine, +/− curvature of the spine	Strain or sprain
Pain in dermatome distribution: pain may go around chest or abdomen as a belt would; history of trauma, cough, or increased physical exertion	Tight paraspinous muscles, +/− change in reflexes in an upper or lower extremity, increased pain with range of motion of spine	Intervertebral disk disease
Pain in dermatome distribution; history of chicken pox	Red base with blisters in a dermatome distribution	Herpes zoster
Life-threatening, overwhelming pain, often described as tearing and unremitting; +/− SOB, +/− weakness, lightheadedness, and often in elderly patients with multiple cardiovascular risk factors	Patient appears scared; +/− difference in pulses between the two sides of the body; CXR shows a widened mediastinum, or the abdominal x-ray shows a widened aorta	Dissecting aortic aneurysm

COMMON DIAGNOSTIC PATTERNS (CONTINUED)

Symptoms	Signs	Diagnosis
Progressive, often severe, unremitting pain; +/− a history of cancer; history of weight loss in an older patient	Point tenderness over a vertebral body or bodies; x-ray shows destruction of a vertebral body or bodies	Bony metastasis
Acute, severe, and unremitting pain usually in a postmenopausal woman	Point tenderness over a vertebral body or bodies; x-ray shows shortening of a vertebral body or bodies	Compression fracture of a vertebral body

Upper Back

Fever, cough, SOB, or dyspnea on exertion	Rhonchi on chest examination, increased respiratory rate, +/− fever	Pneumonia
Sudden onset of pain in one side of the back associated with severe SOB	Increased respiratory rate, hypoxemia, nonspecific ST–T-wave changes on the ECG, +/− rub	Pulmonary emboli
Increased pain with inspiration or expiration; patient able to pinpoint area of pain	Rub may be heard with inspiration or expiration	Pleurisy
Life-threatening feeling, pain, dull ache, or squeezing feeling	+/− S_3 and S_4; a murmur may be heard best in the axilla; ECG changes in leads R and V_1	Ischemia or acute myocardial infarction in the posterior cardiac wall

Lower Back

Pain in the CVA area, dull ache, fever, +/− dysuria	Fever, tenderness when tapping the CVA area, urinary WBC casts	Pyelonephritis
Acute, spasmodic, severe, episodic pain in the CVA area with radiation to the front of the abdomen toward the groin	Patient writhing in pain; tenderness when tapping the CVA area on the same side as the pain; urinalysis may show crystals or RBCs	Renal calculus
Constant mid to left mid-back pain; pain increases with eating; history of gallstones or alcohol abuse; +/− other GI symptoms (e.g., anorexia, vomiting)	Tenderness when palpating left paraspinal area; epigastric tenderness; increased amylase and lipase levels; ultrasound shows edema of the pancreas	Pancreatitis

COMMON DIAGNOSTIC PATTERNS (CONTINUED)

Symptoms	Signs	Diagnosis
GI symptoms; right mid-back pain; constant, dull ache; +/− fever; acute and sometimes recurrent	Tenderness when tapping right mid-back; RUQ tender when palpated; ultrasound shows gallstones or thickened gallbladder wall	Gallbladder disease
Subacute, dull, boring mid-back pain; weakness; weight loss; jaundice	Possible mass in the epigastric area; jaundice	Pancreatic cancer
Acute pain and dull ache in the right lower back, +/− fever, +/− GI symptoms	Rectal examination causes tenderness in the RLQ; rebound tenderness; increased WBC count with a left shift	Acute appendicitis
Acute pain and dull ache in the left lower back, +/− fever, +/− GI symptoms	Rectal examination causes tenderness in the LLQ; rebound tenderness; increased WBC count with a left shift	Acute diverticulitis
Subacute, burning pain in the mid-back; may radiate paravertebrally; may be worse when lying down; may decrease with food	Tender, guarding of the epigastric area; +/− heme-positive stool; mid-back tender to tapping	Posterior peptic ulcer
Intermittent or constant pain and dyspareunia	Mass palpable on pelvic examination	Ovarian or uterine mass
Dyspareunia, +/− fever, +/− vaginal discharge, +/− GI complaints	Tender mass on pelvis	Ovarian abscess or pelvic inflammatory disease

Note. CXR = chest x-ray; SOB = shortness of breath; ECG = electrocardiogram; S_3 = third heart sound; S_4 = fourth heart sound; WBC = white blood cell; CVA = costovertebral angle; GI = gastrointestinal; RUQ = right upper quadrant; RLQ = right lower quadrant; LLQ = left lower quadrant; RBCs = red blood cells.

DIAGNOSIS: LUMBOSACRAL STRAIN OR SPRAIN

CASE 4-2

INITIAL PRESENTATION

A 75-year-old man comes to the office complaining of severe lower back pain, which is unrelieved by heat, aspirin, acetaminophen, or ibuprophen. He is unable to sleep due to the pain. On examination he is exquisitely tender over the L3 and L4 vertebral bodies. There is no paravertebral muscle spasm and no changes in the pain with range of motion. On rectal examination, he has an irregular, firm prostate.

DIAGNOSIS: PROSTATIC CANCER WITH BONY METASTASES

CASE 4-3

INITIAL PRESENTATION

An 85-year-old woman with type II diabetes mellitus is seen in the emergency room. She complains of tearing pain in her upper central back. On physical examination her lungs and heart are normal, but the physician notices +2/+2 pulses in her right arm and 0/+2 pulses in her left arm. Her blood pressure, which was normal on admission, is now 60/palpable mm Hg in her right arm and negligent in her left arm. She is only mildly short of breath. A chest x-ray shows a widened mediastinum.

DIAGNOSIS: DISSECTING THORACIC AORTIC ANEURYSM

CHAPTER 5
Chief Complaint: Abdominal Pain

Marjorie A. Bowman, M.D., M.P.A.

CASE 5-1

INITIAL PRESENTATION

R. Black, a 35-year-old woman, has had recurrent abdominal pain for several years. It seems crampy, rather diffuse, and often is better after a bowel movement. She has intermittent constipation and loose stools. Her examination is normal.

What is the most likely cause of this chronic abdominal pain?

Discussion

Abdominal pain is very common and is usually self-limited, but it can be chronic.

KEY SYMPTOMS, SIGNS, AND OTHER FACTORS

Perhaps the best first question about abdominal pain is the *duration* of the symptoms. Chronic abdominal pain suggests very different medical problems than acute abdominal pain. Common causes of chronic abdominal pain include irritable bowel syndrome, dyspepsia, and reflux esophagitis. Intermittent, severe pain with short-lived relief is common with spasm of the ureter (kidney stones), gallbladder or common bile duct (gallstones), or intestines (constipation, diarrhea).

The *location of the pain* is also important. *Right upper quadrant pain* is more likely to be some form of gallbladder problem or hepatitis. Pneumonia can also present with right upper quadrant pain. *Midepigastric pain* is more often as-

> **Common Causes of Chronic Abdominal Pain**
> Irritable bowel syndrome
> Dyspepsia
> Reflux esophagitis

> **Common Causes of Acute Abdominal Pain**
> Infectious gastroenteritis
> Gastritis
> Reflux esophagitis
> Idiopathic

sociated with stomach problems, such as ulcer or nonulcer dyspepsia, and sometimes reflux esophagitis. *Mid- to left-sided abdominal pain*, particularly if radiating to the back, suggests pancreatitis. *Periumbilical pain* moving to the right lower quadrant is classic for appendicitis. Acute *left lower quadrant pain* is commonly diverticulitis or constipation. *Right or left lower quadrant pain* can be seen with ectopic pregnancy, ovarian disorders, or pelvic inflammatory disease in women or epididymitis in men. *Suprapubic pain* may be associated with bladder infections or gynecologic disorders, such as pelvic inflammatory disease.

> Knowing the duration and location of pain, if there is fever or bleeding, and the patient's age, gynecologic history (women), concurrent symptoms, and medical and drug history can help the physician determine the cause of abdominal pain.

Diffuse pain may precede more specific localization as the disease progresses, such as in appendicitis. Diffuse pain is also common with irritable bowel syndrome or inflammatory bowel disease. Kidney stones are associated with pain radiating from the abdomen to the perineal area.

Fever is a key differentiating symptom. Fever is most common with infection, such as gastroenteritis and appendicitis, but can be seen with other entities, such as inflammatory disease.

Bleeding is important to detect. Blood loss from the upper intestinal tract can appear in vomitus, as black stools (melena), or as hemoccult-positive stools. Blood loss from the upper tract is commonly from ulcer, gastritis, or erosive esophagitis; cancer is much less common. Blood loss from the lower tract can appear as bright-red blood (often mixed with the stools) or hemoccult-positive stools. Blood loss from the lower intestinal tract is associated with inflammatory bowel disease, diverticulitis, diverticulosis, colon cancer, angiodysplasia, Meckel's diverticulum, and local anal problems such as anal fissures and hemorrhoids.

The *age* of the patient is important. Elderly patients tend to present with less specific symptoms than young adults and may be quite ill with few signs or symptoms.

In *women*, the gynecologic history is very important, particularly for lower abdominal pain. Any woman with even a slight chance of pregnancy and lower abdominal pain should have a pregnancy test and pelvic examination. Sexually transmitted diseases can also lead to lower abdominal pain. Intermenstrual lower quadrant pain is common with mittelschmerz, the pain associated with ovulation. Ectopic pregnancy is particularly important to consider.

In *men*, abdominal pain can be associated with hernias, prostatitis, epididymitis, and testicular torsion. Genitalia and rectal examinations are important.

Concurrent symptoms can be helpful. Diarrhea suggests an intestinal disorder. Constipation and vomiting occur with many illnesses and do not differentiate well between diseases. Concurrent pain, prostration, rigid abdomen, and tenderness (often with rebound tenderness) suggest an acute abdomen, which often requires surgery.

Medical and drug histories can provide major clues. For example, a patient with previous arteriosclerosis is much more likely to have ischemic bowel disease. A patient with a history of kidney stones may well have kidney stones again. Many drugs can cause gastritis (alcohol) or ulcers (aspirin, nonsteroidal anti-inflammatory agents).

COMMON DIAGNOSTIC PATTERNS

Symptoms	Signs	Diagnosis
Epigastric Pain		
Burning, nighttime awakening, blood loss, and subacute	Epigastric tenderness and anemia	Ulcer
Burning, pain into chest, worse when lying flat and after big meals, and subacute	Epigastric tenderness	Reflux esophagitis
Acute pain through to back and vomiting	Tenderness and elevated amylase levels	Pancreatitis
Acute pain and alcohol ingestion	Epigastric tenderness and elevated GGT	Alcoholic gastritis
Chronic pain that is poorly characterized	Epigastric tenderness	Dyspepsia
Right Upper Quadrant Pain		
Intermittent, severe, acute pain radiating to back or shoulder, with or without vomiting	Local tenderness and positive Murphy's test	Cholelithiasis
Fever, pain radiating to back or shoulder, malaise, and vomiting	Local tenderness and elevated WBCs	Cholecystitis
Fever, nausea and vomiting, and jaundice	RUQ tenderness and elevated liver function tests	Hepatitis
Fever and cough	Abnormal lung examination	Pneumonia

COMMON DIAGNOSTIC PATTERNS (CONTINUED)

Symptoms	Signs	Diagnosis
Right Lower Quadrant Pain		
Periumbilical pain moving to RLQ and low-grade fever	Localized rebound RLQ tenderness	Appendicitis
Menstrual irregularities	Localized tenderness and a palpable ovarian mass	Ovarian cyst
Pain after menses, vaginal discharge, and fever	Cervical motion tenderness and cervical discharge	Pelvic inflammatory disease
Intermenstrual pain	Localized tenderness and possibly rebound tenderness	Mittelschmerz
Left Lower Quadrant Pain (same as right lower quadrant pain, but appendicitis is unlikely, and diverticulitis is more likely)		
Acute localized pain with change in bowel habits and often fever	Localized tenderness and possibly elevated WBCs	Diverticulitis
Suprapubic Pain		
Acute dysuria and frequent urination with or without fever	Local tenderness and abnormal urinalysis	Urinary tract infection
Vaginal discharge and fever	Cervical motion tenderness	Pelvic inflammatory disease
Fever	Abnormal genitalia and rectal examination or both	Epididymitis or prostatitis
Local or abdominal pain	Testicular tenderness	Testicular torsion
Diffuse Pain		
Acute pain, diarrhea, fever, and vomiting	Abdominal tenderness	Infectious gastroenteritis
Acute pain, diarrhea, fever, vomiting, and others with same food exposure have same symptoms	Abdominal tenderness	Food poisoning
Acute pain, malaise, and fever	Rebound and elevated WBCs	Peritonitis
Acute pain, malaise, fever, and rectal bleeding	Rebound and elevated WBCs	Ischemic bowel

COMMON DIAGNOSTIC PATTERNS (CONTINUED)

Symptoms	Signs	Diagnosis
Chronic pain, varying bowel habits, and relief after having a bowel movement	Normal examination	Irritable bowel syndrome
Chronic pain, recurrent pain, rectal bleeding, and fever	Weight loss, varying abdominal examination, elevated WBCs, and elevated ESR	Inflammatory bowel disease
	Other	
Diffuse pain or pain localized to a specific area	Rectal bleeding and anemia	Colon cancer
Pain from back or abdomen to perineum that is intermittent, severe, and acute	RBCs on urinalysis	Kidney stones

Note. GGT = γ-glutamyltransferase; WBCs = white blood cells; RUQ = right upper quadrant; RLQ = right lower quadrant; ESR = erythrocyte sedimentation rate; RBCs = red blood cells.

DIAGNOSIS: IRRITABLE BOWEL SYNDROME

CASE 5-2

INITIAL PRESENTATION

A 40-year-old man has had pain for 2 hours starting in his back. The pain is severe and intermittent. When he is in pain, he cries out and writhes. His abdominal examination is negative, and there are red blood cells in his urine.

DIAGNOSIS: KIDNEY STONES

CASE 5-3

INITIAL PRESENTATION

A 50-year-old woman has had diffuse abdominal pain for the last 1½ days, although it now seems to be more in the left lower quadrant. She has a mild fever and left lower quadrant tenderness, with a slightly elevated white blood cell count and erythrocyte sedimentation rate.

DIAGNOSIS: DIVERTICULITIS

SUGGESTED READING

Blondell RD: Abdominal pain: what happens in primary care? *Arch Fam Med* 5:287–288, 1996.

Klinkman MS: Episodes of care for abdominal pain in a primary care practice. *Arch Fam Med* 5:279–285, 1996.

CHAPTER 6
Chief Complaint: Fever

David E. Nicklin, M.D.

CASE 6-1

INITIAL PRESENTATION

M. Jones, a 24-year-old woman, has had increasing temperature over several days to 39.5°C (103°F). She complains of right flank pain, urinary frequency, and dysuria. She has vomited twice today. She is sexually active and had a normal period two weeks ago. She has no pelvic pain or vaginal discharge. Physical examination shows an ill-appearing woman with right costovertebral angle tenderness, mild tenderness over the bladder, and no uterine or adnexal tenderness.

What causes a fever and how is the cause of it determined?

Discussion

Fever is a very common complaint. Most patients with fever have acute infections such as upper respiratory infections (URI), pharyngitis, gastroenteritis, or urinary tract infections. However, fever is a nonspecific sign that can be associated with many other types of illness, including chronic infection, neoplasms, autoimmune illness, and drug reactions. The source of a fever can be determined in most patients by a history, physical examination, and simple laboratory testing, which provide the physician with localizing symptoms and signs. Fever of unknown origin (FUO) is defined as a fever persisting for over a week in a hospitalized patient or 3 weeks in an outpatient without diagnosis after careful history, physical, and routine laboratory testing. This chapter focuses on common causes of fever. (The suggested readings contain longer discussions of FUO.)

> The diagnosis in most febrile patients can be determined with a simple history, physical, and office laboratory tests.

It is a common mistake to believe that a fever is a dangerous event requiring treatment. Leukocytes are more effective in fighting

> **Fever is a helpful physiologic response to infection.**

infection at higher temperatures, and a fever is a helpful physiologic response to infection. At times patients may have headache and myalgia with fever and may benefit from antipyretic, analgesic treatment. When patients are uncomfortable or temperature exceeds 40.0°C (104°F), fever should be reduced. This is best done with centrally acting antipyretics (acetaminophen or aspirin and nonsteroidal anti-inflammatories). If necessary these drugs can be used every 4 hours or alternated every 2 hours. Forcibly lowering the fever with cold baths, sponging with rubbing alcohol, or use of cooling blankets cause additional thermal stress, make the patient miserable, and should only be considered for temperatures remaining over 40.5°C (105°F) despite oral antipyretic treatment.

KEY SYMPTOMS, SIGNS, AND OTHER FACTORS

General appearance is hard to quantify, but for experienced physicians it is a critical factor in evaluating febrile patients. Patients with serious infections appear weak, drained, and may be lethargic. Patients with a general healthy appearance usually have minor infections.

Knowing the *duration* of a fever can be helpful in determining the cause of the fever. Fever that is present for several days or less is generally caused by acute bacterial or viral illness or drug reaction. Fever lasting more than a week is often seen with viral hepatitis, mononucleosis, tuberculosis, lymphoma, human immunodeficiency virus (HIV), endocarditis, vasculitis, and occult abscess.

While bacterial infections may cause only low-grade fever and self-limited viral illnesses can cause high fever, in general, patients with a temperature over 39°C (102°F) have a greater likelihood of serious or life-threatening illness. This is particularly true in geriatric patients.

A survey of respiratory, gastrointestinal, and genitourinary symptoms will often suggest a focus of infection. When there are no *localizing symptoms or signs*, acute fever is often due to viral illness, drug reaction, or sinusitis. Subacute or chronic fever may be due to occult abscess, mononucleosis, tuberculosis, hepatitis, occult malignancy, HIV, or endocarditis.

The presence of documented *weight loss* suggests a more long-standing, serious illness such as tuberculosis, lymphoma, endocarditis, HIV infection, or inflammatory bowel disease.

Certain *medications* can also cause a fever. A drug fever can be due to almost any medication but is seen most commonly with sulfanilamide drugs. It is also seen with penicillins, streptomycin, methyldopa, and barbiturates. A diffuse rash may also be seen. The drug fever may occur soon after starting a medication or after the patient has been taking it for days or weeks. In a drug fever, white blood cell (WBC) count differential may show increased eosinophils, and the tachycardia generally seen with fever may be absent.

Myalgia and diffuse aching can be seen with any fever but is more common in any viral illness, including hepatitis. It is also seen in Rocky Mountain spotted fever.

Diffuse adenopathy is suggestive of mononucleosis, HIV infection, or lymphoma.

Primary HIV infection may cause fever, as do many of the opportunistic infections seen in advanced HIV. A history of multiple sexual partners, high-risk sexual practices, or intravenous drug abuse is often present. Patients may be uncomfortable acknowledging these behaviors, and HIV testing should be encouraged in patients with persistent, unexplained fever.

Deep venous thrombosis (DVT) may cause fever. Risk factors include bed rest, obesity, pregnancy, genetic clotting abnormalities, and diagnosis of malignancy. There may be redness, warmth, and tenderness, but these may be absent with pelvic thrombophlebitis. Pleuritic chest pain and shortness of breath suggest DVT with pulmonary embolism.

Valvular abnormality or congenital heart disease should raise suspicion of *bacterial endocarditis*. A new heart murmur may be present. Intravenous drug abuse can cause endocarditis in normal heart valves.

Travel to tropical, underdeveloped areas is associated with malaria or tuberculosis. Histoplasmosis may be seen in patients who have lived in the Ohio River valley.

COMMON DIAGNOSTIC PATTERNS

Symptoms	Signs	Diagnosis
Several days of myalgia, runny nose, sore throat, dry cough, and low-grade fever	Looks well, nasal stuffiness, and clear lungs	Upper respiratory infection
Several days of low-grade or high fever, sore throat without nasal congestion, and cough	May look ill, pharynx has erythema or exudate, and cervical adenopathy	Pharyngitis (bacterial or viral)
Several days of high fever and cough productive of green sputum	Appears ill, and rales over affected lung area	Bacterial pneumonia

COMMON DIAGNOSTIC PATTERNS (CONTINUED)

Symptoms	Signs	Diagnosis
Several days of high fever, dysuria, urinary frequency, flank pain, and more common in women	Appears ill, tenderness of costovertebral angle, and urinalysis shows increased WBCs	Pyelonephritis
Acute, high or low-grade fever, low pelvic pain, sexually active woman, and pain typically several days after menses	Appears ill, shuffling bent over walk, and exquisite tenderness on pelvic examination	Pelvic inflammatory disease
Acute fever, may be high, on sulfa drug for infectious symptoms, which are now resolved (e.g., UTI)	Appears well, no localizing signs, may have diffuse rash, and increased eosinophils	Drug fever
Ill for a week or more, low-grade fevers, sore throat, myalgia, and rare in patients over age 30	May appear ill, diffuse adenopathy with anterior and posterior cervical location, and pharynx may have exudate	Mononucleosis (Epstein-Barr virus)
History of valvular heart disease, days or weeks of fever without localizing signs, and may have lost weight	Appears ill, may have new murmur, and often no localizing signs	Endocarditis
History of tuberculosis exposure (homeless, Third World travel, elderly), chronic cough, and weight loss	Appears ill, lungs show rales or rhonchi, and CXR shows apical infiltrate	Tuberculosis
Fever for weeks, history of unprotected sex with high-risk partner, IV drug use, dry cough, and weight loss	Appears ill, diffuse adenopathy, and lungs generally clear	HIV infection or *Pneumocystis* pneumonia
Fever for weeks, weight loss, and no other symptoms	Appears ill, diffuse adenopathy, and otherwise a normal examination	Lymphoma or sarcoidosis

Note. WBCs = white blood cells; sulfa = sulfanilamide; UTI = urinary tract infection; CXR = chest x-ray; IV = intravenous; HIV = human immunodeficiency virus.

DIAGNOSIS: PYELONEPHRITIS

CASE 6-2

INITIAL PRESENTATION

A healthy 25-year-old man has 2 days of a temperature of 38.3°C (101°F). He reports a scratchy throat, runny nose, and a dry cough. He complains that his muscles ache, and he is fatigued. Physical examination shows a well-appearing patient with mild erythema of the pharynx, nontender sinuses, and clear lungs.

DIAGNOSIS: VIRAL UPPER RESPIRATORY ILLNESS

CASE 6-3

INITIAL PRESENTATION

A 40-year-old man has not felt well for 2 months. He has lost 15 lbs and has felt feverish on and off for the past month. He has no localizing symptoms. He has a lifelong history of a heart murmur of unknown cause. On physical examination the patient appears chronically ill. On cardiac examination there is a III/VI harsh crescendo-decrescendo murmur at the left upper sternal border; otherwise the cardiac examination is normal.

DIAGNOSIS: ENDOCARDITIS

SUGGESTED READING

Cunha BA: The clinical significance of fever patterns. *Infect Dis Clin North Am* 10(1):33–44, 1996.

Johnson DH, Cunha BA: Drug fever. *Infect Dis Clin North Am* 10(1):85–91, 1996.

Simon HB: Hyperthermia. *N Engl J Med* 329(7):483–487, 1993.

Styrt B, Sugarman B: Antipyresis and fever. *Arch Intern Med* 150(8):1589–1597, 1990.

Sullivan M, Feinberg J, Bartlett JG: Fever in patients with HIV infection. *Infect Dis Clin North Am* 10(1):149–165, 1991.

CHAPTER 7
Chief Complaint: Red Eye

Richard A. Neill, M.D.

CASE 7-1

INITIAL PRESENTATION

R. Miller, a 40-year-old woman, presents with a 3-day history of scratchy red eyes accompanied by crusting of her lids each morning. She denies any visual changes and has no fever, runny nose, sneezing, or cough. She states that her symptoms began shortly after one of her children was sent home from school with "pink eye."

When should you worry about red eyes?

Discussion

While viral conjunctivitis is the most common cause of pink eye, many less common but potentially catastrophic conditions can present in a similar fashion. Performing a standard eye examination on all patients presenting with eye complaints will help the physician catch less common causes of red eye. After checking visual acuity in each eye, the physician should check visual fields and extraocular eye movements. From there, the examination proceeds from the outermost to innermost anatomic structures of the eye: lids and lashes, conjunctiva (including lid eversion to check for foreign bodies), sclera, cornea (including fluorescein staining), anterior chamber, pupillary reflex, lens, vitreous, and the fundus.

> An eye examination should always include visual acuity, extraocular eye movements, and visual field testing.

> Ocular pain, photophobia, loss of vision, proptosis, ciliary flush, uneven corneal light reflection, corneal opacity, and unreactive pupils are red flags.

KEY SYMPTOMS, SIGNS, AND OTHER FACTORS

You should always be alert for symptoms or signs that distinguish a benign case of conjunctivitis from a vision-threatening eye condition.

Decreased visual acuity can occur with keratitis (inflammation of the cornea), closed-angle glaucoma, and less commonly with uveitis.

Severe ocular pain is almost always an ominous sign. Acute closed-angle glaucoma, orbital cellulitis, scleritis, and uveitis (inflammation of the iris and ciliary muscle) typically present with pain. Mild pain, itching, and even feeling like there is something in the eye are common with conjunctivitis.

A *ciliary flush* (circumcorneal vascular congestion) suggests closed-angle glaucoma or uveitis.

Lid swelling can be a sign of blepharitis, stye, chalazion, or facial irritant reactions such as poison ivy or a reaction to cosmetics. Swelling can also be seen in orbital and periorbital cellulitis.

Proptosis is often present in periorbital or orbital cellulitis. Orbital tumors can also cause this.

Focal conjunctival redness suggests such conditions as subconjunctival hemorrhage, pterygium, or an inflamed pinguecula.

Purulent discharge can be due to viral or bacterial conjunctivitis or dacryocystitis (infected tear duct).

Itching is characteristic of allergic conjunctivitis.

Pain with blinking is characteristic of scleral foreign bodies or corneal abrasions.

Photophobia can be due to uveitis, keratitis, or a foreign body.

COMMON DIAGNOSTIC PATTERNS

Symptoms	Signs	Diagnosis
History of exposure ~ 1 week prior, monocular or binocular, mild discomfort, and isolated or with URI symptoms	Diffuse conjunctival injection and watery discharge	Viral conjunctivitis
Isolated to eye in adults but in newborns (ophthalmia neonatorum) can be part of systemic infection	Marked and diffuse conjunctival injection and purulent discharge	Bacterial conjunctivitis (adults: *Staphylococcus, Streptococcus, Haemophilus*; infants: *Gonococcus, Chlamydia*)
Itching, sneezing, tearing, and binocular	Mild-to-moderate conjunctival injection and watery discharge	Allergic conjunctivitis
History of trauma and foreign body sensation	Focal or minimal conjunctival injection and foreign body	Conjunctival foreign body, and corneal abrasions

COMMON DIAGNOSTIC PATTERNS (CONTINUED)

Symptoms	Signs	Diagnosis
Photophobia, blurred vision, acute periocular pain, nausea, and binocular	Ciliary flush, corneal clouding, unreactive pupillary reflexes, and elevated intraocular pressure	Acute closed-angle glaucoma
Photophobia, blurred vision, periocular pain, foreign body sensation, and monocular or binocular	Ciliary flush and corneal opacification	Keratitis (corneal inflammation)
Photophobia, periocular pain, normal vision, and binocular	Miotic or irregularly shaped pupil and cellular debris in anterior chamber on slit lamp examination	Uveitis (inflammation of iris, ciliary muscle, or both)
Severe ocular pain, which is often in conjunction with rheumatoid arthritis or systemic vasculitis and monocular or binocular	Focal conjunctival injection and scleral thinning	Scleritis
Mild burning or scratchiness, monocular or binocular, and often in conjunction with rosacea	Crusted lid margins with scaly debris on examination and mild conjunctival injection	Blepharitis (inflammation of the lids)
Focal pain and monocular	Nodule at the lid margin or internal lid surface and mild conjunctival injection	Stye (external hordeolum) or chalazion (internal hordeolum)
Focal pain	Red and swollen medial lower lid, purulent discharge, excessive tearing, and palpebral conjunctival injection	Dacryocystitis
Monocular, periorbital pain, and fever	Proptosis, diminished extraocular movements, mild conjunctival injection, and erythema of lids	Orbital cellulitis
Diplopia, visual loss, pain, monocular, and tearing	Proptosis, conjunctival injection, and diminished extraocular movements	Orbital tumor
Asymptomatic	Focal conjunctival hemorrhage	Subconjunctival hemorrhage
Asymptomatic	Triangular flesh-toned growth pointing to or overgrowing cornea	Pterygium (conjunctival hyperplasia)

Note. URI = upper respiratory infection.

DIAGNOSIS: VIRAL CONJUNCTIVITIS

CASE 7-2

INITIAL PRESENTATION

A 23-year-old man presents with a 3-week history of redness in his left eye. He has no pain, photophobia, visual loss, or history of trauma. Confrontation testing is normal, but he has diplopia when glancing to the affected side.

DIAGNOSIS: ORBITAL TUMOR INVOLVING THE LEFT LATERAL RECTUS MUSCLE

CASE 7-3

INITIAL PRESENTATION

A 45-year-old woman is frantic. She awoke this morning with a large "blood clot" in her right eye. She has no pain, photophobia, or loss of vision. Her extraocular movements are normal. She has been coughing at night due to a recent cold.

DIAGNOSIS: SUBCONJUNCTIVAL HEMORRHAGE

SUGGESTED READING

Trobe JD: *The Physicians' Guide to Eye Care*. San Francisco, CA: American Academy of Ophthalmology, 1993.

Hara, JH: The red eye: diagnosis and treatment. *Am Fam Phys* 54(8):2423–2430, 1996.

CHAPTER 8
Chief Complaint: Dizziness

Katherine C. Krause, M.D.

CASE 8-1

INITIAL PRESENTATION

J. Chambers, a 33-year-old man, complains of dizziness followed by nausea and vomiting for the past 3 days. He has had some difficulty maintaining his balance when walking. This feeling of "loss of balance" is similar to feelings he had as a child when he purposely spun around until he got so dizzy he fell down. He otherwise feels well and has no other medical problems. He remembers having several days of upper respiratory symptoms 2 weeks prior. He has no "ringing in his ears," but he does have some decreased hearing in his right ear.

Is this dizziness or true vertigo?

Discussion

True vertigo is the illusion that either one's own body or the environment is spinning. It is informative for the physician to ask, "What do you mean by dizzy?" and then not provide suggestive words. The physician should ask the patient to substitute another single word for dizzy that best describes the experience: "falling" or "turning" suggests true vertigo while "lightheaded" or "floating" is not true vertigo. True vertigo can be divided into peripheral or central in origin. Peripheral disease involves the end organs (i.e., semicircular canals, cochlea). Balance and hearing may be affected (e.g., labyrinthitis), or only balance may be affected (e.g., benign positional vertigo, vestibular neuronitis). The three main categories of central vertigo are vascular conditions such as basilar artery disease, demyelinating conditions such as multiple sclerosis, and drug-induced conditions. It is helpful to remember the anatomy of the inner ear. The front part (cochlea) involves hearing; the back part (vestibular labyrinth) maintains balance and equilibrium at rest and during motion. The same fluid flows between the cochlea and the labyrinth. Nerve stimuli constantly move from both vestibular labyrinths to the four vestibular nuclei where there are

> **Most vertiginous episodes are benign and self-limited.**

secondary connections to the cerebellum and to the motor nuclei of the eyes and the spinal cord. Normally, these stimuli are balanced. If they are not, vertigo results.

Patients with dizziness describe feeling as though they are lightheaded or about to faint without actually fainting. Usually they feel better when they lie down. This sensation is caused by diffuse cerebral ischemia in most cases except psychogenic. Common causes of presyncopal lightheadedness include vasovagal episodes, postural hypotension (medications), and cardiac disease (dysrhythmias, congestive heart failure, low output states).

> **The most common causes of true vertigo in adults are benign positional vertigo and labyrinthitis.**

Disequilibrium or unsteadiness is a sensation of the body rather than the head and is always more prominent when the patient is standing. Any disturbance of neurosensory structures involved in posture control can cause imbalance in an older person (e.g., peripheral neuropathy, cerebellar disease, deconditioning).

KEY SYMPTOMS, SIGNS, AND OTHER FACTORS

Designating vertigo as episodic or continuous is useful. Central causes tend to be *continuous* (stroke, anxiety, depression), while peripheral causes tend to be *episodic*, occurring in distinct bouts separated by periods when the patient is symptom free. *Continuous vertigo* of several weeks duration, increasing in severity, and accompanied by other neurologic signs and symptoms should signal tumor. Acute onset of unilateral weakness, incoordination, diplopia, and numbness suggest brainstem stroke. Hearing is unaffected, but nystagmus is present. Impacted cerumen and serous otitis also cause continuous vertigo. Recurrent episodes suggest *benign positional vertigo* or *Meniere's disease.*

Duration of these episodes is important. Benign paroxysmal positional vertigo usually lasts less than a minute, transient ischemic attacks (TIA) last from 20 minutes to several hours, and Meniere's disease vertigo lasts from 2 hours to 2 days. The signs and symptoms of brainstem strokes, if survived, last from 1½ weeks to months.

Sudden onset of dizziness suggests a vascular, infectious, cardiac, or traumatic cause.

Medical history is important, particularly for known neurologic disorders, diabetes, or cardiovascular disease. Hypertension is also frequently associated with vertigo, particularly in the elderly.

A *drug history* that elicits use of over-the-counter medications such as aspirin, cold preparations, and sleeping-aid drug combinations should be included as these preparations can cause dizziness. Ototoxic and salt-retaining drugs; steroids or nonsteroidal anti-inflammatory agents; and recreational drugs such as cocaine, amphetamines, heroin, and marijuana also may cause either dizziness or vertigo.

Vertigo or headaches occurring several weeks after a *head injury*, whether the injury caused unconsciousness or not, should alert the physician to potentially unrecognized intracranial injuries.

Vertigo is rarely a prelude to *seizure*.

Vertigo can represent a *migraine* equivalent.

Tinnitus, ear fullness, and *hearing deficit* suggest Meniere's disease. These symptoms are rare in labyrinthitis and are absent in benign positional vertigo. *Nausea* and *vomiting* may be present in all three of these conditions.

Chronic progressive hearing loss coupled with poor speech discrimination, tinnitus, fullness and localized pain, facial numbness, or weakness raises suspicion of an *acoustic neuroma* or a *nasopharyngeal tumor.* Persistent unilateral serous otitis can be seen.

Positional changes (head movement) instigates benign positional vertigo but not Meniere's disease. Lying still or extinguishing the response by repeating the movement relieves the vertigo of benign positional vertigo but not the vertigo of other causes. Dizziness that occurs after standing up may represent orthostatic hypotension.

Nystagmus elicited by caloric testing, Barany testing, or other postural maneuvers occurs in benign positional vertigo, Meniere's disease, and labyrinthitis. The nystagmus is horizontal and abates after a few seconds. In central lesions, the nystagmus is often vertical and does not fatigue.

Age of the patient is significant. New onset lightheadedness in the elderly is likely to be due to cardiac or cerebrovascular insufficiency. Impairment of vision, proprioception, and hearing in the elderly cause vertigo. These sensory losses combined with orthostatic hypotension from antihypertensive drugs, diuretics, and drugs used to treat vertigo significantly increase the risk of falls.

> The most common causes of lightheadedness include stress, anxiety or depression, circulatory problems, arrhythmias, hyperventilation, and idiopathy.

In adults, *psychogenic* dizziness tends to be constant or occurs in repetitive bouts around stressful events. The patient hyperventilates and may develop perioral numbness and tingling.

COMMON DIAGNOSTIC PATTERNS

Symptoms	Signs	Diagnosis
Antecedent viral infection, acute onset vertigo, nausea, vomiting, hearing loss, and lasts 7–14 days	Has nystagmus on gaze away from affected ear suppressed by visual fixation	Labyrinthitis
Same as above without hearing deficit and lasts longer	Same as above	Vestibular neuronitis
Vertigo only in certain head positions and no hearing deficit	Repeating maneuver extinguishes response and has horizontal and positional nystagmus	Benign positional vertigo
Recurrent bouts of vertigo lasting 2 hours to 2 days, tinnitus, ear fullness, hearing loss, and worse during episodes	Has nystagmus during episodes, which is postural in 25% of patients, and progressive low-frequency hearing loss	Meniere's disease
Continuous vertigo, progressive deafness with poor speech discrimination, and +/− localized headache	+/− Unilateral serous otitis, abnormalities of cranial nerves V, VII, X and finger-to-nose test, spontaneous nystagmus, and +/− café-au-lait spots	Acoustic neuroma
Continuous vertigo but less severe, mild nausea, rare vomiting, acute onset unilateral weakness, incoordination, diplopia, and numbness	Vertical nystagmus and abnormal neurologic examination	Vertebrobasilar artery disease
Body unsteadiness and decreased hearing, sight, and touch	Peripheral neuropathy (diabetes, alcohol), decreased hearing, and decreased vision	Multisensory deficit
Dizziness accompanied by hyperventilation with hand tingling, perioral numbness and apprehension	Motor tension and autonomic hyperactivity	Anxiety or depression
Presyncopal lightheadedness and palpitations	Irregular rapid thready pulse, intermittent abnormal ECG, and decreased BP on tilt test	Cardiac dysrhythmias

COMMON DIAGNOSTIC PATTERNS (CONTINUED)

Symptoms	Signs	Diagnosis
Continuous dizziness and wide-based gait	Ataxia and endpoint nystagmus	Anticonvulsant, sedative-hypnotic, or drug toxicity
Vertigo, sudden weakness, blurred vision separated in time occurring over years, and varying neurologic symptoms	Episodes of optic neuritis, flaccid paresis, abnormal vestibular response, and abnormal variable neurologic examination	Multiple sclerosis
Lightheadedness, nervousness, jittery, sweaty, and nausea	Decreased blood glucose levels	Hypoglycemia
Lightheadedness, fatigue, polyphagia, and polydipsia	Increased blood glucose levels	Hyperglycemia

Note. ECG = electrocardiogram; BP = blood pressure.

DIAGNOSIS: VIRAL LABYRINTHITIS

CASE 8-2

INITIAL PRESENTATION

D. Linders, a 73-year-old diabetic hypertensive woman, experienced acute onset of a spinning sensation with blurred vision and difficulty seeing objects on her left side, which lasted 1 week. She attributed these problems to her diabetes, but her symptoms remained after she brought her glucose down to a normal range, so she came to the office. Once there, she described a right-sided headache and numbness in the first three fingertips of her left hand and left upper lip, which came and went during a 3-hour period. During the examination, which revealed a blood pressure of 180/100 mm Hg and a homonymous hemianopsia, her facial numbness expanded to include her entire cheek. She was admitted to the hospital for a stroke in evolution. Her magnetic resonance imaging (MRI) scan showed low flow in her right posterior cerebral artery and an old right occipital stroke. After treatment with intravenous tissue plasminogen activator (t-PA) and antihypertensive medication, her vertigo and sensory symptoms disappeared, and she had partial recovery of her field of vision.

DIAGNOSIS: VERTIGO WITH STROKE

SUGGESTED READING

Drachman DA, Hart CW: An approach to the dizzy patient. *Neurology* 22:1328–1334, 1972.

Sloan PD: Dizziness in primary care: results from the National Ambulatory Medical Care Survey. *J Fam Prac* 29(1):33–38, 1989.

Sloan PD: Evaluation and management of dizziness in an older patient. *Clin Geriatr Med* 12(4):785–794, 1996.

CHAPTER 9
Chief Complaint: Cold

Marjorie A. Bowman, M.D., M.P.A.

CASE 9-1

INITIAL PRESENTATION

A. Little, a 35-year-old woman, has felt bad for 2 days. Specific symptoms include a runny nose, some chills (unknown whether or not she has a fever), a sore throat, and a mild headache. Physical examination is unremarkable except for some clear to cloudy white rhinorrhea, red swollen turbinates, and mild erythema of the throat.

Does this patient have just a cold?

Discussion

Most colds are viral in origin and require only symptomatic treatment, but some patients develop concurrent bacterial infections or reversible bronchial obstruction requiring treatment. Also, other infections (such as Rocky Mountain spotted fever or herpes encephalitis) can start with vague symptoms, such as malaise and body aches, that patients may interpret as "a cold" or "the flu." Thus, "a cold" as a presenting symptom is nonspecific, and additional details are needed to determine if it is a common viral infection or something requiring specific treatment.

> **Common Causes of a Cold**
> Viral upper respiratory infection
> Sinusitis
> Influenza

KEY SYMPTOMS, SIGNS, AND OTHER FACTORS

There are several key symptoms that suggest the need for more than symptomatic treatment.

Double sickness, that is, getting sick, starting to get better, then getting sick again, is a symptom of the development of bacterial infections, such as otitis media, sinusitis, or pneumonia.

A *sore throat* with a fever and not much else may be a "strep throat" requiring antibiotics. Facial pain and tenderness with *purulent rhinorrhea* suggests sinusitis, although green rhinorrhea can

> **Common Symptoms or Signs of Bacterial Infections in Patients Complaining of a Cold**
> Double sickness
> Prolonged green rhinorrhea or sputum
> Red ear drum or drums
> Localized lung rales or rhonchi

occur for a day or two with a routine cold. "*Chest tightness*" suggests wheezing (sometimes not audible on examination) or pneumonia. A *cough* can occur with a cold or with wheezing, but the production of purulent sputum for more than a day or two particularly suggests bronchitis or pneumonia. More generalized *muscle and body aching* and fever out of proportion to the milder rhinorrhea is characteristic of influenza. Concurrent nausea, vomiting, and possibly diarrhea are also common. *Stiff neck* is classically associated with meningitis, but it is not specific. *Seizures* with colds in adults suggest meningitis or encephalitis (such as herpes encephalitis). Similarly, depressed mental status is worrisome for central nervous system infection.

Concurrent *rashes*, if classic, can help make a diagnosis. Many viruses can cause rashes, although this is more common in children. Urticaria can result from allergies to medications taken, *Streptococcus* infection, or herpes virus. Rocky Mountain spotted fever can start with a "cold," and the patient often has a history of a tick bite, headache, and photophobia; the rash (macules on the palms and soles progressing to the extremities and becoming petechial) comes later.

> **Most Common Cause of Chronic Rhinorrhea**
> Allergy

Lyme disease also sometimes starts with myalgias and fever; the rash called erythema migrans (gradually expanding red ring) is present in most patients.

COMMON DIAGNOSTIC PATTERNS

Symptoms	Signs	Diagnosis
Rhinorrhea, +/− fever, and malaise	Swollen, red turbinates and clear to cloudy discharge	Viral URI
Body and muscle aches, fever, mild rhinorrhea, and headache	Mild rhinorrhea, low WBCs and occurs in epidemics	Influenza

COMMON DIAGNOSTIC PATTERNS (CONTINUED)

Symptoms	Signs	Diagnosis
Purulent rhinorrhea, postnasal drip, +/− fever, double sickness, malaise, and facial pain or tenderness	Facial tenderness and abnormal x-rays	Sinusitis
Sore throat and fever with few other symptoms	Red throat, sometimes white spots, and positive strep test	Strep throat
Rhinorrhea, no fever, and chronic	Purplish, pale, boggy turbinates	Allergic rhinitis
Rhinorrhea, fever, double sickness, and earache	Red, bulging ear drum	Otitis media
Rhinorrhea, purulent sputum production, fever, and chest tightness	Clear lungs or wheezing and reduced peak flow	Bronchitis with or without asthma
Rhinorrhea, malaise, double sickness, purulent sputum production, fever, and chest pain	Localized rales, rhonchi, abnormal x-ray, and elevated WBCs	Pneumonia
Upper respiratory symptoms, photophobia, fever, headache, and stiff neck	Stiff neck, drowsiness, and abnormal cerebrospinal fluid	Meningitis

Note. URI = upper respiratory infection; WBCs = white blood cells.

DIAGNOSIS: UPPER RESPIRATORY INFECTION

CASE 9-2

INITIAL PRESENTATION

A 45-year-old woman developed a runny nose, a mild sore throat, malaise, and head stuffiness 6 days ago. She felt really bad the first 2 days, but then she started improving. Yesterday she started to feel bad again with a "worsening" frontal headache, and the nasal discharge became thicker and was dark in color. She has a low-grade fever and "feels lousy." Physical examination is remarkable for thick nasal secretions and tenderness over the maxillary sinuses.

DIAGNOSIS: BACTERIAL SINUSITIS SUPERIMPOSED ON VIRAL UPPER RESPIRATORY INFECTION

CHAPTER 10
Chief Complaint: Cough

Marjorie A. Bowman, M.D., M.P.A.

CASE 10-1

INITIAL PRESENTATION

L. Daniels, a 45-year-old woman, complains of a nagging non-productive cough that has awakened her from sleep for the last 2 months. She does not smoke, has had no upper respiratory infections, and has been remarkably healthy. She denies fever, shortness of breath, wheezing, nasal congestion, or any other associated symptoms. She takes no chronic medications. Over-the-counter cough preparations have failed. On further questioning the physician finds that her cough is quieter during the day. In the review of systems, the physician notes that the patient has occasional heartburn.

Is cough the primary problem?

Discussion

Cough is a reflexive defense mechanism invoked by the body in an attempt to clear the lungs of offending agents. In most cases, cough occurs as one of a constellation of symptoms resulting from a brief self-limited condition such as the common cold, influenza, or sinusitis. In these illnesses, symptoms such as fever, pharyngitis, or rhinorrhea can coexist and even overshadow cough. Even when cough is the most prominent symptom, however, the causative condition can be recognized by the overall symptom pattern accompanying the illness. Symptomatic treatment and reassurance of the self-limited nature of the condition are usually sufficient.

KEY SYMPTOMS, SIGNS, AND OTHER FACTORS

Duration of the cough is important. *Acute cough* lasting a few days to a few weeks is usually due to viral upper respiratory infections. Lingering cough, which persists after other viral symptoms have resolved, is common in infections due to organisms such as *Mycoplasma pneumoniae* and *TWAR Chlamydia*. *Chronic cough* is defined as an isolated cough lasting longer than 4 weeks. Among non-smokers, chronic cough is usually attributable to one of four conditions: gastroesophageal reflux disease (GERD), postnasal drip syndrome (PNDS), cough variant asthma, or iatrogenic cough from angiotensin-converting enzyme (ACE) inhibitors. Together these conditions account for 95% of cases in nonsmoking adults.

Always take a complete *smoking history*. Patients may be reluctant to admit smoking a pipe, cigar, marijuana, or cocaine if asked only about cigarettes. In addition, patients will deny a smoking history if asked only about current use, even if they just stopped smoking yesterday! Smoking-induced chronic bronchitis is the most frequent cause of cough among smokers. This cough is more productive and more persistent, occurring for at least 3 months in each of two successive years. Also, ask about exposure to *second-hand smoke* or *inhaled irritants* at work or home, such as cleaning solutions, paint fumes, or machinery exhaust.

Concurrent symptoms, when present, can give a clue to the diagnosis. *Rhinorrhea* or sinus congestion suggests PNDS caused by allergy or persistent upper respiratory infection. Patients with PNDS clear their throat frequently. Occult foreign bodies should also be suspected, especially in younger patients. *Heartburn, worsening of cough with recumbency*, and *wheezing* occur with GERD. Wheezing in isolation can indicate cough-variant asthma. *Constitutional symptoms* such as weight loss, fever, and night sweats can be seen in tuberculosis, lymphoma, lung cancer, and mixed connective tissue disorders such as sarcoidosis and lupus. These symptoms warrant extensive evaluation. *Blood-tinged sputum* can occur in simple bronchitis, though persistent blood streaking portends more ominous etiologies such as lung cancer. *Hemoptysis* requires evaluation via bronchoscopy with the amount and duration of hemoptysis dictating the urgency of the evaluation.

The character and timing of chronic cough have little predictive value in nonsmoking patients with a normal chest x-ray despite a frequent emphasis on differentiating productive from nonproductive or morning from evening cough.

Most Common Causes of Chronic Cough

Smoking (chronic bronchitis)
PNDS
GERD
ACE inhibitors
Cough-variant asthma
Respiratory infection

COMMON DIAGNOSTIC PATTERNS

Symptoms	Signs	Diagnosis
Smoker with productive cough lasting at least 3 months in each of 2 successive years	Barrel-chested, muscle wasting in the chest and neck, diminished breath sounds, prolonged expiratory phase, and reduced peak expiratory flow	Chronic bronchitis
Minimally productive cough, worsening with recumbency or after meals, and heartburn	None but may wheeze	GERD
Nonproductive cough, rhinorrhea, and history of allergies	Frequent throat clearing	PNDS
Paroxysms of nonproductive cough sometimes interspersed with wheezing	Reduced peak expiratory flow with provocation testing	Cough-variant asthma
Paroxysms of nonproductive cough sometimes interspersed with wheezing after exercise	Reduced peak expiratory flow with provocation testing	Exercise-induced asthma
Nonproductive cough and ACE inhibitor use	None	Medication-induced cough
Blood-tinged sputum, hemoptysis, and a smoker	Weight loss and abnormal CXR	Lung cancer
Productive cough, night sweats, and anorexia	Fever and weight loss	Tuberculosis
Dry cough, night sweats, and fatigue	Nighttime fever and hilar adenopathy on CXR (sarcoid)	Sarcoidosis and SLE
Paroxysmal dry cough lasting less than 2 weeks	+/− fever, and prolonged inspiratory "whoop"	Pertussis
Prolonged dry cough following a prodrome of upper respiratory symptoms	Normal breath sounds with diffuse interstitial markings on CXR (out of proportion to examination findings) and cold agglutinins	Atypical pneumonia due to *Mycoplasma pneumoniae* or *TWAR Chlamydia*
Isolated nonproductive cough	None	Occult sinusitis, foreign body in airway or external auditory canal

Note. GERD = gastroesophageal reflux disease; PNDS = postnasal drip syndrome; ACE = angiotensin-converting enzyme; CXR = chest x-ray; SLE = systemic lupus erythematosus.

DIAGNOSIS: GASTROESOPHAGEAL REFLUX DISEASE

CASE 10-2

INITIAL PRESENTATION

A 32-year-old man complains of debilitating paroxysms of cough with exercise. His lung examination is normal before and after in-office exercise, but he coughs repeatedly and gets mildly short of breath. A diagnostic trial of inhaled beta agonist in the office relieves his symptoms.

DIAGNOSIS: EXERCISE-INDUCED ASTHMA

CASE 10-3

INITIAL PRESENTATION

A 22-year-old female patient with atopic eczema presents with a 3-year history of nagging cough each spring. Her examination reveals boggy nasal mucosa and mucoid exudate covering her pharynx.

DIAGNOSIS: POSTNASAL DRIP SYNDROME

SUGGESTED READING

Ebell MH: Diagnosis of chronic cough. *J Fam Pract* 43(3):231–232, 1996.

Lalloo UG, Barnes PJ, Chung KF: Pathophysiology and clinical presentations of cough. *J Allergy Clin Immunol* 98(5):591–596, 1996.

Mello CJ, Irwin RS, Curley FJ: Predictive values of the character, timing, and complications of chronic cough in diagnosing its cause. *Arch Intern Med* 156(9):997–1003, 1996.

CHAPTER 11
Chief Complaint: Wheezing

Ilene M. Rosen, M.D., and Lisa M. Bellini, M.D.

CASE 11-1

INITIAL PRESENTATION

T. Stephens, a 25-year-old woman, complains of cough and shortness of breath with minimal amounts of activity 10 days after an upper respiratory infection. These symptoms are associated with headache, rhinorrhea, and nasal congestion. She has never used tobacco. Her lung examination is notable for diffuse, high-pitched, continuous sounds heard during inspiration and expiration.

When is wheezing asthma?

Discussion

Wheezes are continuous adventitious lung sounds that are superimposed on the normal breath sounds. Wheezes are defined as high-pitched, continuous sounds with a dominant frequency of 400 hertz (Hz) or more. The word "continuous" means that the duration of a wheeze is longer than 250 msec.

KEY SYMPTOMS, SIGNS, AND OTHER FACTORS

A thorough *history* is very important and should reveal prior diagnoses of asthma, urticaria, eczema, rhinitis, or nasal polyps. A history of longstanding tobacco use may suggest chronic obstructive pulmonary disease, while previous thromboembolic events suggest pulmonary embolism as the cause of wheezing. Recurrent infections may suggest bronchiectasis. Prior surgery or trauma to the trachea can also cause wheezing.

An *exposure history* is also important when differentiating causes of wheezing. Symptoms occurring abruptly after exposure to a specific allergen, cold air, a strong odor, physical exercise, a viral

> Wheezes are clinically noted as musical sounds that can be further characterized by their intensity, pitch, duration in the respiratory cycle, and relationship to the phase of respiration and location.

respiratory infection, or emotional excitement suggest certain types of asthma or reactive airway disease. Chronic exposures, including, exposure to birds, impure cooling and humidification systems, and chemicals such as isocyanates, can also cause wheezing.

Concurrent symptoms should be elicited. *Fever* may indicate an associated infection; although it is important to note that the mechanisms causing airway narrowing are also associated with the release of systemic substances that cause fever independent of infection. *Chest pain*, either substernal or pleuritic, may be useful in elucidating a cardiac or pulmonary etiology. The presence of a *productive cough* suggests acute or chronic bronchitis.

A detailed *medication history* is necessary. Angiotensin-converting enzyme (ACE) inhibitors and beta antagonists may be associated with wheezes. Aspirin sensitivity may be noted in patients with asthma.

Physical examination findings may be helpful in determining an etiology. The evaluation for respiratory distress begins by observing the patient's breathing and speech patterns. A normal breathing pattern is deep and regular at approximately 14–16 respirations/min. Shallow respirations at a rate greater than 20/min are suggestive of respiratory distress. A speech pattern consisting of sentences interrupted by respirations every one to two words as well as the use of accessory muscles, pursed-lip breathing, and a prolonged expiratory phase all suggest respiratory distress. The presence of tachycardia, tachypnea, or a paradoxical pulse is an indication of the severity of airway obstruction. A quiet chest may reflect shallow breathing in a patient with an extremely severe obstruction. Wheezing that is exacerbated in the supine position may be a sign of congestive heart failure (CHF) or an endobronchial lesion that becomes more obstructive with changes in position. CHF may be associated with a third heart sound (S_3) gallop and crackles in addition to wheezes.

The relationship of wheezing to the *phase of respiration* may be a key differentiating symptom. Wheezes heard during inspiration may indicate upper airway obstruction from a foreign body or epiglottitis. Expiratory wheezes may be heard in chronic obstructive pulmonary disease, emotional laryngeal stenosis, and forced expiration in normal adults. Disease processes that may cause wheezing throughout the entire respiratory cycle include asthma, tracheobronchitis, tracheomalacia, and pulmonary edema.

The *location* of the wheezing is also important. Wheezes may be heard diffusely throughout both lung fields in diseases such as chronic obstructive pulmonary disease (COPD), asthma, pulmonary edema, and tracheobronchitis. Wheezes localized to one area of one lung suggest bronchial obstruction, such as a bronchial foreign body aspiration, bronchiectasis, endobronchial tumor, or pulmonary embolus. High-pitched sounds, which are more prominent over the neck during inspiration, are consistent with stridor associated with upper airway obstruction. Emotional laryngeal stenosis or laryngeal asthma is associated with expiratory wheezing that is heard over the neck and appears to be transmitted to the chest.

The *timing* of wheezing is also important. Nocturnal wheezing is suggestive of gastroesophageal reflux disease (GERD) or obstructive lung disease as a result of circadian variations in the circulating levels of endogenous catecholamines and histamine. Wheezing that occurs after physical exertion suggests exercise-induced asthma. The first episode of wheezing after 50 years of age is usually cardiac in origin.

> The most common cause of wheezing is asthma. In older adults, CHF is a common cause of acute wheezing.

COMMON DIAGNOSTIC PATTERNS

Symptoms	Signs	Diagnosis
Cough, dyspnea, and wheezes	Tachypnea, pulsus paradoxus, diffuse inspiratory and expiratory wheezes, prolonged ratio of expiration to inspiration, and accessory muscle use	Asthma
Fever, stridor, shortness of breath, and large amount of secretions	Fever, salivation, "hot-potato" voice, and inspiratory wheezes heard over the neck	Epiglottitis
Dyspnea, cough with blood-tinged sputum, chest pain, orthopnea, and paroxysmal nocturnal dyspnea	Tachycardia, elevated neck veins, diffuse wheezes, rales, S_3, and lower extremity edema	Pulmonary edema
Dyspnea, wheezes, and rapid improvement after bronchodilator therapy	Expiratory wheezes heard over the neck and transmitted to the chest	Emotional laryngeal stenosis (laryngeal asthma)
Paroxysms of cough, wheezes	Localized wheezing which may be position dependent	Endobronchial disease such as foreign body or neoplasm

COMMON DIAGNOSTIC PATTERNS (CONTINUED)

Symptoms	Signs	Diagnosis
Chronic cough productive of sputum with acute attacks of wheezing	Daily sputum production for 3 months of the year for 2 consecutive years, and diffuse wheezes	Chronic bronchitis
Nonproductive cough, dyspnea, and wheezes	Pursed-lip breathing, accessory muscle use, decreased breath sounds, and end-expiratory wheezes	Emphysema
Sudden onset of dyspnea on exertion, pleuritic chest pain, and wheezes	Localized wheezing	Pulmonary embolus
Cough, dyspnea, and wheezes during the work week, but improves over weekend	Tachypnea, accessory muscle use, pulsus paradoxus, diffuse inspiratory and expiratory wheezes, and prolonged ratio of inspiration to expiration	Occupational asthma
Productive cough, wheezes, fever, and pleuritic chest pain	Diffuse wheezes, localized tubular breath sounds and egophany, and fever	Pneumonia
Productive cough, wheezes, and fever	Diffuse wheezes and rhonchi, and fever	Acute tracheobronchitis

DIAGNOSIS: ASTHMA

Discussion

Management Principles

The management of a patient who presents with wheezing is directed by the history and physical examination. If clinical evaluation suggests significant airway obstruction, emergent management of the airway is indicated. Pulse oximetry should be used to assess the degree of hypoxia. An arterial blood gas can be obtained to evaluate the presence of hypercapnia. Bedside spirometry or peak flows can demonstrate obstruction in the acute setting and then can be done serially to monitor improvement. In less acute situations, pulmonary function tests can be obtained to evaluate the presence of airway obstruction or hyperinflation. If there is evidence of obstruction, a flow–volume loop may be helpful in determining whether the obstruction is intrathoracic or extrathoracic. Thyroid function tests should be ordered in any patient who has a neck mass, wheezing, and signs and symptoms consistent with hyperthyroidism. A chest radiograph is indicated in all patients with wheezing to rule out primary pulmonary causes such as pneumonia, foreign body aspiration, pulmonary edema, and other lower airway and thoracic diseases. Lateral radiographs of the neck may be helpful if epiglottitis is expected, as they may reveal a narrowed tracheal air stripe due to epiglottic edema. The presence of thromboembolic disease can be assessed with a ventilation/perfusion (V/Q) scan. Electrocardiograms (ECGs) and other cardiac studies should be undertaken as clinically indicated.

Therapy should be based on clinical suspicion of underlying diseases. Patients with acute symptoms of wheezing and signs of airway obstruction may require nebulized β_2 agonists, hydration, oxygen, and systemic steroids. Patients with chronic symptoms should be evaluated with formal pulmonary function studies prior to the institution of chronic inhaled bronchodilator or steroid therapy. Antibiotic therapy is indicated in patients with signs of a bacterial respiratory infection.

CASE 11-2

INITIAL PRESENTATION

A 55-year-old man presents with dyspnea and chest pain, which is worse with deep inspiration, 2 days after returning from a business trip to Japan. He reports that he remained in his seat to complete paperwork for most of the airplane flight. Physical examination reveals 89% oxygen saturation, which is below normal, and inspiratory and expiratory wheezing heard in the right lower lobe. A V/Q scan is abnormal.

DIAGNOSIS: PULMONARY EMBOLUS

SUGGESTED READING

McFadden ER Jr: Asthma. In *Harrison's Principles of Internal Medicine*, 13th ed. Edited by Isselbacher KJ, et al. New York, NY: McGraw-Hill, 1994, pp 1167–1172.

Meslier NG, Charbonneau G, Racineux JL: Wheezes. *Eur Respir J* 8:1942–1948, 1995.

Szidon JP, Fishman AP: Approach to the pulmonary patient with respiratory signs and symptoms. In *Pulmonary Diseases and Disorders*, 2nd ed, vol 1. Edited by Fishman AP. New York, NY: McGraw-Hill, 1988, pp 313–366.

CHAPTER 12
Chief Complaint: Shortness of Breath

Steven C. Larson, M.D.

CASE 12-1

INITIAL PRESENTATION

M. George, a 50-year-old man with a history of heavy tobacco use, notes a scratchy throat, which seems to have worsened his chronic cough. He now has a low-grade fever and a change in the color of his phlegm from white to yellow. He notes wheezing as well as marked shortness of breath while at rest. Physical examination reveals a thin, middle-aged man breathing rapidly through pursed lips with marked use of accessory muscles. Auscultation of his lungs reveals poor excursion of the chest wall and diffuse expiratory wheezes throughout.

What is the easiest way to approach shortness of breath?

Discussion

Shortness of breath (SOB) can be a harbinger of serious disease. Clinical conditions may deteriorate rapidly. In managing the patient with a complaint of shortness of breath, a focused, rapid assessment of symptoms and signs enables the physician to generate an effective working differential diagnosis.

KEY SYMPTOMS, SIGNS, AND OTHER FACTORS

Cough is relatively nonspecific and is seen in those processes that affect the airways or lung parenchyma, including asthma, bronchitis, tumor, foreign body, congestive heart failure (CHF), and pulmonary embolism.

Fever indicates an inflammatory process, usually an infection involving the respiratory tract. Keep in mind, however, that it can be seen in pulmonary emboli as well as tumors.

Chest tightness may reflect either wheezing in the patient with asthma or acute CHF or cardiac ischemia in the patient with underlying cardiac disease.

Hemoptysis is associated with pulmonary emboli, but blood-tinged sputum also occurs in bronchiectasis, pneumococcal pneumonia, tuberculosis, and CHF.

Knowing the *onset and duration of symptoms* can help the physician diagnose the cause of the symptoms. The acute onset of shortness of breath suggests a process with the capacity for a fulminant course. This is seen in patients with pulmonary emboli, spontaneous pneumothorax, and coronary artery disease, CHF, or both. Subacute or chronic presentations are found in asthma patients, patients with chronic obstructive pulmonary disease (COPD), and those with stable CHF.

Medical and drug histories provide major clues to the etiology of shortness of breath. For instance, a history of extensive tobacco use or occupational exposure to known sensitizing substances and wheezing suggests the possibility of a form of reactive airway disease or COPD. On the other hand, an individual with multiple cardiac risks (hypertension, diabetes, tobacco use, elevated cholesterol, family history) raises concern for a primary cardiac process.

COMMON DIAGNOSTIC PATTERNS

Symptoms	Signs	Diagnosis
Pulmonary		
Progressive cough, wheeze, and SOB	Tachycardia and tachypnea, accessory muscle use, expiratory wheezes, and diminished peak flow	Asthma or emphysema
Chronic cough with sputum production and exertional dyspnea	Overweight; cyanotic; coarse rhonchi and wheezes, which change in location and intensity after a deep cough; and ABG reveals chronic elevated CO_2	COPD
Cough, sputum, fever, and SOB	Tachycardia, tachypnea, cough, dullness to percussion, and crackles on auscultation	Pneumonia, including tuberculosis
Acute onset SOB, cough, and pleuritic chest pain	Tall, thin build; absent breath sounds on one side; and CXR reveals absent lung markings	Spontaneous pneumothorax
Acute onset SOB, cough, and pleuritic chest pain	Tachycardia; tachypnea; hypoxia; swollen, tender calf; and V/Q scan or pulmonary angiogram confirms the diagnosis	Pulmonary embolism

COMMON DIAGNOSTIC PATTERNS (CONTINUED)

Symptoms	Signs	Diagnosis
SOB, chest pain, and weight loss	Cachexia, lymphadenopathy, +/− decreased breath sounds, +/− dullness to percussion, and CXR or CT scan shows mass	Lung cancer
Cardiac		
SOB, chest tightness or heaviness, nausea, sweats, palpitations, orthopnea, edema, and paroxysmal nocturnal dyspnea	Hemodynamic instability, diaphoresis, jugular venous distention, rales or wheezing, S_3, peripheral edema, CXR suggests CHF, and ECG reveals ischemia	Coronary artery disease and CHF
Miscellaneous		
Chest tightness, lightheadedness, palpitations, and perioral numbness	Carpopedal spasm and no hypoxia	Panic attack
Wheezing, soft tissue swelling, and hives	Strider, urticaria, angioedema, and airway instability	Anaphylactic reaction

Note. SOB = shortness of breath; COPD = chronic obstructive pulmonary disease; ABG = arterial blood gas; CO_2 = carbon dioxide; CXR = chest x-ray; V/Q = ventilation/perfusion; CT = computed tomography; S_3 = third heart sound; CHF = congestive heart failure; ECG = electrocardiogram.

DIAGNOSIS: TRACHEOBRONCHITIS SUPERIMPOSED ON CHRONIC OBSTRUCTIVE PULMONARY DISEASE

CASE 12-2

INITIAL PRESENTATION

A 28-year-old man complains of the sudden onset of shortness of breath associated with right-sided pleuritic chest pain. He has been afebrile and notes no cough, diaphoresis, palpitations, or nausea. On examination, he is a thin man, resting comfortably with stable vital signs. He has a midline trachea, a normal cardiac examination, and a notable absence of breath sounds on auscultation of the right upper chest.

DIAGNOSIS: SPONTANEOUS PNEUMOTHORAX

CASE 12-3

INITIAL PRESENTATION

A 65-year-old woman with a history of hypertension, elevated cholesterol, and 40-pack-a-year cigarette use complains of shortness of breath and chest heaviness. The patient noted nausea and lightheadedness associated with the sudden onset of her breathing difficulty. She has no history of similar complaints. On examination, she is an anxious, elderly woman in moderate distress. Her skin is cool and moist. She has a respiratory rate of 30 breaths/min and a heart rate of 110 beats/min. She is sitting upright and has jugular venous distention notable from across the room. Auscultation of her lungs reveals rales in the lower two-thirds of the lungs bilaterally. Her cardiac examination reveals a regular tachycardia with normal first and second heart sounds, and increased third and fourth heart sounds; no murmur is auscultated.

DIAGNOSIS: CONGESTIVE HEART FAILURE AND CORONARY ARTERY DISEASE

SUGGESTED READING

Gillespie D, Staats B: Unexplained Dyspnea. *Mayo Clinic Proc* 69:657–663, 1994.

Smith P, Britt J, Terry P: Common pulmonary problems: cough, dyspnea, chest pain, and the abnormal chest x-ray. In *Ambulatory Medicine*, 4th ed. Edited by Barker L, Burton J, Zieve P. Baltimore, MD: Williams & Wilkins, 1995, pp 637–641.

CHAPTER 13
Chief Complaint: Palpitations

R. Parker Ward, M.D., and Lisa M. Bellini, M.D.

CASE 13-1

INITIAL PRESENTATION

N. Sinclair, a 17-year-old woman, presents after a sudden episode of "pounding and racing" in her chest. Her symptoms began after arriving at the podium for her first presentation in her high school public speaking class. Additional symptoms included severe shortness of breath and sweating. The episode resolved 20 minutes after leaving the classroom. Her physical examination is unremarkable. The patient is with her mother who is concerned that her daughter has had a heart attack.

Are the palpitations a result of significant heart disease?

Discussion

Palpitations, defined as the subjective awareness of one's own heartbeat, are a common presenting complaint to primary care physicians. Palpitations are one of the most difficult symptoms to evaluate and treat because of the numerous possible etiologies ranging from potentially life-threatening arrhythmias to psychiatric illnesses. Healthy individuals may experience palpitations, usually from sinus tachycardia, at times of physical or emotional arousal. Patients experiencing palpitations sense a change in cardiac rate or rhythm or have a heightened somatic awareness brought on by some psychologic disturbance. There is a wide range of sensitivity to cardiac activity, with some patients sensing minor changes in heart rate and others oblivious to very rapid or chaotic rhythms. Common patient descriptions of palpitations include "rapid beating," "fluttering," "irregular beating," "skipped beats," "pauses," "racing," and "pounding." These symptoms cause great concern in patients because they fear that they represent significant underlying heart disease.

The etiology of palpitations can generally be divided into cardiac, psychiatric, and other. A thorough history, physical examination, electrocardiogram (ECG), and selective laboratory tests reveal the etiology of palpitations in most cases. It is important to establish whether there are any factors that trigger symptoms (drinking coffee, smoking, exercise, emotional stress) and whether there are symptoms of an underlying disease (ischemic heart disease, thyrotoxicosis). Age is an important determinant of the etiology of palpitations, as elderly patients are more likely to have significant underlying cardiac disease than younger patients. Prior infarction or angina also raises the likelihood that palpitations are due to a significant cardiac problem. Thorough medication, diet, and drug histories are important because medications such as methylxanthines or sympathomimetics, drugs of abuse such as cocaine and amphetamines, and excessive caffeine can exacerbate or produce palpitations.

KEY SYMPTOMS, SIGNS, AND OTHER FACTORS

> The most common cardiac causes of palpitations are sinus tachycardia, premature atrial and ventricular beats, and atrial fibrillation. The most worrisome is ventricular tachycardia.

Palpitations associated with *lightheadedness* or *syncope* are due to a reduction in cardiac output and should be considered an ominous symptom suggesting significant underlying cardiac disease. *Shortness of breath* or *chest pain* may accompany benign causes of palpitations (anxiety attacks), but in the setting of underlying heart disease they often indicate ischemia. Ischemia can cause arrhythmias, such as ventricular tachycardia resulting from atrial fibrillation. *Situational symptoms* refer to those symptoms that occur repeatedly in the same or similar situations (such as driving in traffic or public speaking) and subsequently resolve when the situation ends. This type of history suggests a psychiatric etiology for palpitations.

> The most common psychiatric causes of palpitations are panic attacks or generalized anxiety disorder.

Cardiac rhythm is important to assess. An *irregular pulse* is found in atrial fibrillation, multifocal atrial tachycardia, and with frequent premature atrial or ventricular contractions. A *regular pulse* is found in sinus tachycardia, paroxysmal supraventricular tachycardia, and ventricular tachycardia. In a young person, *intermittent* palpitations with sudden onset and resolution suggest paroxysmal supraventricular tachycardia. In an older person, intermittent palpitations with sudden onset and resolution, particularly when associated with exercise, are worrisome for ventricular tachycardia. *Skipped beats* in the setting of a history of a tick bite, fever, and rash may suggest the diagnosis of Lyme disease, which can cause skipped beats or palpitations through infection of the myocardium, pericardium, or most commonly the conduction system of the heart.

> The most common "other" causes of palpitations are certain medications, hyperthyroidism, and excessive caffeine ingestion.

History is very important because intermittent arrhythmias are often missed on routine ECG.

Physical signs may reveal evidence of an enlarged thyroid gland (goiter) or heme-positive stool, which may elucidate other causes of palpitations such as hyperthyroidism or anemia, respectively.

Discussion

Management of patients with palpitations is directed by the results of the history and physical examination. An ECG should be part of the initial evaluation for all patients. Each ECG should be evaluated for heart rate, regular or irregular rhythms, presence and morphology of P waves, width of the QRS complex, and the presence of atrial or ventricular extra beats. For sustained cardiac causes of palpitations, a diagnosis can often be made with ECG alone. Laboratory tests such as electrolytes, hematocrit, and thyroid function tests are indicated in all patients in whom there is not an obvious noncardiac cause of palpitations (i.e., Case 13-1). Stress testing should be performed in older patients who are at risk for underlying coronary artery disease, particularly those with symptoms of chest pain or shortness of breath or those with palpitations that occur with exercise. Frequent, intermittent palpitations can best be evaluated with a continuous 48-hour ambulatory Holter monitor. Less frequent palpitations require an ambulatory "event" monitor, which requires the patient to push a button when symptoms occur to record their cardiac rhythm. Echocardiography can be considered if history and physical examination findings suggest congestive heart failure, pericarditis, or mitral valve prolapse. Any patient with palpitations and a true syncopal episode needs immediate hospital admission, telemetry, and cardiac evaluation. Patients with symptoms of anxiety or panic should be evaluated carefully for psychiatric disease and reassured that their symptoms are not life-threatening. Referral to a cardiologist should be considered for young patients with supraventricular arrhythmia, as electrophysiologic studies may indicate the arrhythmia is amenable to ablation. Older patients with ventricular arrhythmia who are at high risk of sudden death should also be referred to a cardiologist.

COMMON DIAGNOSTIC PATTERNS

Symptoms	Signs	Diagnosis
Irregular heartbeat and lightheadedness with or without dyspnea or chest pain	Irregularly irregular pulse, decreased blood pressure from baseline, and ECG with irregularly irregular rhythm and no P waves	Atrial fibrillation
Sudden onset and termination of racing heartbeat, spontaneous rapid resolution, often recurrent at times of stress, and associated with lightheadedness and SOB	Tachycardia that is rapid and regular, diaphoresis, and ECG with rapid regular rhythm	Paroxysmal supraventricular tachycardia
"Skipped beats"	Regular pulse with intermittent irregular beats and ECG with extra beats	Premature atrial or ventricular contractions
Intermittent racing heartbeat, chest pain, and dyspnea	Midsystolic click and ECG often normal but occasionally shows premature ventricular contractions	Mitral valve prolapse
Rapid heartbeat, smoking history, baseline dyspnea on exertion, and swollen lower extremities	Irregular and rapid pulse, palpable P_2, right ventricular heave, elevated neck veins, lower extremity edema, ECG with tachycardia, and P waves of different morphology	Multifocal atrial tachycardia
Rapid heartbeats and lightheadedness, syncope, or chest pain	Very rapid regular pulse, cannon *a* waves, split S_1, ECG with wide QRS complexes, and AV dissociation	Ventricular tachycardia
Fast heartbeat, weight loss, sweating, and heat intolerance	Tachycardia, enlarged thyroid, tremors, and abnormal TFT	Hyperthyroidism
Rapid heart rate and weakness, lethargy, exertional dyspnea, or chest pain	Sinus tachycardia, pallor of skin and conjunctiva, and decreased hematocrit	Anemia
"Pounding" in chest, severe dyspnea, impending sense of doom, and resolves rapidly	Normal examination and normal ECG	Panic attack

COMMON DIAGNOSTIC PATTERNS (CONTINUED)

Symptoms	Signs	Diagnosis
Racing heartbeat associated with nervousness or excessive worry, which impairs daily functions	Normal examination and normal ECG	Generalized anxiety disorder

Note. ECG = electrocardiogram; SOB = shortness of breath; P_2 = pulmonic valve sound; S_1 = first heart sound; AV = atrioventricular; TFT = thyroid function test.

DIAGNOSIS: PANIC ATTACK

CASE 13-2

INITIAL PRESENTATION

A 58-year-old gentleman with a long history of poorly controlled high blood pressure reports a sudden onset of a "fluttering" in his chest 2 days ago. The sensation has continued, and it is worse when he gets up and moves around. Physical examination reveals a heart rate of 120 beats/min and an irregularly irregular pulse. ECG is irregular with no discernible P waves.

DIAGNOSIS: ATRIAL FIBRILLATION

CASE 13-3

INITIAL PRESENTATION

A 60-year-old man with a history of a heart attack 5 years ago develops a "rapid heart rate" while mowing the lawn. Associated symptoms included a tightness in his chest and severe lightheadedness, which caused him to fall to the ground. He does not think he lost consciousness, and all the symptoms resolved with rest.

DIAGNOSIS: VENTRICULAR TACHYCARDIA

SUGGESTED READING

Barsky AJ, Cleary PD, Remy RC, et al: The clinical course of palpitations in medical outpatients. *Arch Intern Med* 155:1782–1788, 1995.

Knudson M: The natural history of palpitations in a family practice. *J Fam Pract* 24:357–360, 1987.

Weber BE, Kapoor WN: Evaluation and outcomes in patients with palpitations. *Am J Med* 100:138–145, 1996.

CHAPTER 14
Chief Complaint: Vomiting

Steven C. Larson, M.D.

CASE 14-1

INITIAL PRESENTATION

L. Green, a 20-year-old male university student, presents with the sudden onset of nausea, vomiting, and crampy abdominal pain. He was previously well; 2 hours earlier he had eaten an egg roll from a fast-food truck outside his English class. His physical examination is benign.

What are the related symptoms that should raise concern for the individual with vomiting?

Discussion

Vomiting in and of itself is a relatively benign process; however, it becomes clinically significant when associated with profound volume loss, the inability to maintain nutritional stores, bleeding, or the manifestation of serious organic illness. When confronted with a patient complaining of emesis, the clinician needs to recognize the potential for serious underlying life-threatening processes.

KEY SYMPTOMS, SIGNS, AND OTHER FACTORS

Fever may indicate a more invasive or systemic process such as acute cholecystitis, pancreatitis, or enteroinvasive gastroenteritis.

Abdominal pain should be noted for location, duration, and type. Constant, gnawing, epigastric pain is suggestive of peptic ulcer disease while crampy, intermittent pain is more common with small bowel obstruction. *Abdominal distention* is commonly noted by patients with small bowel obstruction. *Bloody emesis*, or "coffee grounds" (dark brown-black appearance of emesis), is commonly seen in individuals with upper gastrointestinal bleeding.

Headache associated with vomiting may suggest a migraine or be a sign of increased intracranial pressure. *Lightheadedness* in an individual with ongoing emesis suggests significant volume loss, and care should be taken to ascertain their volume status by checking vital signs while supine and erect.

Medical and surgical history is especially important in the patient with emesis. Individuals with diabetes, for instance, are particularly vulnerable to metabolic changes precipitated by volume loss, stress, and starvation. Vomiting may indicate the presence of diabetic ketoacidosis. Prior intra-abdominal surgery suggests a high likelihood of small bowel obstruction from adhesions.

A chronic history of vomiting can be a sign of a *psychiatric illness*. Vomiting following meals, with no apparent underlying physical etiology, may indicate bulimia and can be associated with somatization disorder.

Medications should be reviewed; an inability to continue on an oral regimen due to vomiting may prove problematic for many patients, such as those with hypertension. Likewise, the individual on a standard insulin regimen needs to be cautioned about monitoring sugars closely and adjusting dosages accordingly.

The *last menstrual period (LMP)* in an otherwise healthy appearing young woman may provide a clue to pregnancy or hyperemesis gravidarum.

COMMON DIAGNOSTIC PATTERNS

Symptoms	Signs	Diagnosis
Acute, intense vomiting, anorexia, nausea, headache, myalgias, +/− diarrhea, and fever	Fever, dehydration, and hyperactive bowel sounds	Viral gastro-enteritis
Acute vomiting and diarrhea	+/− Fever, dehydration, hyperactive bowel sounds, and mild abdominal tenderness	Food poisoning, bacterial gastro-enteritis, or both
Binge eating followed by induced vomiting, depression, and secrecy about the eating–vomiting pattern	Minimal physical findings and laboratory results reveal hypokalemia and metabolic alkalosis	Bulimia
Anorexia, nausea, vomiting, and abdominal pain	Dehydration, tachypnea, metabolic acidosis with ketones present on urinalysis and in the serum, and elevated blood sugar	Diabetic ketoacidosis
Pain precipitated by meal, nausea, vomiting of un-digested food, often diabetic, and subacute presentation	Localized epigastric tenderness, secussion splash, and UGI radiologic examination reveals a dilated stomach with air–fluid levels	Gastroparesis

COMMON DIAGNOSTIC PATTERNS (CONTINUED)

Symptoms	Signs	Diagnosis
Epigastric pain, nausea, and coffee-ground emesis	May have hypotension, tachycardia, localized epigastric tenderness, mass on palpation of the pyloric region, heme-positive stool or emesis, and diagnosis made by UGI or EGD	Peptic ulcer disease
Nausea and vomiting and severe RUQ pain lasting several hours and resolving spontaneously; may have recurrent episodes	Afebrile, localized RUQ pain without peritoneal signs, WBCs normal, RUQ ultrasound reveals gallstones, and pericholic edema	Chronic cholecystitis
Nausea and vomiting, fever, chills, constant RUQ pain lasting greater than 5 hours	Fever, hypoactive bowel sounds, localized RUQ pain with peritoneal signs (Murphy's test), elevated WBCs, and nuclear medicine scan outlines the hepatic and common bile ducts but fails to visualize the gallbladder	Acute cholecystitis
Epigastric pain that radiates to the back, which can be precipitated by alcohol use	Pain localized to the epigastrium, and elevated serum lipase, amylase, or both	Pancreatitis
Severe, intermittent, colicky abdominal pain, and vomiting	Abdominal distention with high-pitched bowel sounds and x-ray confirms dilated small bowel with air–fluid levels	Small bowel obstruction
Nausea, vomiting, anorexia, late menses, and fatigue	Urinalysis reveals elevated ketone and HCG levels	Vomiting of pregnancy
Headache, nausea, vomiting scotoma, and photophobia	Photophobia; focal neurologic abnormalities if complicated	Migraine
Dizziness, nausea, and vomiting	Nystagmus	Vertigo
Headache, nausea, vomiting, +/− stiff neck, photophobia, and focal neurologic examination	Elevated blood pressure, papilledema, and +/− focal neurologic examination	Increased intracranial pressure

Note. UGI = upper gastrointestinal; EGD = esophagogastroduodenoscopy; WBCs = white blood cells; RUQ = right upper quadrant; HCG = human chorionic gonadotropin.

DIAGNOSIS: GASTROENTERITIS CAUSED BY FOOD POISONING

CASE 14-2

INITIAL PRESENTATION

A 17-year-old woman who is sexually active, with no prior medical or surgical history, now complains of 3 days of marked nausea and vomiting. She has been unable to keep liquids down. Examination reveals a weak young woman with an unremarkable examination. Urine ketones are positive.

DIAGNOSIS: PREGNANCY

CASE 14-3

INITIAL PRESENTATION

A 48-year-old man, with a surgical history notable for a cholecystectomy 10 years ago and an appendectomy as a child, has experienced 24 hours of diffuse, intermittent abdominal pain, vomiting, and recent abdominal distention. He has not had a bowel movement for 2 days and presents complaining of repeated episodes of emesis. Examination reveals an uncomfortable, middle-aged man who is tachycardic and afebrile with a distended, tender abdomen and high-pitched hyperactive bowel sounds. His rectal examination was heme-negative.

DIAGNOSIS: SMALL BOWEL OBSTRUCTION

SUGGESTED READING

Friedman L, Isselbacher K: Anorexia, nausea, vomiting, and indigestion. In *Harrison's Principles of Internal Medicine, 12th ed.* Edited by Wilson J, Braunwald E, Isselbacher K. New York, NY: McGraw-Hill, 1991, pp 251–253.

Hanson JS, McCallum RW: The diagnosis and management of nausea and vomiting: a review. *Am J Gastroenterol* 80:210–218, 1985.

CHAPTER 15
Chief Complaint: Constipation

Marjorie A. Bowman, M.D., M.P.A.

CASE 15-1

INITIAL PRESENTATION

H. Brown, a 65-year-old woman, complains of constipation. She recently fell and broke her hip, had surgery, and has reduced mobility. Her stools are firm, and she feels she cannot completely evacuate. She does not require pain medications.

Does this woman have constipation, and if she does, is it functional constipation?

Discussion

When a patient complains of constipation, the first task is to clarify what the patient means. Some patients believe that a lack of a daily bowel movement is constipation, but this can be normal for an individual. In medical terms, constipation is more specifically thought of as having a bowel movement less than twice a week, the passage of firm usually small stools often with straining, and a feeling of a lack of full evacuation. Obstipation is extreme constipation, often the lack of passage of a stool. In general, the United States diet is low in fiber, leading to firmer, less frequent stools than may be ideal.

KEY SYMPTOMS, SIGNS, AND OTHER FACTORS

There are several factors associated with functional constipation. These are: a low-fiber diet, stool withholding (not having a bowel movement at the time of the urge), insufficient fluid intake, lack of exercise, lack of mobility, medications, long-term laxative abuse, pregnancy, and use of certain drugs. Commonly used drugs that can cause

Factors Associated with Functional Constipation
Low-fiber diet
Stool withholding
Insufficient intake
Lack of exercise
Medications
Long-term laxative abuse
Pregnancy

constipation are antidepressants, calcium-channel blockers, opiates, cholesterol-binding resins, aluminum and calcium antacids, and anticholinergics.

A patient experiencing constipation as well as any of the following symptoms, signs, or factors may have an illness other than basic functional constipation.

Bleeding can come from something simple, such as an anal tear from the large hard stool or hemorrhoids, but it can also suggest cancer. Anal tears and hemorrhoids are usually associated with local rectal pain and bright-red blood around the stool, rather than blood mixed with the stool, which suggests a source higher in the colon. Constipation and rectal bleeding can also occur in inflammatory bowel disease.

Acute constipation suggests an intestinal disorder; in older patients, cancer should be suspected, but intestinal ischemia is another consideration. Painful problems of the rectum such as thrombosed hemorrhoids can cause acute constipation.

Total lack of bowel movements suggests obstruction. This can be from a volvulus, obstructive cancer, diverticulitis, and severe constipation. Acute *vomiting* associated with constipation suggests some amount of obstruction. Vomiting and concurrent constipation can also be seen with liver diseases.

Fever suggests inflammation or infection. The most common cause of concurrent fever and constipation would be diverticulitis. Occasionally, a slight fever is associated with severe constipation.

Alternating *diarrhea* and constipation is a hallmark of irritable bowel syndrome. Diarrhea and stool leakage also can occur when constipation is so severe that liquid leaks around a hard portion of stool in the colon.

Acute *weight loss* may accompany constipation with loss of appetite and some obstruction. Subacute weight loss suggests inadequate dietary intake or cancer.

Constipation can occur with *concurrent illnesses* and is particularly associated with hypothyroidism, hypercalcemia (of any cause), multiple sclerosis, and uremia.

COMMON DIAGNOSTIC PATTERNS

Symptoms	Signs	Diagnosis
Chronic constipation, low-fiber diet, and other risk factors	Normal examination	Functional constipation
Subacute constipation and use of a new drug	Normal examination	Drug-induced constipation

COMMON DIAGNOSTIC PATTERNS (CONTINUED)

Symptoms	Signs	Diagnosis
Constipation, alternating with diarrhea, and crampy abdominal pain	Normal examination	Irritable bowel syndrome
Constipation and black stools	Heme-positive stools with or without anemia	Colon cancer
Acute constipation, fever, and LLQ abdominal pain	Regional tenderness, with or without elevated WBCs	Diverticulitis
Vomiting and lack of stool	Diffuse tenderness, distention, and x-ray of abdomen suggests obstruction	Obstruction
Elderly, generalized abdominal pain, and acute constipation	Diffuse tenderness with or without blood in the stool	Ischemic bowel

Note. LLQ = lower left quadrant; WBCs = white blood cells.

DIAGNOSIS: FUNCTIONAL CONSTIPATION SECONDARY TO INACTIVITY

CASE 15-2

INITIAL PRESENTATION

A 55-year-old man has been constipated for 2 days. He also noticed slight chills last night and had a temperature of 101°F. There is left lower quadrant tenderness.

DIAGNOSIS: DIVERTICULITIS

CASE 15-3

INITIAL PRESENTATION

An 87-year-old woman confined to bed after a severe stroke has chronic constipation. She develops leakage of loose brown stool. Rectal examination reveals hard stool in the rectal vault.

DIAGNOSIS: SEVERE CONSTIPATION ASSOCIATED WITH LACK OF ACTIVITY LEADING TO STOOL LEAKAGE

CASE 15-4

INITIAL PRESENTATION

A 58-year-old man complains of gradually increasing constipation over the last few months. Two weeks ago, he passed some bright-red blood mixed with his stool. The physical examination is benign, including anal and rectal examinations.

DIAGNOSIS: COLON CANCER

SUGGESTED READING

Camilleri M, Thompson WG, Fleshman JW, et al: Clinical management of intractable constipation. *Ann Intern Med* 121:520–528, 1994.

CHAPTER 16
Chief Complaint: Diarrhea

Steven C. Larson, M.D.

CASE 16-1

INITIAL PRESENTATION

B. Kaplan, a 28-year-old previously healthy man, presents with a 3-month history of intermittent periumbilical pain and frequent episodes of poorly formed bloody stool. He has noted a decrease in his appetite as well as a mild weight loss. He has had no history of prior gastrointestinal illness and denies any recent travel. He uses no medications, alcohol, or tobacco. On examination, he is resting comfortably, has a low-grade temperature of 100°F, and stable vital signs. His abdominal examination is notable for active bowel sounds; the abdomen is nondistended and nontympanic with diffuse, moderate tenderness throughout. He has no evidence of rebound or guarding. His stool is heme-positive on rectal examination.

What elements in this patient's history enable the physician to gauge the severity of his illness appropriately?

Discussion

Most patients with the acute onset of diarrhea have a benign, self-limited course. Workups in these situations tend to be limited to those individuals with symptoms that raise concern for an enteroinvasive process: fever, significant abdominal pain, bloody stool, or all three. Chronic diarrhea, especially when associated with clinical evidence of failure to thrive and malnutrition, invariably requires a more detailed workup.

KEY SYMPTOMS, SIGNS, AND OTHER FACTORS

The *duration* of the symptoms is an important indicator of the seriousness of the disease. The acute onset of diarrhea, lasting only 2–3 days, is typical of a benign process. Diarrhea of longer duration should raise concerns, especially when associated with weight loss or signs of failure to thrive. This may indicate malabsorption, human immunodeficiency virus (HIV), or malignancy with colonic obstruction.

Diarrhea with *profuse loss of fluid* may lead to symptoms of intra-vascular compromise such as lightheadedness or syncope.

Fever should raise concerns of an enteroinvasive process, especially if associated with abdominal pain or bloody stool.

Flatulence is a common complaint of patients with lactose intolerance, giardiasis, or *Clostridium difficile* infection.

Vomiting, when associated with diarrhea, myalgias, and headache, suggests a viral gastroenteritis.

An uncomplicated course of diarrhea may occur with mild, diffuse, crampy *abdominal pain.* More severe pain, especially if chronic, localized, or associated with systemic symptoms, must be considered an indicator of a potentially life-threatening process.

Weight loss suggests a significant organic etiology. A small amount of weight loss can occur with acute diarrhea.

As noted above, *bloody stool* is indicative of an enteroinvasive process and should alert the physician to a potentially complicated patient. Bloody stool is a common symptom of patients who are infected with organisms such as *Shigella, C. difficile,* invasive *Escherichia coli,* or *Amoeba.* It is also a common clinical finding in patients with ulcerative colitis, pseudomembranous colitis, or diverticulitis.

The *travel history* of individuals with new onset of diarrhea may reveal recent exposure to food- and water-borne infectious pathogens such as *Giardia, Salmonella, Shigella, E. coli,* and *Amoeba.*

Taking a *dietary history* may help the physician determine the cause of a patient's diarrhea. Lactose intolerance is associated with flatulance, diarrhea, and abdominal cramps following the ingestion of dairy products.

A *sexual history* should also be taken from patients complaining of diarrhea. Over half of HIV-positive patients experience diarrhea over the course of their illness. Opportunistic and conventional enteric pathogens in this population include *Isospora, Cryptosporidium, Mycobacterium avium-intracellulare, Giardia, Salmonella,* and *Shigella.* Also, diarrhea can be related to HIV infection alone.

Recent *contact* among individuals with similar complaints suggests food poisoning or infectious diarrhea.

The use of certain *medications* may cause diarrhea. The recent use of drugs such as quinidine, magnesium-containing antacids, colchicine, and broad-spectrum antibiotics may result in diarrhea.

COMMON DIAGNOSTIC PATTERNS

Symptoms	Signs	Diagnosis
Vomiting, diarrhea, abdominal cramps, and others with the same symptoms	Mild, diffuse tenderness and hyperactive bowel sounds	Food poisoning
Fever, abdominal pain, and bloody stool	Fever; hypotension; diffuse mild, abdominal pain; active bowel sounds; methylene blue stain of stool reveals fecal leukocytes; and elevated peripheral WBC count	Invasive gastroenteritis (*Shigella, Amoeba,* enteroinvasive *E. coli*)
Profuse, watery diarrhea with abdominal cramps; occasionally bloody stool; and onset of symptoms follows recent antibiotic use	+/− Fever, diffuse abdominal tenderness, fecal leukocytes, *C. difficile* cytotoxin in stool, and sigmoidoscopy reveals multiple discrete yellowish plaques	*C. difficile* enterocolitis
Explosive, watery diarrhea; foul-smelling, greasy stool; abdominal cramps; abdominal distention and marked flatulence; anorexia; and nausea and vomiting	+/− Abdominal distention and stool examination reveals motile trophozoites	Giardiasis
Diarrhea, gaseousness, abdominal bloating, and cramps following the ingestion of milk products	Hyperactive bowel sounds	Lactose intolerance
Weight loss; large volumes of frothy, malodorous stool; chronic, intermittent diarrhea; no nocturnal episodes; sharp, crampy abdominal pain often localized to the lower quadrants	Anxious demeanor and benign abdominal examination	Irritable bowel syndrome
Constipation, rectal fullness, and oozing stool	Firm stool palpable in the LLQ and KUB x-ray confirms presence of stool	Impaction or colonic obstruction

COMMON DIAGNOSTIC PATTERNS (CONTINUED)

Symptoms	Signs	Diagnosis
Diarrhea, abdominal pain, and weight loss	Diffuse abdominal tenderness; fever; heme-positive stool; elevated sedimentation rate; increased fecal leukocytes with a predominance of lymphocytes; and colonoscopy reveals inflamed, able mucosa	Inflammatory bowel disease
Large volume of diarrhea	Benign examination	Laxative abuse
Marked, diffuse abdominal pain	Clinical evidence of peripheral vascular disease, limited physical findings, heme-positive stool, and angiogram confirms the diagnosis	Ischemic bowel
Fever, weight loss, failure to thrive, diffuse abdominal pain, and HIV risk factors	Cachexia, dehydration, fever, abdominal distention with diffuse tenderness, hepato-splenomegaly, low CD4 count, and HIV positive	HIV disease

Note. WBC = white blood cell; *E. coli* = *Escherichia coli*; *C. difficile* = *Clostridium difficile*; KUB = kidney, ureter, and bladder; LLQ = left lower quadrant; HIV = human immunodeficiency virus.

DIAGNOSIS: INFLAMMATORY BOWEL DISEASE

CASE 16-2

INITIAL PRESENTATION

A 23-year-old woman presents with a 2–3-month history of lower abdominal pain and intermittent diarrhea. She describes the diarrhea as explosive, watery, and most notable in the early morning. She also notes intermittent, crampy lower abdominal pain. She denies any fevers, chills, sweats, or weight loss. Her examination is entirely unrevealing.

DIAGNOSIS: IRRITABLE BOWEL SYNDROME

CASE 16-3

INITIAL PRESENTATION

An 18-year-old man presents with a history of intermittent, crampy lower abdominal pain associated with diarrhea and flatulence. Symptoms frequently occur following the ingestion of ice cream and other dairy products. His examination is unrevealing.

DIAGNOSIS: LACTOSE INTOLERANCE

SUGGESTED READING

Donowitz M, Kokker F, Saidi R: The evaluation of chronic diarrhea. *N Engl J Med* 332:725–729, 1995.

Cheskin L: Constipation and diarrhea. In *Ambulatory Medicine*, 4th ed. Edited by Barker L, Burton J, Zieve P. Baltimore, MD: Williams & Wilkins, 1995, pp 481–491.

Cheney C, Wong RKH: Acute infectious diarrhea. *Med Clin North Am* 77:1169–1196, 1993.

David E. Nicklin, M.D.

CASE 17-1

INITIAL PRESENTATION

A. Murphy, a 25-year-old man, complains of 3 days of rectal bleeding, which started after straining when passing a hard stool. Bowel movements are generally firm. The blood is bright red, and it is on the stool and on the tissue when he wipes. There is also some pain when passing stools since the bleeding began.

How does the physician distinguish between life-threatening and less serious causes of rectal bleeding?

Discussion

Blood in the stool is often due to simple hemorrhoids or an anal fissure. However, it can also be the presentation of colon cancer or life-threatening gastrointestinal bleeding. A careful evaluation is required to separate trivial from potentially life-threatening illness. A thorough history and guided physical examination, including a digital rectal examination and an anoscopy, will provide a diagnosis in the office for many cases and guide additional testing where appropriate.

> Digital rectal examination and anoscopy are the central elements in the evaluation of rectal bleeding. In most cases these procedures will reveal the source of benign rectal bleeding.

Blood in the stool may also be found through screening. The United States Preventive Services Task Force recommends that healthy adults over age 50 have their stool tested for occult blood annually, as well as undergo flexible sigmoidoscopy every 3–5 years, to screen for colorectal cancer. Screening is particularly important for patients at increased risk, including patients with a family history of colon cancer, polyps in first-degree relatives, or a history of familial polyposis. It has been suggested that screening begin in these higher risk patients 5 years

> All patients with guaiac-positive stool who are over age 50 or who have a family history of colon cancer or polyposis require colonoscopy or barium enema with sigmoidoscopy for evaluation.

before the age at which their relative was diagnosed with colon cancer and that colonoscopy or barium enema with flexible sigmoidoscopy may be the preferred screening approach.

KEY SYMPTOMS, SIGNS, AND OTHER FACTORS

All patients who complain of blood in their stool should receive *stool guaiac* testing. Iron tablets, bismuth (Pepto-bismol), and some foods (e.g., beets) result in dark stools, which patients mistake for blood. If an anorectal site of bleeding can be identified and stool obtained through the anoscope above the site is guaiac negative, bleeding at a more proximal site is unlikely.

The *color of the blood* and the *quality of the stool* are important. Anal and rectal bleeding sites result in bright red blood, which coats the stool and mixes with water in the toilet and on the tissue. As the bleeding site becomes more proximal, the blood becomes burgundy colored and mixes with the stool. Bleeding proximal to the colon generally results in melena—black, foul-smelling stool. However, rapid bleeding can result in quick transit through the gut and burgundy or red blood may be seen as it passes through the rectum.

Hard stool and straining during a bowel movement are commonly seen in patients with hemorrhoids and anal fissures. Chronic diarrhea with blood suggests inflammatory bowel disease.

Age and family history are important *risk factors* for *colorectal cancer*. Colorectal cancer is generally a disease of older adults. It is relatively rare under age 50, the exceptions being patients with familial polyposis syndrome or active ulcerative colitis for 10 or more years. In high-risk patients and in any older patient with rectal bleeding, a careful evaluation to rule out colon cancer is required.

Weight loss is suggestive of inflammatory bowel disease or advanced colon cancer.

Patients with a *family history of bleeding problems*, a *history of bleeding from sites other than the rectum* (e.g., gums, nose), or who bruise easily should be evaluated for disorders of the platelets or clotting.

Orthostatic blood pressure changes, if present, suggest active bleeding with volume depletion, a life-threatening problem.

Pale skin and *mucosa* suggest significant anemia—a hemoglobin usually lower than 8 g/dL—and is most often seen with chronic blood loss from colon cancer, ulcer, or inflammatory bowel disease.

Abdominal pain suggests pathology not limited to the rectum, such as colon cancer, inflammatory bowel disease, or peptic ulcer disease. *Rectal* and *anal pain*, particularly with bowel movements, is often seen in external hemorrhoids or rectal fissures.

Tenderness on abdominal examination suggests pathology not limited to the rectum, such as advanced colon cancer, diverticulitis, peptic ulcer disease, and inflammatory bowel disease.

Digital rectal examination and anoscopy are the central elements in the evaluation of rectal bleeding. Palpation for masses and tenderness and a careful visual inspection to 8 cm are possible during these procedures and will reveal the source of most benign causes of rectal bleeding. Regardless of the source, ongoing bleeding can result in anemia, and hemoglobin levels must be checked in all patients with blood in the stool. Coagulation studies and platelet counts are indicated only when history suggests a bleeding disorder (family history; multiple, recurrent sites of bleeding).

When blood is found in a patient's stool, rectal examination and anoscopy may show a bleeding site. If not, further testing, including imaging of the colon and possibly the proximal bowel, is required to find the source of bleeding. Even when a physical examination shows bleeding hemorrhoids or an anal fissure, some patients (based on their risk factors for colorectal cancer or persistent bleeding) require imaging of the colon. These would include patients over age 50 and those at higher risk due to family history. Young, low-risk patients may be managed with repeat testing of stool for occult blood after bleeding from hemorrhoids or fissures has resolved.

COMMON DIAGNOSTIC PATTERNS

Symptoms	Signs	Diagnosis
Hard stool, bright red blood in toilet and on toilet tissue, and younger patients	Visible bleeding site on anoscopy, clot over dilated vein, and stool guaiac test is negative	Hemorrhoids with bleeding
Hard stool, bright red blood in toilet and on toilet tissue, and younger patients	Visible fissure on anoscopy and stool guaiac test is negative	Anal fissure
Older patient (over age 50) and no symptoms	No bleeding site on anoscopy, stool brown, and stool guaiac test is positive	Suspect colon polyp or cancer
Older patient, red or burgundy blood mixed with stool, may be active bleeding, and clots	No bleeding site on anoscopy and stool from guaiac test is positive and bloody	Diverticular bleeding

COMMON DIAGNOSTIC PATTERNS (CONTINUED)

Symptoms	Signs	Diagnosis
Older patient, red or burgundy blood mixed with stool, and generally no active bleeding	No bleeding site on anoscopy and stool from guaiac test is positive and bloody	Colon cancer or polyps
Any age, red or burgundy blood mixed with stool, and may be active bleeding	No bleeding site on anoscopy and stool from guaiac test is positive and bloody	A-V malformation
History of ingesting iron tablets, Pepto-Bismol, or beets, and stools are dark	No bleeding site on anoscopy and stool guaiac test is negative	Diet-induced color change and no pathology
Younger patient, stools loose with mucus and visible blood, and weight loss	No bleeding site seen on anoscopy and stool guaiac test is positive	Inflammatory bowel disease (Crohn's disease, ulcerative colitis)
Burgundy blood mixed in stool or blood only with no stool, acute, and patient dizzy	Orthostatic blood pressure changes, no anal bleeding site, passing of dark blood by rectum, and epigastric tenderness	Peptic ulcer disease

Note. A-V = arteriovenous.

DIAGNOSIS: ANAL FISSURE

CASE 17-2

INITIAL PRESENTATION

A 60-year-old woman with no prior history of rectal bleeding complains of 12 hours of red and burgundy blood mixed with stool, including clots. A screening examination last year was guaiac negative. She has been feeling well until this acute illness. Rectal examination and anoscopy are normal. Stool shows gross blood and is markedly guaiac positive.

DIAGNOSIS: DIVERTICULAR BLEEDING

CASE 17-3

INITIAL PRESENTATION

A 45-year-old man in good health comes to the office for a checkup. He is feeling well, has regular bowel movements, and no history of rectal bleeding. His mother had colon cancer diagnosed at age 48. Because of the positive family history, a rectal examination is performed and shows brown stool that is guaiac positive. He is referred for colonoscopy.

DIAGNOSIS: EARLY (DUKES A) COLON CANCER

SUGGESTED READING

Bono MJ: Lower gastrointestinal tract bleeding. *Emerg Med Clin North Am* 14(3):547–556, 1996.

Friedman LS, Martin P: The problem of gastrointestinal bleeding. *Gastroenterol Clin North Am* 22(4):717–721, 1993.

Hilsden RJ, Shaffer EA: Management of gastrointestinal hemorrhage. *Can Fam Physician* 41:1931–1936, 1939–1941, 1995.

Mujica VR, Barkin JS: Occult gastrointestinal bleeding. General overview and approach. *Gastrointest Endosc Clin North Am* 6(4):833–845, 1996.

Talbot-Stern JK: Gastrointestinal bleeding. *Emerg Med Clin North Am* 14(1):173–184, 1996.

CHAPTER 18
Chief Complaint: Blood in Urine

James A. Nicholson, M.D.

CASE 18-1

INITIAL PRESENTATION

K. Sweeney, a 43-year-old man, notices that while voiding, his urinary stream suddenly becomes reddish in color. One hour later he voids again and "fills the toilet bowl with blood." He also notices mild urinary burning during and just after voiding. Otherwise, he feels healthy. His physical examination is completely benign, including a normal genital and prostate examination. Urinalysis shows a large amount of hemoglobin, moderate leukocyte esterase, and trace protein. Microscopic examination shows many red blood cells, occasional white blood cells, and no casts. A left renal mass is noted on renal ultrasound.

When does blood in the urine mean life-threatening disease?

Discussion

Hematuria is the medical term for blood in the urine. It is commonly separated into gross (blood visible to the naked eye) or microscopic (blood found only on urinalysis) categories. *Gross hematuria* frequently triggers an emergency visit from a very anxious patient who is otherwise asymptomatic. It can signal a life-threatening or major disease. The

> Hematuria may represent a life-threatening disease.

leading causes of gross hematuria include infections, either bacterial or viral; neoplasia, either benign or malignant; and urinary stones. Other important etiologies include vasculitis, coagulopathies, prostatitis, and trauma. *Microscopic hematuria* is less frequently caused by serious life-threatening diseases and is more frequently caused by problems located in the lower urinary tract. It is usually found through screening or in the process of evaluating another problem. Common causes of true microscopic hematuria include urethritis, cystitis, prostatitis, renal calculi, and benign renal cysts. However, because all problems that cause gross hematuria can initially present as microscopic hematuria, most patients testing greater than trace heme-positive on a urine dipstick should be completely evaluated.

The amount of blood required to turn a urine dipstick positive for hemoglobin is quite small, and trace positive heme on a dipstick may deserve minimal attention. Foods such as beets, drugs such as phenazopyridine, and some dyes can turn urine red in color. Povidone-iodine can turn a dipstick falsely positive. In addition, menstrual discharge or myoglobin released from injured muscle will turn a dipstick falsely positive for "blood." Excessive excretion of vitamin C can inactivate the urine dipstick assay for blood and lead to a false-negative dipstick urinalysis.

KEY SYMPTOMS, SIGNS, AND OTHER FACTORS

Suprapubic tenderness suggests urinary tract infection. A culture should be taken in the setting of hematuria prior to starting antibiotics.

Rectal pressure suggests prostate or seminal vesicle pathology.

Flank pain radiating to the groin suggests renal stone disease, tumor, or an obstructive process of the upper urinary tract.

Weight loss, anorexia, and *anemia* suggest the presence of a malignancy of the urinary system.

Unexplained hypertension suggests a renal tumor.

Urinary incontinence suggests an irritable bladder or overflow incontinence. Bladder irritability can come from bacterial infection, urinary stones, or bladder tumor. Overflow incontinence is usually caused by either a bladder outlet obstruction or an atonic denervated bladder.

Joint pain, rash, and *fever* suggest glomerulonephritis related to vasculitis. The erythrocyte sedimentation rate (ESR) and 24-hour urinary protein will be elevated.

Recent severe pharyngitis suggests poststreptococcal glomerulonephritis.

Hemoptysis suggests Goodpasture's syndrome.

Age considerations are important, especially if there is a lack of any specific symptoms other than urinary frequency, dysuria, and gross hematuria. Young adults most commonly have urinary tract infections, and older adults have a higher rate of tumors involving the kidneys, bladder, or prostate. Bladder and renal malignancies frequently present with hematuria as the only initial symptom.

Tobacco abuse is associated with an increased risk of developing bladder cancer.

Gender considerations are sometimes important. Women get urinary tract infections more frequently than men. Hematuria in women must be differentiated from vaginal bleeding. Bladder cancer is more common in men.

COMMON DIAGNOSTIC PATTERNS

Symptoms	Signs	Diagnosis
Suprapubic tenderness associated with dysuria and urinary frequency	Positive leukocyte esterase on urine dipstick, many WBCs on microscopic urinalysis, and bacteriuria	Urinary tract infection and prostatitis
Same as above with fever, chills, malaise, back pain, and prostration	Significant fever, diaphoresis, toxic appearance, leukocytosis, and CVA tenderness	Pyelonephritis
Rectal pressure	Low-grade fever, hesitancy, enlarged tender prostate	Prostatitis
Intermittent flank, lower abdominal, and groin pain	Pain out of proportion to objective findings; no rebound tenderness	Urinary obstruction from ureteral stone, tumor, or blood clot
Recent major trauma (severe fall, motor vehicle accident, gunshot wound)	Unstable vital signs, and evidence of trauma to back or abdomen	Urinary tract injury—renal or bladder laceration or hemorrhage
Weight loss and anorexia	Anemia, elevated ESR, new hypertension, and renal mass	Renal tumor
Skin rash, arthralgia, and fever	Arthritis, proteinuria on 24-hour collection, +ANA, +ASO, +SLE prep; elevated ESR and serum complement	Nephritis or vasculitis involving the kidney, SLE, poststreptococcal GN, polyarteritis nodosa, SBE, Goodpasture's syndrome, and HS purpura
Hematuria following strenuous exercise	Minimal clinical findings	Exercise-induced ("march") hematuria

Note. WBCs = white blood cells; CVA = costovertebral angle; ESR = erythrocyte sedimentation rate; ANA = antinuclear antibody; ASO = antistreptolysin O; SLE = systemic lupus erythematosus; GN = glomerulonephritis; SBE = subacute bacterial endocarditis; HS = Henoch-Schönlein syndrome.

DIAGNOSIS: GROSS HEMATURIA DUE TO RENAL CELL CARCINOMA

CASE 18-2

INITIAL PRESENTATION

A 47-year-old man who has not seen a physician in years presents for an "urgent" complete physical examination. His 43-year-old brother was just diagnosed with renal cell carcinoma. The patient has no major complaints, but for the past year he has noted occasional rectal pressure and difficulty starting his urinary stream. His examination is unremarkable except for an enlarged, boggy, and somewhat tender prostate gland. His urine is clear yellow but tests positive for moderate hemoglobin and trace leukocyte esterase. Microscopic urinalysis shows numerous red blood cells and occasional white blood cells.

DIAGNOSIS: MICROSCOPIC HEMATURIA DUE TO BENIGN PROSTATITIS

CASE 18-3

INITIAL PRESENTATION

A 69-year-old grandmother presents with a 2-week history of intermittent asymptomatic gross hematuria. She has no history of urinary tract problems but reports having had a hysterectomy years ago. Her urinalysis shows 4+ heme, trace leukocyte esterase, and 1+ protein. Microscopic examination shows many red blood cells and occasional white blood cells. Repeat urinalysis the next day shows persistent hematuria, and her urine culture is negative. Polycystic kidneys were noted on intravenous pyelogram (IVP), and the patient was informed that she had a hereditary problem that probably accounted for her hematuria. However, she also underwent a cystoscopy, which found a small transitional cell carcinoma.

DIAGNOSIS: HEMATURIA DUE TO POLYCYSTIC KIDNEY DISEASE AND TRANSITIONAL CELL CARCINOMA OF THE BLADDER

Discussion

The workup of hematuria requires a thorough evaluation of the upper and lower urinary tracts for abnormalities. It is possible, especially in the elderly, to have more than one problem with the urinary tract, and the finding of a single abnormality should not cause the remainder of a workup to be canceled. This patient could have developed a complicated urinary tract infection, a debilitating iron deficiency anemia, or a more invasive bladder cancer had the second diagnosis not been made in a timely manner.

> The finding of hematuria, especially in the elderly, suggests the need for full evaluation of upper and lower urinary tracts for abnormalities.

SUGGESTED READING

Ahmed A, Lee J: Asymptomatic urinary abnormalities. Hematuria and proteinuria. *Med Clin N Am* 81:641–652, 1997.

McCarthy JJ: Outpatient evaluation of hematuria: locating the source of bleeding. *Postgrad Med J* 101:125–128, 1997.

Rockall AG, Newman-Sanders AP, Al-Kutoubi MA, et al: Haematuria. *Postgrad Med J* 73:129–136, 1997.

Sutton J: Evaluation of hematuria in adults. *JAMA* 264:2475–2491, 1990.

CHAPTER 19
Chief Complaint: Painful Urination

Elizabeth M. Datner, M.D.

CASE 19-1

INITIAL PRESENTATION

K. White, a 23-year-old woman, complains of burning and frequency of urination that has been getting worse over several days. She currently feels urgency, as if she will not make it to the bathroom in time, but when she voids, she has only a small amount of urine.

What is the context in which the dysuria is occurring?

Discussion

Dysuria (painful urination) may be an indication of several possible diagnoses. This symptom results from inflammation of the urethra and bladder neck or both, regardless of the cause. Inflammation is usually caused by infectious agents, most commonly bacteria, but may also indicate mechanical problems or noninfectious inflammation due to focal irritation.

KEY SYMPTOMS, SIGNS, AND OTHER FACTORS

Urgency, the compelling need to urinate and sensation of impending incontinence, is a symptom commonly associated with dysuria. Urgency may imply bladder inflammation; however, any distention of the bladder, either internal such as a full bladder or external such as compression from a mass or pregnancy, can also cause urgency. *Frequency* of urination (four to six times a day is normal for most people) without increased urine volume can indicate a decrease in the filling capacity of the bladder. Any cause of irritation of the bladder (e.g., infection, foreign bodies, tumors) can lead to an inflammatory infiltrate and edema, which will cause mild stretching and loss of elasticity of the bladder muscle.

Abdominal pain associated with urinary tract infections is usually described as lower abdominal or suprapubic fullness or a pressure-like sensation. Lower abdominal or pelvic pain may be associated with sexually transmitted diseases in women, particularly those associated with pelvic inflammatory disease.

Back pain associated with dysuria suggests the possibility of kidney involvement such as with pyelonephritis and should prompt the physician to look for systemic signs of infection.

Systemic complaints, particularly *fever*, but also myalgia, arthralgia, nausea, or vomiting indicate a more serious or complicated problem. These symptoms frequently indicate a systemic infection, and patients with these complaints require more detailed evaluation and management. Fever associated with symptoms of a urinary tract infection (UTI) should prompt questions to elicit symptoms of pyelonephritis.

Sexual history is essential in patients complaining of dysuria. Painful urination is frequently the only complaint offered by patients who are subsequently diagnosed with sexually transmitted diseases. Explicit information regarding the presence and type of penile or vaginal discharge, presence of testicular or vaginal pain, use of condoms, dyspareunia (pain with intercourse), or traumatic intercourse should be sought. In women with infectious vaginitis or cervicitis there may be an associated change in vaginal discharge, but this may not be appreciated by the patient. In men, the typical penile discharge of gonococcal or chlamydial urethritis frequently is not present or not noticed by the patient. In either case, the patient may be embarrassed or afraid to alert the physician to these symptoms. A history of exposure to new or multiple sexual partners should be gleaned and will alert the astute physician to look beyond a simple UTI as the etiology of dysuria.

The *age* of the patient should modify the working differential diagnosis for the complaint of dysuria. Young patients in childbearing years are at a higher risk of sexually transmitted diseases. The elderly female patient is prone to develop UTIs but is also at risk for atrophic vaginitis, which may present with painful urination. Middle-aged women are prone to developing interstitial cystitis and bladder inflammation and irritation due to multiple causes, including collagen vascular diseases, autoimmune diseases, and allergic reactions. Similarly, the elderly man is certain to develop prostatic hypertrophy, putting him at risk for developing UTIs as the result of incomplete emptying of the bladder. Prostatic hypertrophy is an important complicating factor to be considered for future treatment. These patients may present to the physician with a complaint of abdominal pain and an inability to void.

Medical history can give the physician a clue to the possible cause of dysuria. The patient with an immunocompromised state for any reason (e.g., diabetes mellitus, human immunodeficiency virus [HIV], chronic steroid use) is predisposed to developing fungal infections such as vaginitis in women or balanitis in men. Previous problems with the urinary tract or recent instrumentation can indicate mechanical or traumatic etiologies for dysuria. Recent use of certain medications (i.e., anticholinergic agents) can precipitate acute urinary retention.

COMMON DIAGNOSTIC PATTERNS

Symptoms	Signs	Diagnosis
Women with Dysuria		
Frequency, urgency, and suprapubic discomfort	Suprapubic tenderness, abnormal urinalysis, and positive culture	UTI
Fevers, back pain, or both	Fever, CVA tenderness, abnormal urinalysis, and positive culture	Pyelonephritis
Middle-aged, hematuria, and recurrent symptoms	Abnormal urinalysis and negative culture	Interstitial cystitis
Sexually active with multiple or recent change in partners	Vaginal discharge	Sexually transmitted disease such as *Chlamydia*, gonorrhea, *Trichomonas*, or herpes simplex infection
Sexually active with multiple or recent change in partners	No vaginal discharge, abnormal urinalysis, and negative urine culture	Urethral syndrome such as *Chlamydia*, gonorrhea, or herpes simplex infection
External burning, itching, or both, and rarely frequency or urgency	Vaginal or perineal inflammation or lesions, fungi or normal vaginal smear	Vaginitis: atrophic in postmenopausal women, fungal in immuno-compromised women, or perineal lesions or local irritation
Men with Dysuria		
Sexually active with multiple or recent change in partners	None or penile discharge	Sexually transmitted disease such as *Chlamydia*, gonorrhea, *Trichomonas*, or herpes simplex infection

COMMON DIAGNOSTIC PATTERNS (CONTINUED)

Symptoms	Signs	Diagnosis
Men with Dysuria		
Frequency and urgency with or without suprapubic discomfort	Suprapubic tenderness, abnormal urinalysis, and positive culture	UTI
Fevers, back pain, or both	Fever, CVA tenderness, abnormal urinalysis, and positive culture	Pyelonephritis
Urinary retention; frequency and urgency; and low back pain, perineal pain, or both	Prostatic tenderness and fevers	Prostatitis
Testicular pain, frequency and urgency, and +/− penile discharge	Tenderness, swelling, and redness of scrotum; +/− fevers; and penile discharge	Epididymitis with or without orchitis
Suprapubic pain, hesitancy, straining to void, decreased size and force of stream, terminal dribbling, and nocturia	+/− palpable bladder and +/− enlarged prostate	Acute urinary retention with or without UTI
Men or Women with Dysuria		
Frequency and urgency with or without suprapubic discomfort	Abnormal urinalysis and negative culture	Local bladder irritation (e.g., chemotherapeutic agents, radiation)
Contact with new substance (e.g., soaps, lotions, creams)	None	Contact or allergic reaction
Recent trauma (including sexual)	Focal evidence of injury	Traumatic urethritis

Note. UTI = urinary tract infection; CVA = costovertebral angle.

DIAGNOSIS: URINARY TRACT INFECTION

CASE 19-2

INITIAL PRESENTATION

A 65-year-old woman with a history of type I diabetes mellitus (type I DM) complains of painful urination. She has had similar episodes since the onset of her diabetes 35 years ago. She has no fevers or abdominal pain but admits to a whitish vaginal discharge. She has not been sexually active since the death of her husband 2 years ago.

DIAGNOSIS: CANDIDAL VAGINITIS

CASE 19-3

INITIAL PRESENTATION

A 21-year-old man with no significant medical history complains of a burning sensation when he urinates, which has been present for 1 week but has gotten significantly worse over the past 2 days. He has also noticed yellowish stains in his underwear. He denies fevers and testicular or abdominal pain but admits to multiple sexual partners.

DIAGNOSIS: GONOCOCCAL URETHRITIS

SUGGESTED READING

Hamilton-Miller JM: The urethral syndrome and its management. *J Antimicrob Chemother* 33 (Suppl A):63–73, 1994.

Lander DV: Vaginitis/cervicitis: diagnosis and treatment options in a limited resource environment. *Women's Health Issues* 6(6):342–348, 1996.

Milsom I: Rational prescribing for postmenopausal urogenital complaints. *Drugs Aging* 9(2):78–86, 1996.

Weissenbacher ER, Reisenberger K: Uncomplicated urinary tract infections in pregnant and nonpregnant women. *Curr Opin Obstet Gynecol* 5(4):513–516, 1993.

CHAPTER 20
Chief Complaint: Testicular and Scrotal Pain, Swelling, or Mass

James A. Nicholson, M.D.

CASE 20-1

INITIAL PRESENTATION

C. Black, a 25-year-old man, presents to the office to have a lump on his right testicle evaluated. It was found by his wife the prior evening, and she has insisted that he have it checked. The testicle is not painful, and there are no urinary tract or systemic symptoms. Examination confirms a firm, 1-cm diameter, nontender nodule that is firmly attached to the right testicle. Urinalysis is normal.

When is a mass in the scrotum not caused by cancer?

Discussion

Disorders of the scrotum can present as a focal mass of the testicle, epididymis, or spermatic cord, or they can present as generalized swelling or pain in a single testicle, both testicles, or the entire scrotum. A mass lesion of the testicle itself raises the possibility of cancer. Abnormalities not coming directly from the testicle are rarely malignant. Pain in a testicle or in the scrotum may indicate infection, testicular torsion, or a problem in the abdomen or pelvis that is referring pain to the scrotum. Recurrent concerns about the scrotum or testicles can also be an indication of a patient's need to talk about a personal problem such as impotence or sexual orientation.

KEY SYMPTOMS, SIGNS, AND OTHER FACTORS

A *focal testicular mass* is usually cause for serious concern. Testicular cancer is the most common solid tumor in young men 15–40 years of age. Benign tumors of the testicle are rare.

Acute tenderness of a single testicle in a younger man, especially when it does not hang like its nonpainful partner, is suggestive of testicular torsion around the spermatic cord. Testicular torsion occurs more frequently on the left side and in the morning hours. In an older man, solitary testicular tenderness is more likely to be caused by epididymitis or orchitis.

A *small area of pain on a single testicle* suggests torsion of the testicular appendix. This small structure may twist and undergo ischemic necrosis. The result is a very tender spot on the side of the testicle, which usually resolves after several days.

Bilateral testicular swelling and pain suggests the presence of an infectious etiology, although infections can be limited to a single testicle. Bacterial epididymitis, with or without orchitis, causes swelling and pain of the epididymal tissue below and to the side of the testicle. Mumps orchitis may present as testicular swelling and pain along with the classical triad of fever, diffuse rash, and parotitis.

Enlargement of nontesticular structures within the scrotum can involve the epididymis (epididymitis or spermatocele), tunica surrounding the testicle (hydrocele), or veins of the spermatic cord (varicocele). Almost all nontesticular lesions are benign. Prior vasectomy can lead to a congestive epididymitis, which occurs on the testicular side of the transected vas deferens. This problem can occur months or years after the time of the vasectomy.

Scrotal pain without scrotal physical findings occurs most often with prostate problems or urinary tract stone disease. It can also come from indirect inguinal hernias; appendicitis; or tumors affecting the bladder, ureter, or kidney. The pain in these situations is referred from the primary site to the scrotum, the testicle, or both.

COMMON DIAGNOSTIC PATTERNS

Symptoms	Signs	Diagnosis
Nonpainful solitary mass of a testicle, usually of recent onset	Hard, irregular, or diffuse mass that does not transilluminate; attached directly to or coming directly from the testicle	Testicular tumor, often malignant
Nonpainful solitary mass within the scrotum involving a structure beside or above the testicle	Smooth nontender mass, separate from the testicle; may transilluminate (hydrocele), disappear in the supine position (varicocele), or be manually reducible (inguinal hernia)	Hydrocele, varicocele, spermatocele, or inguinal hernia
Sudden onset of severe unilateral testicular swelling and pain in a relatively young man; may have history of previous similar episodes that resolved spontaneously	Testicle hangs in a way unlike its partner and is somewhat retracted, tender to palpation, swollen, and elevation of the affected testicle *increases* the pain	Testicular torsion

COMMON DIAGNOSTIC PATTERNS (CONTINUED)

Symptoms	Signs	Diagnosis
Diffuse testicular enlargement and pain, unilateral or bilateral	Fever associated with epididymal inflammation (bacterial infection); diffuse rash, parotid gland swelling (mumps); elevation of the affected testicle reduces the pain	Epididymitis (bacterial infection), or mumps orchitis (viral)
Focal swelling and pain of a small area of one testicle	Pain out of proportion to the physical findings, very focal area of inflamed tissue	Torsion of the testicular appendix
Testicular or scrotal pain with rectal pressure	Tender enlarged prostate with pyuria	Prostatitis
Testicular or scrotal pain without other symptoms	Inguinal mass	Inguinal hernia

DIAGNOSIS: TESTICULAR MASS THAT SUGGESTS MALIGNANCY

Discussion

After referral to a urologist, a testicular ultrasound, and an orchiectomy, this patient's final diagnosis was malignant seminoma. Treatment with radiation therapy makes his prognosis for long-term survival very good. Testicular cancer carries a less favorable prognosis if the diagnosis is delayed. Many men will, for personal or cultural reasons, ignore or delay evaluation of a testicular problem.

CASE 20-2

INITIAL PRESENTATION

The mother of a 15-year-old boy calls to describe her son's severe left scrotal pain that started acutely as he was getting ready to go to school and has become steadily worse ever since. In the emergency room the left testicle is very tender, lies higher in the scrotum than the right, and is moderately swollen. Gentle elevation of the

> Scrotal pain almost always warrants immediate medical attention.

affected testicle worsens the young man's pain. There is no fever and urinalysis is normal. Doppler ultrasound identifies lack of blood flow to the left testicle.

DIAGNOSIS: ACUTE TESTICULAR TORSION

Discussion

Unilateral testicular pain and swelling in a young man raises the possibility of testicular torsion, which is a medical emergency. The diagnosis should not be missed, as delay in definitive treatment for more than 6 hours can lead to ischemic loss of the involved testicle. This patient underwent an emergency orchiopexy with resolution of his pain and preservation of the testicle.

CASE 20-3

INITIAL PRESENTATION

A 41-year-old man develops a left testicular ache, which increases over the next 6 hours. He is very uncomfortable and complains bitterly about left groin pain. He has no other new symptoms except for mild urinary frequency. His physical examination is remarkable for a completely normal testicular and scrotal examination and mild left costovertebral angle tenderness. Urinalysis shows significant microscopic hematuria.

> Scrotal pain should not be discounted because of a normal scrotal examination.

DIAGNOSIS: LEFT URETERAL CALCULI WITH REFERRED PAIN TO THE LEFT TESTICLE

Discussion

Problems that occur in the abdomen and pelvis can cause referred pain to the testicle. Ureteral calculi, prostatitis, bladder tumors, and inguinal hernias are the most common examples. Pain in the scrotum should not be discounted just because the scrotal examination is normal. Appropriate workup might include an intravenous pyelogram (IVP) or renal ultrasound, urine cytology, rectal examination, and referral to general surgery, urology, or both. If a diagnosis is not forthcoming, a pelvic computed tomography (CT) scan could be considered.

SUGGESTED READING

Baum N, Defidio L: Chronic testicular pain. A workup and treatment guide for the primary care physician. *Postgrad Med* 98:151–153, 156–158, 1995.

Gottesman J, Baum N: Common urologic disorders. When to treat and when to refer. *Postgrad Med* 102:235–240, 1997.

Richie JP: Detection and treatment of testicular cancer. *Cancer J Clin* 43:151–175, 1993.

Siegel MJ: The acute scrotum. *Radiol Clin North Am* 35:959–976, 1997.

Son KA, Koff SA: The evaluation and management of the acute scrotum. *Prim Care* 12:637–645, 1985.

CHAPTER 21
Chief Complaint: Swollen Glands

James T. Whitfill, M.D., and Lisa M. Bellini, M.D.

CASE 21-1

INITIAL PRESENTATION

J. Brown, an 18-year-old college student, complains of fatigue, a sore throat, and "lumps" in her neck for the last week. Her boyfriend was diagnosed with mononucleosis 1 month ago. Her physical examination reveals swollen tender cervical and posterior auricular lymph nodes and an erythematous throat.

Is this cancer or a viral infection?

Discussion

"Swollen glands" represent a common problem in clinical practice. Enlarged lymph nodes can be recognized by the patient or the physician during a physical examination. Lymphadenopathy can be the presenting symptom or sign of an inflammatory process or a malignancy. Lymphadenitis is the infiltration of inflammatory cells into lymph nodes. In the acute setting, it represents acute viral or bacterial infection. In the chronic setting, it represents ongoing antigenic stimulation found in human immunodeficiency virus (HIV), autoimmune disorders, tuberculosis, histoplasmosis, sarcoidosis, and drug reactions.

Lymphadenopathy related to malignancy may reflect malignant transformation of cells within the lymph nodes as with lymphoma or infiltration of the lymph nodes with malignant cells. The latter is seen in acute leukemia as well as in metastatic epithelial and sarcomatous tumors.

KEY SYMPTOMS, SIGNS, AND OTHER FACTORS

Age is a very important factor in differentiating causes of lymphadenopathy. Lymphadenopathy is typically benign and caused by infection in patients younger than 30 years of age. Lymphadenopathy is much less likely to be benign in patients over the age of 50, and malignancy must be aggressively excluded.

It is important to determine if a patient with generalized

lymphadenopathy also has *HIV risk factors* (high-risk sexual activity, prior transfusions, intravenous drug use). If so, the patient may have HIV.

Alcohol and *tobacco use* in a patient with localized adenopathy of the head and neck suggests the need to search for a cancer.

The *physical characteristics* of a lymph node are important to note during the physical examination, as they can suggest certain underlying disease states. The four characteristics that should be noted are *consistency, tenderness, mobility,* and *size.* Normal adult lymph nodes are less than 1 cm in diameter, soft, and mobile. Acute infections can result in large, tender nodes that are asymmetric. Chronic infections tend to cause more symmetric and less tender nodes. Metastatic disease typically causes hard, immobile nodes that are asymmetric, while lymphoma causes large, rubbery, and nontender nodes (single or multiple).

> The four characteristics that should be noted during a lymph node examination are consistency, tenderness, mobility, and size.

Localized adenopathy includes cervical, submental, submandibular, supraclavicular, axillary, epitrochlear, and inguinal node enlargement.

Cervical node enlargement accompanied by localizing signs of infection most often suggests infection, especially if tender. The involvement of anterior cervical nodes suggests acute viral or bacterial pharyngitis, while involvement of the posterior nodes alone suggests mononucleosis or viral illness. In an older patient with a history of tobacco and alcohol use, unilateral cervical involvement suggests a head and neck malignancy.

Submental and *submandibular node* enlargement suggests infection when the nodes are tender and associated with poor dentition and mouth pain. If the nodes are hard and fixed, a malignancy is likely.

Supraclavicular node enlargement suggests neoplastic or infectious processes upstream from the lymphatic drainage, such as the esophagus, thorax, or abdomen.

Axillary node enlargement suggests infection or malignancy of the chest wall, breast, thorax, or arm. If axillary lymph node enlargement is unilateral, tender, and associated with signs of infection like cellulitis of the arm, then it is likely benign. The presence of firm or rubbery nodes raises the suspicion of lymphoma or breast cancer.

Epitrochlear node involvement suggests infection of the hand or arm if the nodes are small and tender, sarcoid if they are nontender, and lymphoma if they are rubbery.

Inguinal enlargement is common and can be found bilaterally in healthy patients. If the nodes are less than 1 cm and nontender, they are typically benign. Larger nodes that are tender suggest sexually transmitted diseases, if bilateral, and infection of the lower extremity, if unilateral. The presence of firm, fixed nodes suggests malignancy.

Generalized adenopathy suggests systemic illnesses such as HIV infection, mononucleosis, toxoplasmosis, cytomegalovirus, sarcoidosis, lymphomas or leukemias, immunologic disorders, or drug reactions.

Fever can be seen with infectious and malignant causes of lymphadenopathy. If fever is associated with localizing signs of infection such as pharyngitis or otitis media, then infection is the likely cause. If fever is associated with systemic symptoms such as weight loss, night sweats, or extreme fatigue then it is more likely to be associated with tuberculosis, HIV, or malignancy.

Constitutional symptoms such as fever, weight loss, and night sweats suggest lymphoma, tuberculosis, or HIV.

Persistent adenopathy for weeks or months generally suggests a less benign cause.

COMMON DIAGNOSTIC PATTERNS

Symptoms	Signs	Diagnosis
Sore throat and tender cervical mass	Cervical adenopathy, exudative pharyngitis, and fever	Viral or bacterial pharyngitis
Tender preauricular mass and eye pain	Tender preauricular adenopathy and nonpurulent conjunctivitis	Adenoviral conjunctivitis
Otalgia and tender cervical mass	Cervical adenopathy, red tympanic membrane, and fever	Otitis media
Night sweats, fever, weight loss, cough, and cervical mass	Nontender firm cervical nodes, lymphadenopathy, low-grade fever, and often +PPD	Tuberculosis
Sore throat, tender posterior cervical masses, and extreme fatigue	Tender posterior cervical masses, adenopathy, fever, and elevated atypical lymphocytes	Infectious mononucleosis, toxoplasmosis, or cytomegalovirus
Cervical, axillary, and inguinal masses and HIV risk factors	Nontender, firm, diffuse adenopathy	HIV infection
Supraclavicular, epitrochlear, or axillary adenopathy and cat exposure	Nontender nodes, +/− lesion at site of scratch	Cat-scratch disease

COMMON DIAGNOSTIC PATTERNS (CONTINUED)

Symptoms	Signs	Diagnosis
Fatigue, night sweats, fever, weight loss, and diffuse masses	Localized or generalized adenopathy that is large, nontender, and rubbery	Lymphoma
Painless neck mass	Hard, fixed, greater than 1 cm, nontender cervical adenopathy	Metastatic disease
Nontender mass in axilla and breast mass	Nontender, firm, axillary adenopathy and breast mass	Metastatic breast cancer
Tender groin mass, dysuria, and penile discharge	Tender inguinal adenopathy and purulent penile discharge	Gonococcal urethritis
Persistent cough, SOB, and elbow mass	Firm, nontender epitrochlear adenopathy	Sarcoidosis
Persistent cough with blood streaks and supraclavicular mass	Hard, fixed, nontender nodes and supraclavicular adenopathy	Lung cancer

Note. PPD = purified protein derivative; HIV = human immunodeficiency virus; SOB = shortness of breath.

DIAGNOSIS: INFECTIOUS MONONUCLEOSIS

Management Principles

The management of patients with lymphadenopathy is based on the history and physical examination. There is no common battery of tests that applies to all patients with lymphadenopathy. Ancillary tests such as a monospot or throat culture can confirm the diagnosis of infectious mononucleosis or streptococcal pharyngitis, respectively. HIV testing should be considered for those patients with persistent generalized lymphadenopathy. Any concern for tuberculosis requires placement of a purified protein derivative (PPD) and a chest radiograph. Antibiotic therapy should be considered for those patients with localized lymphadenopathy and the presence of localizing symptoms or signs of infection. If the lymph nodes have characteristics of malignancy or if adenopathy persists unexplained, patients should undergo a lymph node biopsy.

CASE 21-2

INITIAL PRESENTATION

A 62-year-old man with a history of tobacco abuse presents with a lump in his neck. He notes that it has grown larger over the last 4 months, and he occasionally coughs up blood. Physical examination revealed a firm, nonmobile 4-cm node in the anterior cervical chain. Laryngoscopy reveals an ulcerative mass on the left anterior vocal cord.

DIAGNOSIS: METASTATIC SPREAD OF LARYNGEAL CARCINOMA

CHAPTER 22

Chief Complaint: Weight Loss

Matthew H. Rusk, M.D.

CASE 22-1

INITIAL PRESENTATION

K. Singer, an 84-year-old previously healthy woman, noted a 25-lb weight loss over the last 3 months. She is brought in by her son who is concerned that her skin appears yellow. She lives alone, and her husband died 2 years ago. She has no complaints other than feeling weak and having a poor appetite. Her physical examination is normal other than for jaundice and a wasted appearance.

Does this patient's age increase the likelihood that cancer is a cause of her weight loss?

Discussion

The complaint of unexplained weight loss is commonly encountered in primary care settings. While it is difficult to pick an absolute value that marks a significant weight loss, a loss of 5% of total body weight within 6 months or 10% within 1 year is generally considered significant. There are a large number of possible causes, and the key to evaluating the patient productively is a good history and physical examination. Many patients with unexplained weight loss are afraid that they have some serious underlying disease such as cancer. Most of these patients will have another cause for their weight loss and can be reassured after an evaluation. Even after a thorough evaluation, however, the cause of weight loss remains unexplained in many patients.

It is helpful to divide the many possible causes for weight loss into four categories: decreased intake, decreased absorption, increased metabolic demand, and mixed.

KEY SYMPTOMS, SIGNS, AND OTHER FACTORS

A mnemonic phrase developed by L. J. Robbins describes weight loss in *the elderly* as resulting from problems related to the "nine d's": *dentition, dysgeusia, dysphagia, diarrhea, disease* (chronic), *depression, dementia, dysfunction,* and *drugs* (e.g., medication side effects). *Cancer* is a more common cause of unexplained weight loss in the elderly. Older patients are particularly vulnerable to the effects of *poverty* and *social isolation*, both of which make it difficult to obtain sufficient calories. In taking a history from an elderly patient with unexplained weight loss, one should inquire about who does their food shopping and preparation.

In *younger patients*, the differential diagnosis for weight loss is different. Psychiatric causes tend to predominate. In young women, for example, anorexia nervosa is much more common. In this disorder, patients are *obsessively concerned about being thin*. Their sense of self-worth is highly dependent on their weight. In a variant form of this disease, bulimia, patients may eat excessively, and then force themselves to vomit to help relieve the feelings of guilt associated with binging. An important physical sign of bulimia is *premature destruction of dental enamel* and a *red throat* related to the acidity of the patient's vomit. Male athletes may also lose excessive weight as a consequence of *excessive exercise* or caloric restriction. Other patterns or symptoms of weight loss may occur in patients of *any age*. Psychologic causes for weight loss are common in elderly and younger patients. *Poor sleep, loss of appetite*, and a *mood disturbance* may all suggest a serious underlying *depression* with concomitant weight loss.

Diarrhea usually indicates a disease of the gastrointestinal tract. Patients with pancreatic insufficiency often complain of diarrhea with *bloating* and *greasy stools*. They may have an *aversion to fatty foods*, which results from the pain associated with eating them. Characteristically, *bloody diarrhea* and abdominal pain suggest inflammatory bowel disease, though the disease may present in the early stages with weight loss alone.

Diarrhea with flatulence and *crampy abdominal* pain is commonly caused by giardiasis. Infection with this parasite is most often seen in patients who present after a history of outdoor activities, such as camping, where they have consumed water from contaminated lakes or streams. Urban

> One of the most common causes of unexplained weight loss in the elderly is simply a lack of adequate access to food. It is important to ask elderly patients if they prepare their own meals and if they do their own shopping. Problems with access to food may include poverty and social isolation.

> Elderly patients are especially vulnerable to side effects from prescribed medication. Side effects may include nausea, vomiting, or loss of taste. Common culprit medications interfering with taste include digitalis, quinidine, and angiotensin-converting-enzyme (ACE) inhibitors.

outbreaks related to contaminated water supplies have occurred as infections in day-care centers.

Abdominal pain is an important symptom in patients presenting with weight loss. *Abdominal pain that is relieved by eating* may indicate a duodenal ulcer. Gastric ulcers and gallstones typically cause *abdominal pain that is worsened by eating*. *Abdominal pain with jaundice* can denote either a pancreatic or hepatobiliary carcinoma obstructing the common bile duct. In either cancer, patients may present with a *palpable abdominal mass* and profound weight loss. Nonspecific abdominal pain is also found in a variety of other intra-abdominal cancers.

Difficulty swallowing or dysphagia suggests a gastrointestinal cause, including tumors of the mouth or esophagus, strokes, or motility disorders. Strictures of the esophagus caused by reflux may also cause a sensation of food "*sticking in the chest*" after swallowing. Patients with strictures often have a history of *severe heartburn* and an *acid taste*, which suggests gastroesophageal reflux disease (GERD). Patients with these symptoms may avoid eating and as a result suffer weight loss.

Rectal bleeding with weight loss suggests colon cancer or inflammatory bowel disease.

In patients with the appropriate *risk factors*, infection with *human immunodeficiency virus* (HIV) should be considered. While this disease tends to affect younger patients disproportionately, risk factors for HIV should be determined in all patients with occult weight loss. Patients with HIV infection lose weight through multiple and different mechanisms. Decreased intake may be due to odynophagia from esophageal infections or nausea from multiple medications. Dysphagia, malabsorption, and decreased appetite are all common. Many of the specific causes are related to opportunistic infections suggested by the patient's symptoms and physical examination. In later stages of HIV infection, it is not uncommon to see a wasting syndrome characterized by the loss of more than 10% of the patient's weight.

Anxiety, insomnia, and *weight loss* are symptoms that suggest hyperthyroidism. On physical examination these patients may have *velvety skin, hair loss*, and a *resting tachycardia*. In the elderly, excess thyroid hormone production may cause apathetic hyperthyroidism. In this disease, patients appear paradoxically *lethargic* and are often mistaken for having depression. While the diagnosis can be difficult to make on the basis of the history and physical examination alone, thyroid function tests can easily establish the diagnosis. A thyroid-stimulating hormone level should be measured in all patients presenting with weight loss in whom another explanation is not readily identified.

A *history of smoking* suggests the possibility of lung cancer.

Cough would be consistent with lung cancer, tuberculosis, or chronic lung disease.

A *complete review of systems* may also suggest other symptoms, which lead one to suspect the cause of the weight loss.

Abnormal physical examination findings should lead to evaluation based on the finding; for example, generalized lymphadenopathy would make one think of HIV or lymphoma, and a palpable mass would make one suspicious of other cancers.

Role of Testing in Unexplained Weight Loss

Laboratory and radiologic studies should be directed by the results of the physical examination and history. When the history and physical examination do not give a clear explanation for the cause of weight loss, it is reasonable to do certain basic laboratory studies. These would include a complete blood cell count, serum electrolytes, liver function tests, and a thyroid-stimulating hormone assay. Screening tests should include those recommended by the United States Preventive Services Task Force, according to the patient's sex and age. If no diagnosis is clear, the patient should be followed carefully.

COMMON DIAGNOSTIC PATTERNS

Symptoms	Signs	Diagnosis
Decreased Intake		
Young woman preoccupied with weight	Can have damaged dental enamel	Anorexia nervosa or bulimia
Depressed mood, difficulty sleeping, fatigue, and feelings of guilt	None	Depression
Difficulties with personal life and work	May have evidence of liver disease	Alcoholism
Decreased Absorption		
Chronic abdominal pain and greasy foul-smelling stool	May have abdominal tenderness	Pancreatic insufficiency
Crampy diarrhea and recent outdoor activities or travel	None	Giardiasis
Bloody diarrhea and abdominal pain	Blood in stool and increased ESR	Inflammatory bowel disease

COMMON DIAGNOSTIC PATTERNS (CONTINUED)

Symptoms	Signs	Diagnosis
Increased Metabolic Demand		
Change in bowel habits	Blood on rectal examination	Colon cancer
Cough and a smoker	Occasionally lymphadenopathy or abnormal lung examination	Lung cancer
Diarrhea, heat intolerance, and palpitations	Velvety skin and rapid heart beat	Hyperthyroidism
Cough, history of exposure to tuberculosis, living in homeless shelter or prison, and fever	None	Tuberculosis
Fever, rash, and sore joints	Heart murmur, painful nodules on hands, inflamed joints, and rash	Subacute bacterial endocarditis
Mixed		
Fever, opportunistic infections, and diarrhea	Often related to opportunistic diseases	HIV infection
Nausea and fatigue	Swollen legs and may have hypertension	Kidney failure
Shortness of breath and swelling of the legs	Elevated neck veins, crackles on lung examination, and extra heart sound	CHF
Shortness of breath and wasting	Rapid breathing, distant heart sounds, and hyperexpanded chest	COPD
Excessive thirst and increased urination	Poor skin turgor and orthostatic hypotension	Diabetes

Note. ESR = erythrocyte sedimentation rate; HIV = human immunodeficiency virus; CHF = congestive heart failure; COPD = chronic obstructive pulmonary disease.

DIAGNOSIS: PANCREATIC CANCER

CASE 22-2

INITIAL PRESENTATION

A 56-year-old man presents with a 20-lb weight loss over the last 6 months. He has had little interest in his work and usual hobbies since his wife died 1 year ago. He has had difficulty sleeping and feels like he never performs adequately at work.

DIAGNOSIS: DEPRESSION

SUGGESTED READING

Greene HL, Johnson, WP, Maricic, MJ: *Decision Making in Medicine.* St. Louis, MO: Mosby-Year Book, 1993, pp 6–7.

Marton KI, Sox HC Jr, Krupp JR: Involuntary weight loss: diagnostic and prognostic significance. *Ann Intern Med* 95(5):568–574, 1981.

Reife CM: Involuntary weight loss. *Med Clin North Am* 79(2):299–313, 1995.

Robbins LJ: Evaluation of weight loss in the elderly. *Geriatrics* 44:31–37, 1989.

CHAPTER 23
Chief Complaint: Weight Gain

Marjorie A. Bowman, M.D., M.P.A.

CASE 23-1

INITIAL PRESENTATION

B. Rosen, a 23-year-old woman, comes to the office complaining of weight gain, which she attributes to the birth control pills she started taking 10 months ago, 1 month prior to her marriage. She has gained 15 lbs. Her husband has not gained weight. She does not exercise much and cooks all of their meals. Her history and physical examination are otherwise negative.

Could the birth control pills be the cause of her weight gain?

Discussion

Weight gain is a common complaint, although it is usually not the chief complaint, since most people realize the most common reasons for weight gain are eating too much food and exercising too little. As our United States society becomes increasingly obese, food intake and often fat intake are overwhelmingly the primary causes. Another common reason for weight gain is edema.

KEY SYMPTOMS, SIGNS, AND OTHER FACTORS

The *diet history* can quickly provide evidence of overeating. The patient can recount what has been eaten in the last 24 hours or keep a record of everything eaten for later review. Patients often underestimate the portions of food eaten, and it is often helpful for patients to measure or weigh their food for a day. They can also read labels for calorie counts. *Exercise levels*, particularly the low exercise levels of a common sedentary life style, contribute to weight gain.

The rate of development of the weight is important. *Quick weight gain* is often from *edema. Sudden weight gain with marked peripheral edema* is often from right-sided congestive heart failure (CHF). Other associated findings would be ascites, enlarged liver, and jugular venous distention. Left-sided CHF can also be present, with shortness of breath, dyspnea on exertion, paroxysmal nocturnal dyspnea, third heart sound (S_3), and pulmonary rales.

Subacute weight gain developing over several days is also usually from *edema*, often from CHF, cirrhosis, or renal failure.

Slow weight gain is the type seen with overeating but can be seen with drugs, hypothyroidism, hyperadrenocorticism, and diabetes. In the case of diabetes, it is often unclear if the weight gain results from the diabetes or if the obesity causes the diabetes.

Fatigue is very common with weight gain and can be found with almost all of the causes of weight gain, including a sedentary life style. A new onset of *sudden fatigue* may suggest an organic illness, such as renal failure or CHF. While chronic fatigue syndrome (CFS) is often suspected with sudden fatigue, it is not particularly associated with weight gain.

Fatigue, slow weight gain, possibly *edema, constipation*, and *high thyroid-stimulating hormone* (TSH) are consistent with hypothyroidism.

Concurrent *amenorrhea* or menstrual changes should make the physician think of pregnancy in a woman. While a woman often knows that she is pregnant before there is substantial weight gain, this is not always true.

Recurrent monthly *premenstrual weight gain* of 3–5 lbs is considered to be normal and occurs in full-blown premenstrual syndrome.

Life changes (e.g., the new marriage in Case 23-1) suggest concurrent eating and exercise changes causing weight gain. *Depressive symptoms* with weight gain make depression a significant possibility.

Drug history can reveal medications that cause weight gain, including steroids (prescription or illicit), antidepressants (particularly the tricyclics), and phenothiazines. Nonsteroidal anti-inflammatory agents and calcium channel blockers cause edema. Birth control pills can cause weight gain, but stopping the pills usually does not cause weight loss, and the true cause is often overeating. Although many patients think hormone replacement causes weight gain, it is actually associated with less weight gain during menopause.

Family history can be suggestive for obesity, diabetes, depression, and hypothyroidism.

COMMON DIAGNOSTIC PATTERNS

Symptoms	Signs	Diagnosis
Gradual weight gain and excess food intake	Weight high compared with height	Obesity, sometimes drug-induced
Gradual weight gain, swelling, constipation, and fatigue	Slow reflexes, increased TSH, mild edema, and bradycardia	Hypothyroidism

COMMON DIAGNOSTIC PATTERNS (CONTINUED)

Symptoms	Signs	Diagnosis
Subacute weight gain, swelling, and fatigue	Hypertension, abnormal urinalysis, and mild-to-marked edema	Renal failure
Subacute weight gain, swollen abdomen, and leg swelling	Ascites, usually a small liver, prolonged PT, and peripheral edema	Cirrhosis
Subacute weight gain, swelling, and sometimes psychologic symptoms	Hypertension, striae, buffalo hump, and mild edema	Hyperadreno-corticism from Cushing's syndrome or taking steroids
Subacute weight gain, depressive symptoms, and sleep disturbance	Depressed affect	Depression
Subacute weight gain and amenorrhea	Enlarged uterus and positive pregnancy test	Pregnancy
Acute weight gain, swelling, and acute fatigue	Jugular-venous distention, large liver, and peripheral edema	Right-sided CHF
Recurrent monthly premenstrual weight gain of 3–5 lbs	Normal examination	Premenstrual syndrome

Note. TSH = thyroid-stimulating hormone; PT = prothrombin time; CHF = congestive heart failure.

DIAGNOSIS: WEIGHT GAIN SECONDARY TO ENERGY IMBALANCE

CASE 23-2

INITIAL PRESENTATION

A 75-year-old man has a new weight gain and leg swelling. There are a few lung rales, an enlarged liver, jugular-venous distention, and 3 + peripheral edema.

DIAGNOSIS: CONGESTIVE HEART FAILURE

CASE 23-3

INITIAL PRESENTATION

A 43-year-old woman has gained 10 lbs in the last few days, and her legs seem swollen. Except for a blood pressure of 150/105 mm Hg, her examination is nonspecific. Her urinalysis is markedly abnormal.

DIAGNOSIS: ACUTE RENAL FAILURE

CHAPTER 24
Chief Complaint: Insomnia

Amy J. Behrman, M.D.

CASE 24-1

INITIAL PRESENTATION

L. Watkins, a 68-year-old woman, complains of difficulty sleeping for several weeks. She lies awake for at least an hour before falling asleep, wakes frequently during the night, and is unable to fall back to sleep until after 4 A.M. She has lost 10 lbs and complains of feeling sad and anxious. Her husband of 40 years died suddenly 2 months ago. She responds slowly to questions and becomes tearful as the interview progresses. Physical examination is otherwise normal.

What is the most likely cause of this sleep disturbance?

Discussion

Insomnia is a common symptom in the general population for which patients often seek treatment from primary care providers. It affects all ages but is more frequent and problematic among the elderly. In addition to the distressing subjective experience of poor quality sleep, insomnia may worsen a patient's functional status and is associated with higher rates of motor vehicle accidents. Insomnia is frequently multifactorial. It may be caused by minor problems or by potentially dangerous medical conditions. While many cases can be handled simply with behavioral interventions directed toward better sleep habits, some patients need medication to improve sleep, and some require treatment directed at a serious underlying medical or psychiatric condition. Identifying the underlying cause of insomnia is crucial

> Many patients self-medicate for insomnia before seeking medical advice.

> Formal sleep studies with EEGs are not necessary for the diagnosis and management of most patients with insomnia.

to safe and effective treatment. Patients may contribute to diagnosis by keeping a "sleep log" chronicling time to sleep onset, sleep duration, waking times, medication use, and associated symptoms.

KEY SYMPTOMS, SIGNS, AND OTHER FACTORS

Depression is a common, serious, and treatable cause of insomnia. Patients may admit to *sadness, appetite loss, weight loss, decreased libido, decreased social interactions, inability to enjoy normally pleasant activities* (anhedonia), *hopelessness, fatigue, irritability,* or *suicidal ideation*. A history of recent bereavement (death of a spouse, job loss, new physical disabilities) suggests a reactive depression. A history of major depression is a risk factor for recurrent illness. Patients with a bipolar (manic–depressive) syndrome may also present with insomnia.

> History is the key to diagnosing the underlying cause of insomnia. It should include a complete review of symptoms, a medical history, psychiatric history, medication use, work history, and sleep habits.

Anxiety is another common symptom associated with insomnia. Patients typically describe using time in bed before sleeping or on waking to ruminate on problems or concerns.

Visual or auditory *hallucinations* may be associated with disturbed sleep in patients with major psychotic disorders.

Cardiac conditions may cause nocturnal symptoms of *dyspnea, orthopnea,* and *chest pain*. It is critical to elicit this history since the disturbed sleep resulting from these symptoms may occasionally be the initial complaint in patients with congestive heart failure (CHF) or unstable angina.

Wheezing and *dyspnea* may indicate serious obstructive pulmonary disease such as asthma or emphysema. These patients frequently have increased symptoms at night, which may cause difficulty falling asleep, frequent waking, and disordered sleep cycles.

Loud snoring, occasional periods of *absent respirations*, and *frequent waking* are characteristics of sleep apnea, usually due to recurrent upper airway obstruction by soft tissues during sleep. It is most common in obese patients. Patients with this disorder may have severe difficulty staying awake during the day. Nocturnal symptoms may be recognized principally by the patient's sleeping partner. The sleeping partner may also report episodes of confusion in the patient on waking, due to intermittent hypoxemia. If sleep apnea is left untreated, it may progress to pulmonary hypertension and cardiac arrhythmias.

Urinary frequency and *nocturia* from prostatic enlargement, CHF, diuretic use, or urinary tract infection may cause frequent waking and poor sleep quality.

Pain from any underlying cause may cause insomnia. Common conditions causing chronic pain that may be worse at night include degenerative joint disease, reflux esophagitis, and diabetic neuropathy.

A history of *current medications* and drug use should always be obtained. Nonprescription and commonly prescribed drugs associated with insomnia include beta-blockers, calcium channel blockers, clonidine, inhaled bronchodilators, aminophyllines, decongestants, oral contraceptives, appetite suppressants, thyroid hormone, phenytoin, and cortisone. Caffeine is, of course, notorious for producing insomnia. Alcohol and nicotine may also produce insomnia with poor sleep quality despite what may appear to users to be calming effects. Illicit stimulant drugs such as cocaine and amphetamines can cause insomnia, as can withdrawal from sedative agents.

Phase shifting can cause delayed sleep onset, early waking, and poor sleep quality. Common causes of this include "jet lag," alternating or changing work shifts, and irregular sleep habits. Endogenous disruptions of circadian rhythm can produce the same symptoms.

Environmental factors such as noise, light, temperature, roommate habits, and changes in sleep location may cause or contribute to insomnia. Persons with seasonal affective disorder are particularly prone to developing phase-shifted insomnia during times when they are relatively deprived of early morning light.

Restless legs syndrome is a condition in which patients perceive lower extremity discomfort at rest, which is relieved by moving around. It is associated with renal failure and nutritional deficiencies but is usually idiopathic.

> Primary *idiopathic insomnia* is a diagnosis of exclusion.

Although *exercise* has been shown to improve sleep quality in several populations, overtraining and intensive evening exercise may cause insomnia.

COMMON DIAGNOSTIC PATTERNS

Symptoms	Signs	Diagnosis
Decreased appetite, libido, and energy	Psychomotor retardation	Depression
Increased energy	Grandiose thoughts, pressured speech, and delusions	Manic phase of bipolar disorder

COMMON DIAGNOSTIC PATTERNS (CONTINUED)

Symptoms	Signs	Diagnosis
Anxiety and hallucinations	Delusional thought	Acute psychosis
Nocturnal chest pain, pressure, or both; exertional chest pain; and palpitations	Abnormal ECG	Ischemic heart disease
Dyspnea at night and with recumbency, leg swelling, and exertional dyspnea	Abnormal CXR, rales, and pedal edema	CHF
Snoring, frequent waking, severe daytime sleepiness, and weight gain	Obesity, increased P_2, S_4 gallop, pedal edema, abnormal CXR, decreased oxygen saturation, and abnormal sleep EEG	Sleep apnea with pulmonary hypertension
Dyspnea (worse with exertion and recumbency), cough, and "allergies"	Wheezing and decreased peak expiratory flow	Asthma
Frequent urination, nocturia, and decreased stream	Prostatic enlargement and urinary retention	Benign prostatic hypertrophy or prostate cancer
Weight loss, increased appetite, tremor, and diarrhea	Hyperreflexia, exophthalmos, and thyroid nodule	Hyperthyroid disease
Burning nocturnal lower leg pain, frequent urination, thirst, and visual blurring	Elevated blood glucose	Uncontrolled diabetes
Leg discomfort relieved by walking, weight gain, and nausea	Elevated creatinine	Restless legs syndrome associated with renal failure
Recent history of wheezing and congestion controlled by medication	Mild wheezing and coryza	Drug-related insomnia due to bronchodilators and decongestants
Anxiety, sweating, nausea, tremor, muscle cramps, and recent admission to a detoxification clinic	Tachycardia, tremor, hypertension, and rhinorrhea	Withdrawal syndrome
Patients feel the need to keep their legs moving while at rest	Normal examination	Restless legs syndrome

Note. ECG = electrocardiogram; CXR = chest x-ray; CHF = congestive heart failure; P_2 = pulmonic valve sound; S_4 = fourth heart sound; EEG = electroencephalogram.

DIAGNOSIS: MAJOR DEPRESSION FOLLOWING BEREAVEMENT

CASE 24-2

INITIAL PRESENTATION

A 55-year-old man complains of worsening daytime sleepiness, which is interfering with his work and social life. He feels that this is due to "sleeping poorly," although he falls asleep easily and remains in bed 8–9 hours a night. Physical examination is notable for morbid obesity, fourth heart sound, and occasional wheezing in all lung fields. His wife, who accompanies him, states that she frequently wakes at night because of his loud snoring.

DIAGNOSIS: SLEEP APNEA

CASE 24-3

INITIAL PRESENTATION

A 29-year-old physician complains of worsening fatigue and difficulty falling asleep. His new job includes alternating day and night shifts in an emergency department. He drinks large amounts of coffee to stay alert through the end of each shift and frequently drinks several beers "to relax" when he gets home.

DIAGNOSIS: SLEEP PHASE SHIFT FROM ALTERNATING WORK SHIFTS COMPLICATED BY DRUG-RELATED INSOMNIA FROM EXCESSIVE USE OF CAFFEINE AND ALCOHOL

SUGGESTED READING

Gallup Organization: *Sleep in America: 1995*. Princeton, NJ: The Gallup Organization, 1995.

Kupfer DJ, Reynolds CF: Management of insomnia. *N Engl J Med* 336:341–346, 1997.

Medelson WB: A 96-year-old woman with insomnia. *JAMA* 277:990–996, 1997.

Medelson WB: Insomnia. In *Conn's Current Therapy*. Edited by Rakel RE. Philadelphia, PA: W. B. Saunders, 1995, pp 33–35.

Strollo PJ, Rogers RM: Obstructive sleep apnea. *N Engl J Med* 334:99–104, 1996.

Weilburg JB: Approach to the patient with insomnia. In *Primary Care Medicine*. Edited by Goroll AH, May LA, Mulley AG. Philadelphia, PA: J. B. Lippincott, 1995, pp 1062–1066.

CHAPTER 25
Chief Complaint: Malaise and Fatigue

Marjorie A. Bowman, M.D., M.P.A.

CASE 25-1

INITIAL PRESENTATION

B. Jones, a 38-year-old woman, complained of 3 days of feeling "lousy and tired." She expected her menstrual period "any day now," and her last period was approximately 1 month ago. She and her husband use condoms but would not be upset if a pregnancy occurred.

How can the multiple causes of fatigue be differentiated?

Discussion

Malaise and fatigue are common chief complaints among adult patients (approximately 1 out of 5 people complain of chronic fatigue). The most common cause of acute malaise is an infectious illness, such as a viral syndrome. The most common causes of more chronic or subacute malaise and fatigue are lack of adequate sleep, depression or other psychologic problems, hypothyroidism, cancer, chronic fatigue syndrome, or other chronic illness. In women of childbearing age, pregnancy is a common cause of fatigue. Cancer is a more common cause of fatigue in elderly patients than in younger patients. However, most significant illnesses can cause fatigue; thus, the evaluation must be driven by the history and physical findings.

Malaise and fatigue can be considered different entities; however, a patient's descriptions often make differentiation between the two difficult. Fatigue is often thought to refer to a tired state, whereas malaise is considered a general lack of energy.

KEY SYMPTOMS, SIGNS, AND OTHER FACTORS

Depressive feelings, particularly if accompanied by anhedonia (lack of interest in usual activities), crying, or sleep disturbances, suggest depression as the primary cause of the fatigue. Fatigue improved by exertion is more likely to be psychologic in origin. Other common psychologic causes of fatigue are dysthymia, panic disorder, and somatization disorder. Fatigue that is worsened *with exercise* is more likely to be organic in origin.

Weight loss makes psychologic illness (e.g., depression) or significant organic illness (e.g., cancer) more likely. Multiple *trigger (tender) points* are consistent with the diagnosis of fibromyositis (also called fibromyalgia).

The sudden onset of diffuse fatigue associated with increased sleep, sore throat, myalgia, nausea, and lymphadenopathy that is at least 3 months in duration and has no other known cause is consistent with chronic fatigue syndrome. The same symptoms, but usually presenting within 2 to 3 weeks, occur with infectious mononucleosis.

> **Most Common Causes of Chronic Fatigue**
> Lack of adequate sleep
> Depression
> Chronic illness
> Cancer
> Hypothyroidism
> Chronic fatigue syndrome

Nausea or a *late menstrual period* suggests pregnancy. Many women complain of fatigue and are very tired in the first trimester of pregnancy.

Fever suggests infections (basically any kind of infection but remember to consider human immunodeficiency virus [HIV] infection), inflammatory diseases (e.g., inflammatory bowel disease), or cancers (e.g., kidney, liver, hematopoietic cancers).

Insidious onset with new *constipation*, heavy menstrual flow, and skin or hair changes is a pattern seen in hypothyroidism. *Snoring* and falling asleep during routine daytime activities is associated with sleep apnea, which is more common in obese patients. *Polydipsia* and *polyuria* suggest diabetes. *Hyperpigmentation, hyponatremia,* or *orthostatic hypotension* should suggest adrenocortical insufficiency.

Fatigue of a *specific muscle group* with use is found in myasthenia gravis. In this circumstance, the muscle group that is used becomes acutely fatigued, although the patient may complain of overall weakness. Thus, using the arm leads to fatigue there, then using a leg causes it to get fatigued; both recover with a period of rest.

Erratic sleep patterns, "sleeping in" when the opportunity arises, and shift work suggest *inadequate sleep*, a common cause of fatigue in the United States.

COMMON DIAGNOSTIC PATTERNS

Symptoms	Signs	Diagnosis
Erratic sleep pattern and shift work	None	Inadequate sleep
Fatigue, depressive symptoms, crying, and sleep difficulties	Appears sad	Depression or dysthymia

COMMON DIAGNOSTIC PATTERNS (CONTINUED)

Symptoms	Signs	Diagnosis
Fatigue and multiple unexplainable body symptoms	None	Somatization disorder
Attacks of anxiety and fatigue possibly with depression	None except during attacks	Panic disorder
Muscle pain and fatigue and sleep difficulties	Multiple trigger (tender) points	Fibromyositis
Fatigue, sore throat, myalgias, sleep difficulties, nausea, and swollen glands	Perhaps pharyngitis, adenopathy, and normal laboratory tests	Chronic fatigue syndrome
Subacute fatigue and swollen glands	Positive monospot test	Infectious mononucleosis
Fatigue, nausea, and late menses	Positive pregnancy test	Pregnancy
Fatigue, constipation, heavy menses, and skin and hair changes	Goiter	Hypothyroidism
Fatigue, snoring, and falling asleep during routine activities	Abnormal sleep study and obesity	Sleep apnea
Polydipsia, polyuria, and fatigue	High glucose and glycosylated hemoglobin	Diabetes
Specific muscle fatigue, weakness, hoarseness, ptosis, and difficulty swallowing	Muscle fatigue with exertion and positive Tensilon test	Myasthenia gravis
Hyperpigmentation, fatigue, and orthostatic hypotension	Hyponatremia and low morning cortisol	Adrenocortical insufficiency

DIAGNOSIS: PREGNANCY

CASE 25-2

INITIAL PRESENTATION

A 55-year-old woman has gradual onset of malaise, slowed thinking, and swelling of her legs. Her thyroid-stimulating hormone is elevated.

DIAGNOSIS: HYPOTHYROIDISM

CASE 25-3

INITIAL PRESENTATION

A 40-year-old man complains of fatigue, does not feel like participating in his usual woodworking, and is sleeping poorly. He has some trouble falling asleep and often awakens 2 hours early and cannot get back to sleep. This started about 2 months ago. He was demoted at work shortly before the onset of the fatigue.

DIAGNOSIS: MAJOR AFFECTIVE DISORDER, DEPRESSION

CASE 25-4

INITIAL PRESENTATION

A 30-year-old woman originally presented 3 months ago with a low-grade fever, pharyngitis, and anterior cervical adenopathy associated with marked malaise. Since then these symptoms have come and gone, and the fatigue means that she is able to do less than half of what she previously did. She does not have substantial symptoms of depression, her physical examination is normal (except small anterior cervical nodes), and her laboratory studies are normal.

DIAGNOSIS: CHRONIC FATIGUE SYNDROME

SUGGESTED READING

Buchwald D, Umali P, Umali J, et al: Chronic fatigue and the chronic fatigue syndrome: prevalence in a Pacific Northwest health care system. *Ann Intern Med* 123:81–88, 1995.

Katerndahl DA: Differentiation of physical and psychological fatigue. *Fam Pract Res J* 13:81–91, 1993.

Wessely S, Chalder T, Hirsch S, et al: Psychological symptoms, somatic symptoms, and psychiatric disorder in chronic fatigue and chronic fatigue syndrome: a prospective study in the primary care setting. *Am J Psych* 153:1050–1059, 1996.

CHAPTER 26
Chief Complaint: Nerves

Marjorie A. Bowman, M.D., M.P.A.

CASE 26-1

INITIAL PRESENTATION

K. Sanders, a 32-year-old woman, complained that her nerves were getting to her. She stated that she was irritable, jumped at the least little thing, and did not seem to get things done at work. She felt that she had always been a nervous person and that she takes after her mother, who was also nervous and took tranquilizers.

What differentiates psychiatric and physical causes of anxiety?

Discussion

The most common causes of the chief complaint of nervousness are psychiatric (often short-term) stresses, generalized anxiety disorder, panic disorder, major affective disorder (depression), and drug or alcohol abuse. The most common medical cause is hyperthyroidism.

> **Most Common Causes of Anxiety**
> Psychiatric problems
> Hyperthyroidism

KEY SYMPTOMS, SIGNS, AND OTHER FACTORS

Long-standing anxiety is associated with the diagnosis of *generalized anxiety disorder*. These patients often have difficulty falling asleep and worry a lot. There is frequently a family history of anxiety disorders. Attacks of anxiety, chest pain, a feeling of impending doom, increased heart rate, and shortness of breath are consistent with *panic attacks*. Panic attacks often do not have an identifiable precipitant.

Early morning awakening, crying, and a lack of interest in usual activities (*anhedonia*) suggest that the feeling of nervousness is associated with *depression. Obsessive thoughts* or *compulsions* (e.g., checking locks, washing hands) suggest *obsessive-compulsive disorder.*

Changes in life circumstances (e.g., divorce, pregnancy or birth of a child, death of a spouse or loved one, loss of job) can lead to anxiety or the combination of anxiety and depression. Specific stressful events often lead to short-term anxiety.

Alcohol or *illegal drug intake* can lead to a variety of problems, including anxiety directly (e.g., cocaine abuse) or *withdrawal syndromes* that include anxiety. *Goiter; exophthalmos; atrial fibrillation; smooth, shiny skin;* or *hyperreflexia* suggest hyperthyroidism as the cause. *Shortness of breath*, lateralizing chest pain, leg edema, swelling, and *low oxygen levels* suggest pulmonary embolism. Shortness of breath and chest pain associated with hyperresonance, diminished breath sounds, and an abnormal radiograph suggest *pneumothorax*.

Palpitations, weight loss, and *tachycardia* do not help differentiate among the potential causes of nervousness. Caffeine intake can cause symptoms of anxiety (e.g., nervousness, tachycardia, palpitations), but it is often consumed in large quantities by individuals who also have psychologic syndromes. Weight loss is a common symptom of depression, but weight gain may also occur in depressed patients. Acute anxiety may accompany other severe sudden illnesses, such as congestive heart failure, myocardial infarction, and asthma.

> **Anxiety is worsened by:**
> Caffeine intake
> Other drugs such as over-the-counter pseudoephedrine, ephedrine, or many illegal substances

COMMON DIAGNOSTIC PATTERNS

Symptoms	Signs	Diagnosis
Recent anxiety and change in life circumstances	Appears anxious and has slight tachycardia	Stress
Chronic anxiety, difficulty falling asleep, and positive family history	Appears anxious and has slight tachycardia	Generalized anxiety disorder
Anhedonia, sleep difficulties, and depressive symptoms	Appears sad	Major affective disorder; depression
Attacks of anxiety, palpitations, SOB, and tachycardia	None except during attacks	Panic disorder
Obsessive thoughts and compulsive acts	Chapped hands	Obsessive-compulsive disorder
Nervousness and alcohol or drug intake	Tachycardia	Alcohol or drug abuse
Nerves, tachycardia, and shiny skin	Goiter, sinus tachycardia, atrial fibrillation, shiny skin, and hyperreflexia	Hyperthyroidism
Anxiety, SOB, lateralizing chest pain, and leg pain or swelling	Low oxygen level and leg swelling or tenderness	Pulmonary embolism

COMMON DIAGNOSTIC PATTERNS (CONTINUED)

Symptoms	Signs	Diagnosis
Anxiety, SOB, and lateralizing chest pain	Decreased breath sounds, hyperresonance, and abnormal chest radiograph	Pneumothorax

Note. SOB = Shortness of breath.

DIAGNOSIS: GENERALIZED ANXIETY DISORDER

CASE 26-2

INITIAL PRESENTATION

A 32-year-old woman complains of her nerves. She feels jumpy and shaky. Mild exophthalmos and a goiter are noted.

DIAGNOSIS: HYPERTHYROIDISM

CHAPTER 27
Chief Complaint: Depression

Kevin S. Ferentz, M.D.

CASE 27-1

INITIAL PRESENTATION

S. Fitzgerald, a 34-year-old woman, comes into the office with a number of complaints. She has been having frequent headaches, difficulty sleeping, and is worried that "something is terribly wrong" with her. She states she had been "feeling a little down" for the past month. On further questioning, she reports that her appetite "is not as good as usual." Her energy level is low, and she wonders if she might have a "thyroid problem" since this runs in her family. The patient appears somewhat sad. Physical examination is unremarkable except for a 5-lb weight loss since her last visit for a routine gynecologic examination 6 months prior.

When is sadness "depression"?

How can the physician determine whether a patient's symptoms are medical?

Discussion

All people get sad at times. Patients who experience bouts of sadness that pass after a few days usually do not have depression, which is an illness with specific diagnostic criteria called major depressive disorder. However, many patients that have daily sadness or a "depressed mood" for more than 2 weeks are suffering from depression.

> Ten percent of the population has an episode of depression in any one year.

While physicians use the history and physical examination to look for clues of a medical illness causing symptoms of depression, they do not have to "rule out" all physical illnesses before making a diagnosis of depression. In their examinations, physicians should learn to incorporate questions about depressive symptoms when dealing with patients who present with many somatic symptoms. If the patient meets the criteria for depression, they are diagnosed with depression.

Depression occurs in any age group, and it occurs twice as often in women. Women in their childbearing years have the highest prevalence rate. Even after depression is treated, it is likely to recur in most patients. Depression also runs in families so the physician should ask about symptoms of depression in other family members, particularly parents, siblings, and children. Sometimes depression is associated with substance abuse, particularly alcoholism. Patients may use substances to self-treat their depression. Such "dual-diagnosis" patients require treatment for both their substance abuse and their depression. Medications such as reserpine, glucocorticoids, and anabolic steroids have been implicated as causes of depression.

KEY SYMPTOMS, SIGNS, AND OTHER FACTORS

A number of areas must be explored whenever a patient is suspected of having depression (see Chap. 79 on depression in Section II for a complete list of the diagnostic criteria).

> Anxiety can also occur in a depressed patient. If a physician observes that a patient has symptoms of anxiety, the physician should ask that patient about depressive symptoms.

Sleep disturbances, typically waking in the middle of the night and not being able to fall back to sleep; *appetite change*, either eating too much or too little; *lack of energy*; and *suicidal thoughts* can all be signs of depression. Depressed patients also often have *anhedonia*. A good way to ask about anhedonia is "What do you do for fun?" A patient with depression may tell you they have done nothing for fun in some time. While depression is extremely common in the primary care setting, there are other disorders that can be confused with depression.

Depressed mood that develops during a time of stress, such as after switching jobs or buying a new house, is usually due to an *adjustment disorder*. Patients with this problem will usually not have the appetite change or anhedonia seen in depression.

It is normal for people to have a depressed mood after the death of a loved one. This is known as bereavement. Most of these patients will not meet the criteria for depression. Grief reactions usually last 2–6 months and gradually improve. Patients with depressive symptoms that last more than 2 months after the death of a loved one should be treated for depression.

Patients with years of low-grade symptoms of depression (that do not meet full criteria for major depressive disorder) are suffering from *dysthymia*. This relatively chronic condition is often difficult to treat. Patients with dysthymia often state that they were "born depressed."

Women who experience depressed mood prior to their menses may be suffering from *premenstrual syndrome (PMS)* or premenstrual dysphoric disorder. PMS is common, and while the symptoms are often uncomfortable, they are rarely disabling. Premenstrual dysphoric disorder is characterized by significantly more severe symptoms, which lead to some degree of impairment. Symptoms remit in both conditions within a few days of the beginning of menstruation. Antidepressants are sometimes used to treat premenstrual dysphoric disorder. It is also important to note that patients with depression can have exacerbations during the premenstrual period.

Patients with depression may use substances to "self-medicate." In these patients, treatment of the mood disorder may significantly impact the *substance abuse*. In other patients, the substance abuse leads to depression, which may remit with abstinence. All patients with depressive symptoms should be asked about their drug and alcohol use.

Patients who present with fatigue as their major complaint may be suffering from *chronic fatigue syndrome (CFS)*. This highly publicized but little understood illness is characterized by fatigue, sometimes low-grade fever and sore throat, and often symptoms of depression. The Centers for Disease Control has published specific criteria needed to make a diagnosis of CFS (see Chap. 71). Some patients labeled as having CFS may actually be suffering from depression. Anemia should also be considered in patients with fatigue as their main complaint.

Patients who suffer from depressive symptoms along with multiple aches and pains that are tender to the touch (known as *"trigger points"*) may be suffering from fibromyositis. There is often an overlap between depression and fibromyositis, the latter of which is probably overdiagnosed. Interestingly, fibromyositis is often successfully treated with small doses of antidepressant medication.

Recurring abdominal pain with alternating diarrhea and constipation is characteristic of *irritable bowel syndrome (IBS)*. This is a common disorder that shares many symptoms with depression.

Patients with *hypothyroidism* can present with symptoms of depression, but they will usually also have other signs and symptoms of hypothyroidism, which can include constipation, weight gain, and cold intolerance.

Many *medications* have been implicated in causing depressive symptoms. It is critical to take a medication history in patients with symptoms of depression.

COMMON DIAGNOSTIC PATTERNS

Symptoms	Signs	Diagnosis
Depressed mood, sleep disturbance, appetite change, anhedonia, trouble concentrating, decreased energy, and symptoms lasting for more than 2 weeks	Sad affect and poor eye contact	Major depressive disorder
Depressed mood and worries during a stressful life event	Sad or anxious affect	Adjustment disorder
Sadness, crying 3 months after the death of a loved one, and appetite and sleep not affected	Sad affect	Bereavement
Chronic "low-grade" depression for more than 2 years	Sad affect	Dysthymia
Irritability, depressed mood, breast tenderness, and headaches for 1 week prior to menses	Mild edema	Premenstrual syndrome
Markedly depressed mood, marked lability, anhedonia, lack of energy, and appetite change for 1 week prior to menses	Normal examination	Premenstrual dysphoric disorder
Profound fatigue lasting at least 6 months, muscle weakness, and depressed mood	Low-grade fever and cervical or axillary adenopathy	Chronic fatigue syndrome
Morning pain and stiffness, fatigue, and depressed mood	Multiple tender spots (trigger points) and normal sedimentation rate	Fibromyositis
Abdominal pain with alternating diarrhea and constipation, fatigue, and anxiety	Normal	Irritable bowel syndrome
Weight gain, decreased energy, depressed mood, and constipation	Diminished reflexes and lid lag	Hypothyroidism

- -

DIAGNOSIS: DEPRESSION

CASE 27-2

INITIAL PRESENTATION

A 45-year-old businessman comes in complaining of feeling "overwhelmed." He reports having trouble sleeping, especially falling to sleep. He reports recently taking on a new job along with buying a new house. He has had no appetite change. He has been trying to relax by reading, although he is having some trouble concentrating. His energy level is normal.

DIAGNOSIS: ADJUSTMENT DISORDER

SUGGESTED READING

American Psychiatric Association: *Diagnostic and Statistical Manual of Mental Disorders*, 4th ed. Washington, DC: American Psychiatric Association, 1994.

U. S. Department of Health and Human Services: *Depression in Primary Care: Detection, Diagnosis, and Treatment. Clinical Practice Guidelines*. Washington, DC: U. S. Department of Health and Human Services, 1993 (AHSPR publication #93-0050-vol 1, #95-0051-vol 2).

CHAPTER 28

Chief Complaint: Numbness or Tingling

Marjorie A. Bowman, M.D., M.P.A.

CASE 28-1

INITIAL PRESENTATION

C. Jenkins, a 38-year-old female patient who eats a vegan diet, complains of tingling in her hands and feet. Physical examination, including neurologic examination, is normal.

What are the causes of tingling in the hands and feet?

Discussion

Numbness, tingling, and the typical medical term, paresthesias, are not synonymous in terms of how the patient feels but are basically caused by the same entities. Thus, physicians often use the terms interchangeably. Patients describe the feelings in many ways, from an absence of feeling to painful burning and pinprick sensations. When painful, these feelings are termed dysesthesias. All people get positional numbness (basically a mild pressure neuropathy) that quickly resolves when the position is changed. This chapter focuses on the individual with the chief complaint of numbness, rather than motor neurologic difficulties.

KEY SYMPTOMS, SIGNS, AND OTHER FACTORS

The *pattern of numbness* is generally one of three types:

1. Numbness in the *distribution of a peripheral nerve* (e.g., carpal tunnel syndrome, myalgia paresthetica, lumbar disk disease, cervical disk disease) suggests some form of pressure on the nerve (called pressure or compression neuropathy). Neuropathies can be verified with peripheral nerve conduction studies. Patients with disk disease usually complain of pain while many mild pressure neuropathies result in numbness or painful paresthesias only. Another common cause of paresthesias in the distribution of a peripheral nerve is herpes zoster, where paresthesias may precede or be concurrent with a dermatomal rash.

2. Numbness in the *distribution of a central lesion* (e.g., stroke, transient ischemic attack, multiple sclerosis, brain tumor).

3. Numbness of the hands and feet (often called *stocking–glove*

distribution or peripheral neuropathy) is more common with alcoholism, nutritional deficiencies, uremia, arterial insufficiency, and metal toxicities and is also seen transiently with hyperventilation.

Other types of numbness are the ascending numbness and associated motor difficulties of Guillain-Barré syndrome or the foot peripheral neuropathy that is common in diabetes.

Nutritional inadequacies can lead to vitamin B_{12} deficiency, which in turn causes paresthesias.

Upper gastrointestinal (GI) symptoms can also be associated with paresthesias. Patients with *atrophic gastritis* are more likely to develop vitamin B_{12} deficiency. Alcoholism causes both peripheral neuropathy and GI symptoms.

A medical history can sometimes reveal the likely cause of paresthesias. Diabetes is a common cause of peripheral neuropathy, usually evidenced by painful paresthesias in the feet. Many drugs can cause paresthesias, including phenytoin, isoniazid, metronidazole, and several chemotherapy agents. Human immunodeficiency virus (HIV) infection is associated with peripheral neuropathy.

Occupational and recreational activities and exposures can also cause paresthesias. Carpal tunnel syndrome is associated with repetitive activities of the hands and forearms. Heavy metal exposure can occur in many ways but is more common for those who work in battery plants or radiator shops (lead), those who make moonshine alcohol (lead exposure through radiators), or those who work with pesticides (organophosphates). Alcohol is also associated with peripheral neuropathy.

Inability to reproduce the areas of numbness described by the patient during the neurologic examination does not mean that there are no problems but suggests less complete sensory involvement. Also remember that the anatomy of the peripheral nerves and their related sensory distribution vary somewhat among individuals. *Hyporeflexia* or areflexia are found in peripheral neuropathy. *Hyperreflexia* suggests a more central origin. Concurrent motor problems change the likelihood of the causes substantially. With predominance of the *motor symptoms*, more significant compression of peripheral nerves, various myelopathies, mononeuritis multiplex, central lesions, and inherited problems become more likely.

> The most common causes of paresthesias without major motor symptoms in practice are various pressure neuropathies, diabetic neuropathy, alcoholism, vitamin B_{12} deficiency, hypothyroidism, and somatization disorder.

Common Diagnostic Patterns

Symptoms	Signs	Diagnosis
Tingling of the hands, often worse at night, and often use hands extensively at work	Positive Tinel's sign, positive Phalen's test, and possibly muscle wasting	Carpal tunnel syndrome
Numbness in upper outer thigh, may wear tight pants, or keep wallet in front pocket, and often obese	Decreased light touch in the lateral femoral cutaneous nerve	Meralgia paresthetica
Low back pain shooting into the leg and numbness in the leg	Anatomically consistent neurologic examination, and positive straight leg-raising test	Lumbar disk disease
Cervical pain shooting into arm and numbness in shoulder or arm	Anatomically consistent neurologic examination	Cervical disk disease
Dermatomal dysesthesias usually on face or trunk	Vesicular rash may occur after paresthesias	Herpes zoster
Paresthesias of the feet in a diabetic	Usually decreased vibration sense	Diabetic neuropathy
Recurrent variable paresthesias, blurred vision, ataxia, and stiffness	Neurologic signs variable at different visits and consistent MRI of the head	Multiple sclerosis
Tingling of hands and feet	Usually nonspecific examination, may have macrocytosis, and dementia	Vitamin B_{12} deficiency
Tingling of hands and feet	Early examination often normal and positive heavy metal screen	Heavy metal toxicity
Tingling of hands and feet, coldness, and possibly intermittent claudication	Decreased arterial pulses and decreased capillary refill	Arterial insufficiency
Tingling of hands and feet, and history of alcohol intake	Examination varies from normal to signs of advanced alcoholism	Alcoholism
Tingling of hands and feet, constipation, mental dullness, and edema	Decreased reflexes and increased TSH levels	Hypothyroidism
Multiple symptoms in multiple organ systems	Normal examination	Somatization disorder

Note. MRI = magnetic resonance imaging; TSH = thyroid-stimulating hormone.

DIAGNOSIS: VITAMIN B_{12} DEFICIENCY FROM DIETARY INSUFFICIENCY

CASE 28-2

INITIAL PRESENTATION

A 62-year-old woman complains of numbness and painful tingling in both feet, more at night and when she walks. She has had diabetes for 10 years and hypertension for 15 years. There is decreased vibration sense in the lower extremities.

DIAGNOSIS: DIABETIC PERIPHERAL NEUROPATHY

CASE 28-3

INITIAL PRESENTATION

A 32-year-old woman complains of numbness and painful tingling in her fingers of both hands, occurring mostly at night. Three months ago she started working as a sewing machine operator.

DIAGNOSIS: CARPAL TUNNEL SYNDROME

CHAPTER 29
Chief Complaint: Paralysis

Victor Caraballo, M.D.

CASE 29-1

INITIAL PRESENTATION

L. King, a 74-year-old man with a medical history of hypertension and diabetes, presents with onset of left-sided weakness. The patient denies headache, fever, or trauma. On physical examination the patient's left arm and leg are numb and weak with more pronounced symptoms in the upper extremity.

What would be the most likely cause of one-sided weakness?

Discussion

Paralysis is defined as a total loss of muscle contractility, whereas weakness implies diminished muscle strength. Patients usually complain of varying degrees of weakness or inability to move with paralysis representing the end point of the spectrum. Weakness can be a nonspecific complaint of many illnesses, but this chapter focuses on how to differentiate actual loss of muscle function (from a neurologic problem) from other weakness, which tends to be generalized. When secondary to an underlying systemic pathologic process, patients often complain of generalized and vague weakness. In addition, they may have other complaints suggesting a systemic process. Physical examination would reveal no objective focal weakness but may give clues to the patient's underlying disease process. Weakness secondary to neurologic disease is associated with objective signs of focal weakness and is quantified on physical examination as follows:

0 = No muscle contraction
1 = Trace muscle contraction
2 = Movement with gravity eliminated
3 = Movement against gravity only
4 = Movement against gravity and resistance
5 = Normal strength

KEY SYMPTOMS, SIGNS, AND OTHER FACTORS

Overactive deep tendon reflexes, clonus, and the presence of a *Babinski's sign* characterize upper motor neuron lesions arising from problems with either the brain or spinal cord. The most common cause of upper motor neuron lesions is stroke. The probable site of the lesion can often be determined by careful physical examination.

Loss of deep tendon reflexes, muscle wasting, and *fasciculations* characterize lower motor neuron lesions, arising from the anterior horn cell, peripheral nerves, neuromuscular junctions, or muscle. The level of a given patient's lesion may be localized with the use of history, physical examination, electromyogram (EMG), muscle biopsy, and laboratory markers such as creatine phosphokinase (CPK) and antibody titers. See Chap. 28 for a discussion of compression neuropathies, the very common type of lower motor neuron lesions.

Medical history can provide clues to the underlying etiology. For example, patients with a history of vascular disease, smoking, hypertension, diabetes, atrial fibrillation, or previous transient ischemic attacks are at increased risk of stroke. Headache may be a clue to an intracranial process such as tumor or hemorrhage. History of seizure may be a clue to Todd's paralysis.

The *time course of onset* of symptoms may be a clue to etiology. For example, weakness secondary to cerebral vascular occlusion or stroke occurs suddenly while weakness secondary to multiple sclerosis can be more subacute.

Pattern or location of paralysis can provide clues to underlying etiology. For example, central nervous system (CNS) or upper motor neuron disease such as stroke syndromes usually cause paralysis in unilateral large areas of muscle groups while spinal cord lesions cause weakness bilaterally below the level of the lesion. Lower motor neuron disease may be limited to one individual nerve, such as compression neuropathy, or be generalized as in Guillain-Barré syndrome.

COMMON DIAGNOSTIC PATTERNS

Symptoms	Signs	Diagnosis
Upper Motor Neuron		
Acute onset of weakness, numbness, difficulty with speech or gait, and +/− headache	Focal weakness, and/or numbness, hyperactive reflexes on affected side, and hypertension	Stroke syndromes
Same as stroke; transient defined as from seconds to less than 24 hours	Same as stroke; transient defined as from seconds to less than 24 hours	TIA

COMMON DIAGNOSTIC PATTERNS (CONTINUED)

Symptoms	Signs	Diagnosis
Gradual onset of weakness or numbness, headache, and +/− seizure activity	Focalized numbness, weakness, and +/− papilledema	Brain tumor
Weakness associated with back pain, urinary retention, trauma, and cancer	Numbness, weakness localized to a "cord level," point spinal tenderness, and +/− fever	Spinal cord syndrome
Weakness, numbness that is often vague and intermittent, visual symptoms, bladder dysfunction, and spontaneous relapses and remissions	Patients who are 20–50 years old, +/− extraocular movement limitation, and variable neurologic examination often not localizing to a discrete lesion	Multiple sclerosis
Unilateral throbbing headache, +/− visual symptoms, nausea, and migraine headache history	Focalized weakness, numbness, usually transient, and intracranial lesion ruled out	Complicated migraine
Facial asymmetry and weakness, drooling, and inability to close eye	Weakness of *upper and lower* muscles of face, no sensory loss; sparing of the muscles of the forehead and upper lid differentiate central seventh nerve lesion from the peripheral nerve Bell's palsy syndrome	Bell's palsy
Localized weakness after a seizure	Trauma and other intracranial lesions ruled out	Todd's paralysis
Diffuse weakness in upper and lower extremities beginning in hands asymmetrically, gait abnormality, no sensory abnormalities, and +/− difficulty with speech or eating	Combined upper and lower motor neuron signs	Amyotrophic lateral sclerosis
Lower Motor Neuron		
Asymmetric weakness affecting facial and ocular muscles more than limb muscles, visual blurring and double vision, and weakness is worse with continued use of muscle	Extraocular movement limitation, drooped eyelids, drooling, difficulty speaking or swallowing, any combination of truncal or extremity weakness, and normal sensory examination and reflexes	Myasthenia gravis

COMMON DIAGNOSTIC PATTERNS (CONTINUED)

Symptoms	Signs	Diagnosis
Viral illness 2–4 weeks preceding symptoms, history of cancer, exposure to live vaccines in the recent past, and ascending weakness beginning in the legs and progressing to the trunk, arms, and face	Usually symmetric weakness, distal weakness greater than proximal weakness, sensory abnormalities one-third of the time, deep tendon reflexes absent, spinal tap with albuminocytologic dissociation (elevated CSF protein with few to no cells)	Guillain-Barré syndrome
Intermittent episodes of weakness of varying degrees occurring after rest or sleep, more common after high-carbohydrate meal, and +/− positive family history	Weakness usually spares oropharyngeal and respiratory muscles, variable reflex and sensory examination, and abnormal serum potassium	Familial periodic paralysis
Ascending paralysis or weakness and tick bite	Afebrile, sensory abnormalities are uncommon, absent or markedly diminished reflexes, and removal of attached tick is curative	Tick paralysis
Weakness associated with ingestion of canned foods, an infected wound, infant ingestion of honey, or intravenous drug abuse	Symmetric descending weakness beginning with facial muscles, usually no sensory abnormalities, and reflexes are either normal or slightly depressed	Botulism
Muscular		
Male child with difficulty walking, standing, and climbing stairs; abnormal posture; family history of muscular dystrophy often present	Diagnosis by elevated CK levels, muscle biopsy, EMG, and genetic analysis	Muscular dystrophy
Diffuse muscle aches, weakness and malaise, +/− fever, dark urine, history of medication or illicit drug or alcohol use, and may have history of trauma or several days of sitting or lying without change in position	Signs of infection or trauma, diffuse muscular tenderness and weakness, possible signs of renal failure, urinalysis is dip-positive for heme and microscopic-negative for RBCs, and high serum CPK	Rhabdomyolysis

COMMON DIAGNOSTIC PATTERNS (CONTINUED)

Symptoms	Signs	Diagnosis
Rash and proximal muscle weakness, patients have difficulty climbing stairs and raising arms, and significant muscle ache and tenderness	Red, raised rash on face, knuckles, knees, and elbows may precede weakness by several weeks; may have associated malignancy; and increased ESR	Dermatomyositis
Proximal muscle weakness and tenderness with no rash, joint pains, and no systemic symptoms	Absence of rash, usually underlying autoimmune disease, and increased ESR	Polymyositis
Proximal muscle weakness, pain, and tenderness; subacute onset; and may have history of tryptophan or other herbal ingestion	Elevated CPK and muscle biopsy with histologic evidence of myositis with an eosinophilic inflammatory infiltrate	Eosinophilic myositis

Note. TIA = transient ischemic attack; CSF = cerebrospinal fluid; CK = creatine kinase; EMG = electromyogram; RBCs = red blood cells; CPK = creatine phosphokinase; ESR = erythrocyte sedimentation rate.

DIAGNOSIS: MIDDLE CEREBRAL ARTERY STROKE

CASE 29-2

INITIAL PRESENTATION

A 45-year-old diabetic man presents with acute confusion and right-sided weakness. There is no history of trauma, fever, or headache. Physical examination is difficult to complete secondary to patient's confusion. Fingerstick glucose is 20 mg/dL. Symptoms are completely and immediately reversed with administration of intravenous glucose.

DIAGNOSIS: HYPOGLYCEMIA

Discussion

Patients with a variety of medical disorders may present with weakness as a primary complaint. When weakness is secondary to a systemic disease the weakness is generalized, and there is often no objective evidence of focal weakness on physical examination. Examples of systemic diseases that may present with weakness include: anemia, sepsis, hypoglycemia, hypoxemia, electrolyte dis-

Hypoglycemia is the one metabolic disorder that can cause focal weakness.

orders, hypothyroidism, hypoadrenalism, hyperparathyroidism, depression, occult malignancy, congestive heart failure, infectious mononucleosis, and organophosphate poisoning.

SUGGESTED READING

Fulgham JR, Wijdicks EF: Guillain-Barré syndrome. *Crit Care Clin*, 13(1):1–15, 1997.

Pourmand R: Myasthenia gravis. *Disease-A-Month* 43(2):65–109, 1997.

Rowland LP (ed): *Merritt's Textbook of Neurology*, 9th ed. Baltimore, MA: Williams & Wilkins, 1995.

Vallee PA, Reilly KM: Peripheral neuropathies. In *The Clinical Practice of Emergency Medicine*, 2nd ed. Edited by Harwood-Nuss AL, Linden CH, Luten RC, et al. Philadelphia, PA: Lippincott-Raven, 1996, pp 879–883.

Walter JJ: Myopathies and disorders of neuromuscular transmission. In *The Clinical Practice of Emergency Medicine*, 2nd ed. Edited by Harwood-Nuss AL, Linden CH, Luten RC, et al. Philadelphia, PA: Lippincott-Raven, 1996, pp 883–888.

CHAPTER 30
Chief Complaint:
Joint Pain or Swelling

Steven C. Larson, M.D.

CASE 30-1

INITIAL PRESENTATION

T. Ross, a 52-year-old man, presents with 24-hour onset of low-grade fever associated with pain and swelling of his right great toe. Examination of the patient reveals a tensely swollen right metatarsophalangeal joint with overlying warmth and erythema. Range of motion is limited by pain.

How does the physician distinguish a septic joint from the acute crystal flare of gout or acute arthritis?

Discussion

This can be difficult to ascertain. While both conditions are acute in onset and present with similar clinical symptoms, crystal disease is a relatively benign process that can be treated on an outpatient basis. However, the "missed" septic joint can result in eventual joint space destruction and significant morbidity.

KEY SYMPTOMS, SIGNS, AND OTHER FACTORS

The acute onset of joint pain suggests trauma, crystal disease, or a septic joint. Chronic pain is found in rheumatoid arthritis and osteoarthritis.

Fever is a clinical feature found commonly in crystal disease and septic arthritis. It may also be present in rheumatoid arthritis. Crystal disease, septic arthritis, and trauma frequently are *monoarticular* on presentation. *Polyarticular* complaints are a prominent feature of rheumatoid arthritis, osteoarthritis, Lyme disease, and systemic lupus erythematosus.

The pattern of joint pain can indicate the cause. Prolonged morning stiffness with gradual improvement over the course of the day suggests rheumatoid arthritis. Insidious, gradual pain worsened with use is consistent with osteoarthritis. *Peak intensity* of pain is common in septic joints and crystal disease.

An acutely infected joint can be a medical emergency; if undetected or if treatment is delayed, joint destruction is imminent. Any immunocompromised individual with a swollen, hot joint (e.g., alcoholic, diabetic) should be considered infected until a definitive diagnosis is determined.

COMMON DIAGNOSTIC PATTERNS

Symptoms	Signs	Diagnosis
Acute onset of joint pain and swelling with peak intensity at 24–36 hours and +/− low-grade fever	Joint swelling with surrounding warmth and erythema and tenderness on palpation of the joint with limited range of motion; large toe most commonly affected, and synovial fluid contains leukocytes and negative birefringent crystals	Crystal disease (gout)
Acute onset of joint pain and swelling and +/− low-grade fever	Joint swelling with surrounding warmth and erythema; most commonly affects the knees and wrists; x-rays may show calcification in the affected joint and synovial fluid contains leukocytes and weakly positive birefringent calcium pyrophoshate crystals	Crystal disease (pseudogout)
Acute onset of joint pain and swelling with limited range of motion and fever	Monoarticular joint swelling with surrounding warmth and erythema, tenderness on palpation of the joint, and limited range of motion; synovial fluid contains leukocytes, and Gram's stain may reveal organisms	Septic arthritis (nongonococcal)
Fever, chills, migratory polyarthralgias, polytendinitis, and rash	Scattered painless hemorrhagic macules or papules distributed on the extremities and trunk; early disease manifested by polyarthritis and tenosynovitis of the knee, shoulder, wrist, and hand joints; may progress to a purulent monoarticular arthritis; synovial fluid has WBC count of less than 50,000; and culture and Gram's stain may be positive for *Neisseria gonorrhoeae*	Gonococcal septic arthritis

COMMON DIAGNOSTIC PATTERNS (CONTINUED)

Symptoms	Signs	Diagnosis
History of tick bite, rash, fever, fatigue, lethargy, myalgias, arthralgias, headache, intermittent musculoskeletal pain with movement, and arthritis	Red macular rash with expanding border and central clearing, initially self-limiting bouts of asymmetric oligoarthritis, later bouts of arthritis that last weeks to months with the knees most commonly involved; serologic tests are unreliable, and diagnosis is based on clinical findings and response to therapy	Lyme disease
Insidious and slow onset, peak intensity occurs with use and is relieved with rest, and affects only one or a few joints	No warmth or erythema; later crepitance and limited range of motion develop; bony enlargement and irregularity may become prominent; possibly an effusion; and x-ray confirms loss of cartilage space, sclerosis, or loose bodies	Osteoarthritis
Morning stiffness, low-grade fever, and fatigue are prominent; pain is a deep, gnawing discomfort with variable joint involvement	Weakness, soft tissue swelling and deformity in involved joints, +/− erythema but marked tenderness with limited range of motion, and positive rheumatoid factor	Rheumatoid arthritis
Fatigue, fever, weight loss, light-sensitive rash, myalgias, and arthralgias	Symmetric fusiform swelling of joints—most frequently the proximal interphalangeal and metacarpophalangeal joints of the hands, wrists, and knees; fixed erythematous rash over the cheeks and nose; and elevated sedimentation rate and positive antinuclear antibodies in the serum	Systemic lupus erythematosus

COMMON DIAGNOSTIC PATTERNS (CONTINUED)

Symptoms	Signs	Diagnosis
Soft tissue swelling with limited range of motion due to pain and antecedent history of trauma	Point tenderness with limited range of motion due to pain and effusion; synovial fluid may contain blood and fat cells if a coexistent fracture is present, and x-ray will not delineate an injury to cartilage	Trauma

Note. WBC = white blood cell.

DIAGNOSIS: ACUTE GOUTY FLARE

CASE 30-2

INITIAL PRESENTATION

A 22-year-old man complains of right knee pain, which he noted while playing in a recent basketball game. He does not recall direct trauma but thinks the pain began when he landed after dunking the ball. He notes a "locked sensation," resulting in limited range of motion. On examination he is a healthy young man resting comfortably. His right knee is swollen with a visible effusion. The examination of the knee's ligamentous stability appears normal but is limited by pain. He has mild point tenderness on palpation of the medial tibial plateau. X-rays reveal only a moderate knee effusion.

DIAGNOSIS: TRAUMA WITH MENISCAL TEAR

CASE 30-3

INITIAL PRESENTATION

A 53-year-old woman with longstanding diabetes presents with fevers, chills, and a 2–3 day history of a swollen right ankle. She is now unable to bear weight. On examination she is ill-appearing with a temperature of 101°F orally. Her examination is notable for a swollen right ankle with no visible trauma. On palpation the joint is tender, and there is limited range of motion due to pain. The overlying skin is warm and erythematous. X-rays of the ankle are negative.

DIAGNOSIS: SEPTIC JOINT

SUGGESTED READING

Baker D, Schumaker R: Acute monoarthritis. *N Engl J Med* 329:1013–1020, 1993.

Pinals R: Polyarthritis and fever. *N Engl J Med* 330:769–774, 1994.

CHAPTER 31
Chief Complaint: Leg Swelling

Marjorie A. Bowman, M.D., M.P.A.

CASE 31-1

INITIAL PRESENTATION

M. Smith, a 35-year-old woman, is seen for a physical examination. She complains of swelling, which is worse before her period such that she gains 5 lbs and cannot remove her rings. The edema is not visible to the physician.

When is leg edema a sign of serious illness?

Discussion

Edema is often not a chief complaint but one that is brought up as an issue by women. Women often note total body swelling in the premenstrual period and will complain that their rings and shoes are tight.

Edema is often of the lower extremities, but it can also be throughout the body. Mild edema can result from prolonged standing, prolonged heat exposure, or immobility and is common during pregnancy. Edema is more significant if it is the chief complaint that brings the patient to the visit, if it

> **Organs Associated with Marked Lower Extremity Edema**
> Heart
> Liver
> Kidney

is pitting (i.e., finger pressure creates a lasting impression), or if it is visible. Most edema of the lower extremities will improve with elevation of the legs (such as occurs at night).

KEY SYMPTOMS, SIGNS, AND OTHER FACTORS

Weight gain. Acute weight gain with visible pitting edema suggests a significant cause of the edema. This can happen with congestive heart failure (CHF) and cirrhosis. The edema of CHF often starts in the feet and proceeds symmetrically up the legs. It can even proceed to the abdomen and the chest. A subacute weight gain and obvious swelling is also possible with nephrotic syndrome, in which case there would be proteinuria or frank renal failure (acute or chronic leg swelling).

Leg pain. If the patient has *unilateral* leg pain and swelling, the most common causes are thrombophlebitis, muscle tear (plantaris or a portion of the gastrocnemius), and ruptured Baker's cyst (synovial cyst of the knee). Thrombophlebitis is also sometimes bilateral.

Medications That Cause Edema
Nonsteroidal anti-inflammatory agents
Steroids
Calcium-channel blockers
Vasodilators
Phenothiazines

Shortness of breath should raise the suspicions of CHF or thrombophlebitis with pulmonary embolism. History of *alcoholism, spider veins,* or *palmar erythema* should suggest cirrhosis with ascites and peripheral edema. *Recent surgery* should make one think immediately of thrombophlebitis, which is sometimes nonpainful. Lower extremity edema is often associated with "venous stasis" (*varicose veins*), which often results from obesity. This edema is diffuse and sometimes becomes nonpitting.

COMMON DIAGNOSTIC PATTERNS

Symptoms	Signs	Diagnosis
Pitting edema, fatigue, and weight loss	Enlarged liver, spider veins, palmar erythema, and ascites	Cirrhosis
Tight rings or shoes during the premenstrual period	Edema not visible	Premenstrual edema
Leg edema, fatigue, and shortness of breath	Cardiomegaly, S_3, and right ventricular heave	CHF
Leg edema, calf pain, and acute	Local tenderness, warmth, +/– Homan's sign, and +/– palpable cord	Thrombophlebitis
Chronic leg edema	Varicose veins and stasis pigmentation, dermatitis, or both	Venous stasis
Subacute leg edema	Abnormal urinalysis	Nephrotic syndrome or renal failure
Subacute leg edema	Varying by source	Cancers creating ascites or lymphatic obstruction (such as with ovarian cancer)

Note. S_3 = third heart sound; CHF = congestive heart failure.

DIAGNOSIS: PREMENSTRUAL FLUID RETENTION

CASE 31-2

INITIAL PRESENTATION

A 65-year-old man complains of leg swelling over the last several days. He is 15 lbs heavier than usual. His liver is enlarged and slightly tender. There is a third heart sound. There is pitting edema on his abdomen, lower body, and lower extremities.

DIAGNOSIS: CONGESTIVE HEART FAILURE

SECTION II
Recognition and Treatment of Common Adult Medical Problems

CHAPTER 32
Sinusitis

William H. Hubbard, M.D.

PATIENT

R. Wells, a 39-year-old female cigarette smoker, complains of nasal congestion, runny nose, headaches, coughing (especially at night), mild fevers, and generalized weakness for 3 weeks. Several over-the-counter decongestants have been used without lasting results. Besides having a family history of allergies, she usually has more nasal congestion with coughing in the fall and spring of each year.

CLINICAL PRESENTATION

Acute sinusitis is often preceded by an upper respiratory viral infection or a severe allergic inflammatory response.

Initially, the patient may present with a double illness with worsening symptoms for 2 or 3 days followed by improvement, and then the return of symptoms and escalation of illness. Nevertheless, the key symptom pattern would consist of fever, facial fullness or pain, purulent rhinorrhea with posterior nasal drip, and nasal congestion. Other helpful symptoms, if present, would be increased pain while moving the head forward or with mastication, sore throat, hoarseness, and increased coughing while lying down. A headache between and behind the eyes is common for ethmoid sinusitis. Persistent or recurrent bloody discharge can suggest a tumor.

> **Key Symptoms of Acute Sinusitis**
> Fever
> Facial pain
> Purulent nasal drainage

Physical examination reveals red, swollen nasal turbinates with yellowish-green mucus especially on top of the inferior turbinate from the middle meatus, mild-to-moderate posterior pharyngeal lymphoid hyperplasia, and tender moderate anterior cervical lymphadenopathy. Ear examination may show signs of serous otitis media with fluid behind the tympanic membrane and decreased light reflexes. Palpation of the face may reveal tenderness over the cheeks (maxillary sinuses) or above the medial aspect of the eyebrows (frontal sinuses). Occasionally, transillumination of the maxillary sinuses from the outside through the cheeks or from the inside through the mouth can be helpful with a strong light and a darkened examination room. If the frontal sinuses are well developed, these may also be transilluminated through the medial aspect of the orbital ridge. Decreased transillumination of these sinuses suggests the presence of fluid in any of these cavities. An elevated temperature will be helpful in making a diagnosis. Proptosis, extraocular muscle paralysis, or significant eyelid swelling are ominous signs of serious complications.

> **Key Signs of Acute Sinusitis**
> Purulent nasal drainage
> Red, swollen turbinates
> Tenderness over the maxillary or frontal sinuses

EPIDEMIOLOGY

Sinusitis is an ubiquitous disease affecting millions of Americans. It is often associated with a common cold, flu-like illnesses, allergic rhinitis, and cigarette smoking. The recurrent or relapsing infections may involve allergies or obstructions, such as narrowed drainage openings, polyps, or tumors. Potential complications of sinusitis can be the spreading of the infection intraorbitally or intracranially with serious sequelae if not treated with antibiotics.

Most cases of acute sinusitis in adults are due to *Streptococcus pneumoniae, Haemophilus influenzae*, or *Moraxella catarrhalis*. Chronic sinusitis, however, involves different bacteria as a result of stagnation of fluids with hypoxia and a lower pH. These bacteria may be anaerobic as well as aerobic, such as anaerobic *Streptococci, Bacteroides*, and *Corynebacterium* species.

DIAGNOSIS

A thorough history and examination of head, eyes, ears, nose, throat, and neck should give good clues to make a clinical decision in the treatment of a sinus infection. If there is doubt as to whether a patient has a viral infection or a severe allergic rhinitis, a complete blood count (CBC) with a differential blood test and a nasal smear for Wright's stain for eosinophils might be useful. An elevated white blood cell (WBC) count with a marked granulocyte shift would point towards an acute bacterial infection. An increase of eosinophils on the nasal smear greater than 15% would suggest an allergic response. If both of these tests were positive, then an allergic response may have led to edema with obstruction and a secondary bacterial infection. If symptoms do not improve substantially after 2 weeks of treatment or clear by 4 weeks of treatment, a modified or mini-computed tomography (CT) of the sinuses will be needed to reveal any air–fluid levels, to reveal complete opacification of any of the paranasal sinuses, or to detect obstruction of the osteomeatal complexes. An ears, nose, throat (ENT) consultation may be needed to determine if nasal endoscopic surgery to relieve the obstruction is necessary. An ENT consultation should also be considered for unresponsive sinusitis.

TREATMENT

Main goals of treatment are to control infection and to reduce tissue edema to facilitate drainage. Usually, ampicillin or amoxicillin can be used unless there is a high incidence of resistance to these drugs in the local area, or the patient has had recent antibiotic treatment. Other options include amoxicillin/clavulanate, a macrolide, trimethoprim/sulfamethoxazole, doxycycline, or a cephalosporin. Drugs to be considered for chronic sinusitis would be clindamycin, sulfamethoxazole, doxycycline, or cefuroxime. Treatment lengths are highly variable, but 10–14 days are common.

Oral systemic decongestants (pseudoephedrine, phenylephrine, phenylpropanolamine) might be useful to improve the nasal airway passages by decreasing tissue edema. If there are coexisting allergic symptoms, topical corticosteroid nasal sprays (beclomethasone, flunisolide, triamcinolone) might provide relief. There is no reason to use antihistamines for sinusitis, even with coexisting allergies, as these drugs do not reduce edema. Oral steroids are occasionally used for patients with severe, recurring sinusitis.

A follow-up visit in 2–3 weeks might be appropriate to evaluate the need for further antibiotic therapy. The presence of purulent nasal drainage or continued symptoms might indicate another week of antibiotic treatment. Remaining edema of the mucosa of the nostrils is an indication for oral decongestant therapy for a longer period or nasal steroids. In addition, discussions can be carried out for possible testing for seasonal rhinitis and referral for smoking cessation programs.

> **Basic Treatment for Sinusitis**
> Antibiotics
> Oral decongestants
> Topical steroid nasal spray

PROGNOSIS

The duration of this illness is variable, with acute or subacute infections lasting for 1 week to 3 months, chronic infections lasting over 3 months, and recurrent infections lasting variable lengths. Patients with allergies, anatomic, or smoking risk factors have more problems with recurrences.

SUGGESTED READING

American Academy of Otolaryngology-Head and Neck Surgery Foundation: *Common Problems of the Head and Neck Region*. Philadelphia, PA: W. B. Saunders, 1991.

Josephson JS, Rosenberg SI: Sinusitis. *Clinical Symposia*, vol 46, no 2, Summit, NJ: Ciba-Geigy, 1994.

CHAPTER 33
Otitis Media

Judith A. Fisher, M.D.

PATIENT

M. Ross, a 35-year-old female executive, returns from a business trip and immediately seeks medical attention due to severe right ear pain. The patient started her trip with a bad "cold," which consisted of severe upper respiratory tract congestion. On her return air flight she developed the feeling of fullness associated with decreased hearing in her right ear during takeoff. This was followed by severe right ear pain. The stewardess suggested that she yawn successively and chew gum, but the ear pain was not relieved. In the emergency room, she was noted to have an intact, red, bulging tympanic membrane associated with a low-grade fever.

CLINICAL PRESENTATION

Otitis media is uncommon in adults but very common in children. The name otitis media implies a problem in the middle ear. There are two different types of otitis media.

Serous otitis media (SOM) is due to fluid in the middle ear. SOM presents on a more subacute or chronic basis with the patient complaining of a full feeling or decreased hearing in the affected ear. SOM is often precipitated by conditions that cause upper respiratory tract congestion such as "allergies" or "colds." SOM is often self-correcting without treatment.

> SOM is more subacute and has a more redolent course. AOM is painful. The pain is often relieved after several doses of antibiotics.

Acute otitis media (AOM) is due to an infection in the middle ear space. In AOM, patients have acute onset of severe, unremitting, boring pain associated with decreased hearing in the affected ear. In adults these complaints may or may not be associated with a low-grade fever. Upper respiratory tract congestion often precedes AOM.

> Otitis media of either type is associated with decreased hearing.

The patient may have started with SOM secondary to her upper respiratory tract infection. With severe pain, enough to encourage her to seek immediate medical attention, a low-grade fever, and a red bulging eardrum, she had developed AOM.

EPIDEMIOLOGY

SOM and AOM seem to recur in the same adults. It is hypothesized that these individuals have an unusual anatomy of the middle ear, floppiness of the eustachian tubes, or other chronic conditions that cause upper respiratory tract congestion. Any or all of these situations impede the flow of the normal middle ear fluid to the back of the throat. Problems with the immune system could predispose one to recurring AOM.

The usual infectious agents in acute AOM are *Steptococcus pneumoniae, Haemophilus influenzae, Moraxella catarrhalis*, and viruses.

DIAGNOSIS

On physical examination, otoscopy is the most useful diagnostic tool. In AOM the eardrum will appear red and may bulge toward the scope. The redness may be fiery, dull, or appear in red streaks.

SOM can be more difficult to diagnose. The otoscopist may see an obvious fluid level or bubbles of air behind the eardrum. Otherwise, the drum may appear bulging but not red or dull without a light reflex. The eardrum may also appear retracted. A retracted eardrum is the sign of chronic SOM or "glue ear." A sensitive test for detecting SOM is pneumatoscopy. An eardrum that does not move with air pressure is abnormal. The diagnosis is SOM if a nonmoving eardrum has no redness. Some physicians rely on tympanometry to help with difficult diagnoses.

TREATMENT

Antibiotics are used to treat AOM. Common first-line antibiotics are amoxicillin or trimethoprim-sulfamethoxazole given orally for 10 days. Alternatively, one dose of intramuscular ceftriaxone can be administered. Erythromycin sulfisoxazole or erythromycin alone are used in penicillin or sulfa- and penicillin-allergic individuals. Local resistance patterns of the most common etiologic agents will dictate the choice of antibiotic. Physicians often empirically use decongestants and antihistamines, although the literature has never supported the efficacy of these agents in enhancing treatment outcomes. Antibiotics are prescribed for a 10-day course after which the symptoms should be relieved. For continued symptoms associated with a still abnormal tympanic membrane, a second course of antibiotics is prescribed. Some physicians prescribe the same antibiotic for the second course while others change to a new antibiotic. There are positives and negatives to each approach.

SOM often resolves without treatment, and the treatment of SOM is controversial. Some physicians prescribe decongestants and antihistamines, others believe in ear popping exercises (e.g., drinking liquids through a straw while holding your nose or blowing up balloons) several times a day. There have been gadgets developed that are reported to open the eustachian tubes. These treatments are not supported in the literature but are thought to open the eustachian tubes so that the middle ear fluid can drain. Intranasal steroid sprays or oral steroids are thought to be of benefit. Whether treated or not, most bouts of SOM clear in 3 months. If SOM persists after 3 months, surgical intervention consisting of myringotomy (opening a small hole in the eardrum to allow fluid to drain or suctioning the fluid through the same hole) with or without tube insertion is often considered. Any time that a "glue ear" is appreciated, surgical intervention is paramount. Unilateral SOM in an adult of greater than 1-month duration should receive further workup.

> Unilateral SOM lasting more than 1 month in an adult could be a sign of nasopharangeal carcinoma.

SUGGESTED READING

Bluestone C: Diseases and disorders of the eustachian tube—middle ear. In *Otolaryngology*, vol 2, 3rd ed. Edited by Paparella M, Shumrick D, Gluckman J, et al. Philadelphia, PA: W. B. Saunders, 1991, pp 1289–1315.

Giebink G, Quie P: Microbial aspects of otitis media. In *Otolaryngology*, vol 2, 3rd ed. Edited by Paparella M, Shumrick D, Gluckman J, et al. Philadelphia, PA: W. B. Saunders, 1991, pp 1377–1380.

Goycoolea M, Jung T: Complications of suppurative otitis media. In *Otolaryngology*, vol 2, 3rd ed. Edited by Paparella M, Shumrick D, Gluckman J, et al. Philadelphia, PA: W. B. Saunders, 1991, pp 1381–1403.

Paparella M, Jung T, Goycoolea M: Otitis media with effusion. In *Otolaryngology*, vol 2, 3rd ed. Edited by Paparella M, Shumrick D, Gluckman J, et al. Philadelphia, PA: W. B. Saunders, 1991, pp 1317–1342.

Proctor B: Chronic otitis media and mastoiditis. In *Otolaryngology*, vol 2, 3rd ed. Edited by Paparella M, Shumrick D, Gluckman J, et al. Philadelphia, PA: W. B. Saunders, 1991, pp 1349–1376.

Shambaugh G, Girgis T: Acute otitis media and mastoiditis. In *Otolaryngology*, vol 2, 3rd ed. Edited by Paparella M, Shumrick D, Gluckman J, et al. Philadelphia, PA: W. B. Saunders, 1991, pp 1343–1348.

CHAPTER 34
Acute Bronchitis

Kent D. W. Bream, M.D., and Judith A. Fisher, M.D.

PATIENT

T. Smith, a 27-year-old woman, presents to the office with a 9-day history of a "deep" cough productive of a mucous-like sputum, which has changed from white to green over the past week. She reports mild shortness of breath as well as an occasional temperature that rises as high as 101°F. She states that she is tired all the time and "just does not feel well." She works in an office setting and has a 5-year-old child in kindergarten. Over the past week she has tried various over-the-counter formulations with only minimal relief. She denies any headaches, rhinorrhea, or ear symptoms. She requests an antibiotic because she "just wants to feel better."

CLINICAL PRESENTATION

Bronchitis may be acute or chronic. Chronic bronchitis is usually seen in patients with chronic obstructive pulmonary disease (see Chap. 39) or other chronic lung problems. Acute bronchitis may be acute in otherwise healthy lungs or acute as a superimposed illness in chronic lung illness.

Acute bronchitis is one of the most frequently made diagnoses in the office setting. It always presents with a cough and frequently presents with general "cold" symptoms. While the cough may be nonproductive, it frequently is productive of purulent sputum, which may be green or yellowish. A patient may also report fever, chills, myalgias, and mild hemoptysis.

On physical examination, there may be normal breath sounds or fine and coarse rhonchi. These adventitial sounds represent secretions in the bronchial tree. Occasionally, there is wheezing, depending on the patient's proclivity towards reactive airway disease. If not clinically overt, a wheeze may be elicited by forced expiration, or the patient's peak flow may be diminished. The wheeze represents bronchoconstriction due to airway inflammatory secretions. It is crucial to consider this reactive airway component as it can influence prescribed treatment and the success of that treatment. If wheezing is ignored, symptoms may persist. The moist, inflamed environment may also lead to greater susceptibility to secondary infection. Additionally, on auscultation the patient may have diminished air movement secondary to atelectasis or mucous plugging. The physician may also observe purulent sputum. Finally, fever (~101°F) and rhinorrhea may be present.

ETIOLOGY

Bronchitis is more common in parents with children in day care or school, cigarette smokers or passive smokers, and individuals with environmental allergies or asthma. Bronchitis is more common in the winter months when viruses and other infectious agents are more active. Though environmental etiologies are possible, infectious etiologies are most often seen. Outbreaks often occur in epidemics and are most frequently caused by viruses. Viral species include influenza A and B, adenovirus, rhinovirus, coxsackievirus, parainfluenza virus, respiratory syncytial virus, herpesvirus, and echovirus. Bacteria may also be causative agents. More common bacterial species include the usual respiratory tract pathogens *Haemophilus influenzae, Streptococcus pneumoniae,* and *Moraxella catarrhalis.* Less common bacterial species include *Mycoplasma pneumoniae, Chlamydia pneumoniae,* and *Bordetella pertussis.* Rare pathogens include *Mycobacterium tuberculosis, Salmonella,* various fungi, and parasites. These rarer species are more likely to occur in the compromised host. Seasonal variation in prevalence, mechanism of transmittal (i.e., fomite, droplet, contact), and individual patient susceptibility determine the infectious etiology of each episode of bronchitis. Chemical and environmental causes are determined by exposure and individual susceptibility.

DIFFERENTIAL DIAGNOSIS

Bronchitis represents just one aspect in the varied spectrum of respiratory tract inflammation with or without infection. In diagnosing bronchitis, the physician must differentiate it from its close neighbors: upper respiratory tract infection, sinusitis, otitis media, pharyngitis, laryngitis, reactive airway disease, and pneumonia. Gastroesophageal reflux disease (GERD), a mass lesion, or congestive heart failure (CHF) can masquerade as bronchitis as well. Ambiguity in diagnosis may be caused by the overlapping symptoms and concurrent presence of different respiratory tract pathologies. Bronchitis can cause airway reactivity; pharyngitis can coexist or precede bronchitis. Pneumonia can proceed from a poorly treated bronchitis especially in a debilitated patient, or pneumonia can occur at the site of a mass lesion in the bronchial tree or lungs. One must carefully consider the conglomeration of symptoms to arrive at the diagnosis of bronchitis. Due to differences in morbidity, potential mortality, and therapeutic options, it is important to exclude other diagnoses when suspecting bronchitis.

A patient with an "upper respiratory tract infection" usually presents with milder complaints than bronchitis. The patient may complain of cough and fever. The cough will be accompanied by additional symptoms involving parts of the respiratory tract including the nose, ears, pharynx, and lungs. Cough tends to be the primary complaint in bronchitis while in an upper respiratory tract infection, cough is one of many complaints.

Pneumonia and sinusitis with cough are frequently confused with bronchitis. Pneumonia usually has a high fever and more respiratory distress and may be accompanied by chest discomfort. In general, the patient appears more ill and may appear septic with pneumonia. On physical examination a patient with pneumonia may have asymmetric tactile and vocal fremitis. The physician should auscultate for the classic signs of pneumonia, which may include signs of segmental consolidation such as decreased or absent breath sounds with or without egophany. While bronchitis has small areas of decreased breath sounds often localized centrally in the chest, pneumonia will present with an entire segment of decreased or absent breath sounds. If pneumonia is suspected, a diagnostic chest x-ray may be considered. In sinusitis, patients often complain of more facial and head symptoms. Due to postnasal drainage, a cough or wheeze may develop. The patient with sinusitis may present with a productive, purulent cough. The drainage may additionally cause the patient to bronchoconstrict and wheeze. A patient suspected of having sinusitis or bronchitis, purulent nasal discharge, maxillary tooth pain, and cobbling in the pharynx should decrease the physician's suspicion of bronchitis.

Pharyngitis or laryngitis may be present with bronchitis. They may also represent the initial loci of infection that subsequently spreads to the bronchi. These conditions when associated with bronchitis are more likely due to viral or chemical etiology.

GERD may present as a chronic cough and wheeze. A history of GERD in a well-appearing patient with cough and wheeze makes bronchitis a less likely diagnosis. It is important to note, though, that the acid reflux, as well as other chemical and environmental irritants (such as cigarette smoke), can inflame the bronchi enough to lead to bronchitis.

A mass lesion of the lungs may cause a productive or nonproductive cough. If productive, the cough may produce blood-tinged (hemoptysis) or brownish sputum. These patients may present with fever or shortness of breath. On examination they may have no physical findings or evidence of lung consolidation or collapse. Patients with a mass lesion may develop postobstructive pneumonia. A chest x-ray is sometimes diagnostic. If a patient fails to improve as expected, further workup may be indicated, particularly for a patient with a smoking history.

In CHF, patients usually complain that their cough is worse at night or on recumbence. There is no fever, and shortness of breath is more likely to be associated with effort. On examination the patient may have jugular venous distention, hepatojugular reflux, a third heart sound (S_3) on the cardiac examination, and rales or wheezes in the lungs. The rales and wheezes usually occur first in the dependent areas of the lung.

DIAGNOSIS

There is no diagnostic gold standard for bronchitis. Diagnosis is made by history, physical examination, and clinical suspicion. Laboratory studies are not routinely done. A chest x-ray is used only if pneumonia, a mass lesion, or CHF is suspected. In the compromised patient, a sputum Gram's stain and culture may guide the diagnosis and treatment. It has been suggested that a predominance of mononuclear cells in the sputum indicates a viral etiology; a predominance of polymorphonuclear cells in the sputum indicates a bacterial etiology. It is important to remember that the normal oral flora contains *H. influenzae*, *S. pneumoniae*, and *M. catarrhalis*. Therefore, cultures can also be misleading.

TREATMENT

Antibiotics are frequently used to treat bronchitis, but there is no evidence that antibiotic use in acute bronchitis in an uncompromised host decreases morbidity, mortality, or complications. The only exception to this is the treatment of pertussis with erythromycin. The only pharmacotherapy that has repeatedly been shown to improve the symptoms of bronchitis in some patients is bronchodilators. Bronchodilators decrease the reactive airway response to the inflammatory agent. Theoretically, the secondary inflammatory response of reactive airway disease may be decreased.

Pharmacotherapy for symptoms may increase patient comfort. Acetaminophen, aspirin, and nonsteroidal anti-inflammatory agents aid in defervescence and pain relief. Several studies show that there is no good treatment or reason to treat cough, although many physicians continue to prescribe dextromethorphan, codeine, or both especially at bedtime to improve the patient's sleep. Fluids (hydration) as well as a humidified environment (vaporizer or humidifier) may help alleviate symptoms by decreasing the viscosity of sputum, which may facilitate clearance.

SUGGESTED READING

MacKay DN: Treatment of acute bronchitis in adults without underlying lung disease. *J Gen Intern Med* 11:557–562, 1996.

Nennig ME, Shinefield HR, Edwards KM, et al: Prevalence and incidence of adult pertussis in an urban population. *JAMA* 275:1672–1674, 1996.

Orr PH, Scheer K, MacDonald A, et al: Randomized placebo-controlled trials of antibiotics for acute bronchitis: a critical review of the literature. *J Fam Pract* 36:507–512, 1993.

Shapiro BA, Kacmarek RM, Cane RD, et al: *Clinical Application of Respiratory Care*, 4th ed. Philadelphia, PA: Mosby-Year Book, 1991, pp 357–359.

Wright SW, Edwards KM, Decker MD, et al: Pertussis infection in adults with a persistent cough. *JAMA* 273:1044–1046, 1995.

SUGGESTED READING

CHAPTER 35
Pneumonia

Richard A. Neill, M.D.

PATIENT

K. Blackwell, a 52-year-old man, presents to the office complaining of fever, productive cough, and right-sided pleuritic chest pain. He was in his usual state of health until 5 days prior to the visit, when he developed malaise followed by shaking chills, fever, and cough. His sputum was initially green but has turned rust colored over the last 2 days. He has smoked 1 pack of unfiltered cigarettes a day for 20 years and continues to smoke. On examination he has reduced breath sounds and egophony in the right posteroinferior chest. Sputum Gram's stain is unremarkable. A chest x-ray reveals a lobar consolidation of the right lower lobe.

CLINICAL PRESENTATION

The clinical presentation of pneumonia is dramatically influenced by a host of patient and pathogen-specific characteristics. The traditional picture of fever with productive cough, dyspnea, fatigue, and pleuritic chest pain describes the classic presentation of community-acquired streptococcal pneumonia in an immunocompetent host, which is still the most common form of pneumonia.

TABLE 35-1
COMMON PATHOGENS IN COMMUNITY-ACQUIRED PNEUMONIA

Pathogen	Prevalence (%)
Streptococcus pneumoniae	20–60
Viruses (influenza A, respiratory syncytial virus)	2–15
Haemophilus influenzae	3–10
Anaerobic bacteria (especially due to aspiration)	3–10
Pneumocystis carinii	Up to 15% in urban centers
Mycoplasma pneumoniae	4–6
Chlamydia pneumoniae	4–6
Legionella pneumophila	2–8
Moraxella catarrhalis	~1
Staphylococcus aureus	~1
Mycobacterium tuberculosis	~2–5 depending on location and host factors

Patient factors such as age, coexisting illness, immune status, and respiratory mechanics predispose patients to characteristic pathogens. These same factors can explain why different patients manifest differing symptom complexes despite suffering from pneumonias caused by the same pathogen.

Patients at the extremes of age typically present with fewer localizing symptoms. Elderly patients may exhibit nonspecific mental status changes, while young children may present with nonspecific abdominal pain or malaise.

Coexisting illness, whether congenital (e.g., cystic fibrosis) or acquired (e.g., chronic obstructive pulmonary disease [COPD], diabetes, heart failure), alters host response to respiratory pathogens.

Patients with *swallowing dysfunction* (including edentulous patients and anyone with impaired oral sensation, depressed mental status, or oropharyngeal muscle dysfunction) are at risk for aspiration pneumonia, which manifests through the sudden onset of coughing followed by spiking temperatures and infiltrates on chest x-ray.

Immunocompromised patients are at risk for all of the usual pathogens, but additionally they are more prone to opportunistic infections with organisms such as *Pneumocystis carinii* and atypical mycobacteria.

Patients with *impaired respiratory mechanics* due to iatrogenic causes (e.g., ventilator) or congenital or acquired mechanical problems (e.g., scoliosis, paralysis victims) are prone to a variety of infections because of gram-negative and anaerobic organisms. This is due to these patients' inability to clear pathogens from the respiratory tract adequately.

DIAGNOSIS

The diagnosis of pneumonia is largely empiric. Although symptoms of pneumonia can overlap those of bronchitis substantially, the presence of an infiltrate on chest x-ray confirms the diagnosis. However, because many patients develop an infiltrate only after rehydration, an initial diagnostic chest x-ray may be normal in some patients who eventually receive a diagnosis of pneumonia.

Sputum Gram's stain and culture are of dubious value in establishing the identity of causative organisms. Inadequate sputum generation, contamination by oral flora, and pretreatment with antibiotics greatly limit their usefulness. Not unexpectedly, induced sputums performed by trained technicians taken from patients prior to initiation of antibiotic therapy increase the diagnostic yield substantially. Still, stains and cultures remain useful only for a subset of pathogens, as many laboratories do not culture for organisms such as *Mycoplasma* or *Chlamydia* as a result of the inadequacy of culture techniques. Augmenting sputum cultures with concurrent blood and urine cultures increases recovery of bacterial pathogens.

TREATMENT

Therapy should be directed at the causative pathogen and contemporaneously determined antibiotic sensitivities whenever possible. Indiscriminate use of broad-spectrum antibiotics results in antibiotic-resistant strains, which are growing more prevalent year by year. In the absence of a confirmed agent, empiric therapy can be based on patient characteristics, according to guidelines recommended by the American Thoracic Society.

Indications for inpatient management of pneumonia include:

- Age greater than 65
- Unstable vital signs
- Altered mental status
- PO_2 less than 60 mm Hg
- Severe underlying disease (COPD or other lung disease, diabetes, heart failure, liver disease, renal failure)
- Immune compromise (human immunodeficiency virus [HIV] infection, chemotherapy, corticosteroid use)
- Complicated pneumonia (effusion, empyema, extrapulmonary infection, cavitation, multilobar involvement)
- Severe electrolyte, hematologic, or metabolic abnormalities
- Failure to respond to outpatient therapy within 48 to 72 hours

TABLE 35-2
EMPIRIC ANTIBIOTIC TREATMENT OF PNEUMONIA

Clinical Situation	Primary Choice	Alternate Choices
Empiric Outpatient Therapy		
Young, otherwise healthy	Erythromycin	Doxycycline, azithromycin, clarithromycin, and dirithromycin
Less than 60 years old or co-morbid condition	Trimethoprim-sulfamethoxazole plus erythromycin or doxycycline	Azithromycin, clarithromycin, oral second- or parenteral third-generation cephalosporin, or amoxicillin-clavulanate plus erythromycin or doxycycline
Aspiration suspected	Clindamycin	Amoxicillin-clavulanate

Table 35-2 (Continued)

Clinical Situation	Primary Choice	Alternate Choices
Empiric Inpatient Therapy		
Moderately ill	Parenteral second- or third-generation cephalosporin plus erythromycin or doxycycline	Parenteral β-lactam/β-lactamase inhibitor agent plus erythromycin or doxycycline
Moderately ill and aspiration suspected	Parenteral β-lactam/β-lactamase inhibitor agent plus erythromycin or doxycycline	Parenteral clindamycin plus third-generation cephalosporin plus erythromycin or doxycycline
Severely ill	Piperacillin-tazobactam or ticarcillin-clavulanic acid plus aminoglycoside plus parenteral erythromycin	Ceftazidime, cefepime, imipenem-cilastatin, or ciprofloxacin plus aminoglycoside plus parenteral erythromycin

PREVENTION

The United States Preventive Services Task Force (USPSTF) recommends one time vaccination with 23-valent pneumococcal vaccine for all persons over age 65 and for patients with medical and living conditions putting them at high risk for pneumococcal disease (including being immune compromised). The USPSTF also recommends that revaccination be strongly considered for patients who received the 14-valent vaccine or who received the 23-valent vaccine 6 or more years ago and who are at highest risk of serious or fatal pneumococcal infections (such as patients with surgical or functional asplenia).

The USPSTF recommends yearly influenza A vaccine for all patients age 65 and older and adults and children at least 6 months of age who are at an increased risk for influenza-related complications due to certain medical conditions, such as chronic pulmonary and cardiovascular disorders, or who may transmit influenza to individuals at increased risk, such as healthcare workers and household members.

The Advisory Committee on Immunization Practices (ACIP) recommends immunizing children at 2, 4, 6, and 12–15 months of age with *H. influenzae* type b (HIB) conjugate vaccine to prevent sequelae of HIB infection.

SUGGESTED READING

Bartlett JG, Mundy LM: Current concepts: community acquired pneumonia *N Eng J Med* 333(24):1618–1624, 1995.

Fine MJ, Smith MA, Carson CA, et al: Prognosis and outcomes of patients with community-acquired pneumonia: a meta-analysis *JAMA* 275(2):134–141, 1996.

Niederman MS, Bass JB, Campbell GD, et al: Guidelines for the initial management of adults with community-acquired pneumonia: diagnosis, assessment of severity, and initial antimicrobial therapy *Am Rev Respir Dis* 148:1418–1426, 1993.

King DE, Pippin HJ: Community acquired pneumonia in adults: initial antibiotic therapy. *Am Fam Phys* 56(2):544–550, 1997.

CHAPTER 36
Urinary Tract Infection

Eileen E. Reynolds, M.D.

PATIENT

R. Clark, a 23-year-old woman, complains of frequent, painful urination for 2 days. She feels like she has to keep running to the bathroom but urinates only a small amount of dark yellow urine each time. Once there may have been some blood in the urine. This is the first time she has had these symptoms. She does not have a vaginal itch or discharge, fever, nausea, or back pain. She is sexually active with one partner; they usually use condoms.

CLINICAL PRESENTATION

The primary symptoms of urinary tract infections (UTIs) are painful urination, or dysuria, and urinary urgency and frequency. If the infection is confined to the bladder, those are the only symptoms; if the infection involves the kidneys (upper tract infection), then the patient has pyelonephritis, and she will often complain of fever and flank pain. Men with prostatitis may have vague abdominal pain, low back pain, or urinary hesitancy.

> **Clinical Presentation**
> Dysuria
> Urgency
> Frequency
> Absence of discharge

Diabetes, advancing age, and urinary tract obstruction and stones can predispose an individual to infection. Risk factors that increase a woman's chance of getting a bladder infection include sexual activity, diaphragm use, childhood history of UTIs, and adult history of UTIs within the last 2 years. Men who are uncircumcised or who have intercourse with other men are also predisposed.

Many patients, particularly young women, have recurrent bladder infections. They often say that their symptoms are exactly the same as the last time they had a UTI.

EPIDEMIOLOGY

UTI is very common. Dysuria accounts for more than 7 million office visits to healthcare providers each year, with estimated costs of care reaching one billion dollars; the diagnosis for over 60% of these visits is UTI.

The majority of patients with bladder infections are women. Anatomically, women are predisposed to UTI, with a short urethra in proximity to perirectal bacterial colonization. One-half of all adult women will experience a UTI in their lifetimes; 20% will have more than one episode, and 3%–6% of women will go on to have recurrent UTIs. Twenty percent of women over 65 and up to 50% of those over 80 have asymptomatic bacteriuria, which rises with age, disability, and number of medical problems. Pregnant women are also predisposed to asymptomatic bacteriuria. Isolated cystitis is rare in men under age 50. Prostatitis is the most common urinary tract infection in men with the chronic form predominating.

SCREENING

Screening for asymptomatic urinary tract infection or bacteriuria is recommended in pregnant women. Bacteriuria in pregnancy has been associated with a markedly increased risk for pyelonephritis and premature labor and delivery. Asymptomatic bacteriuria is common in the elderly, but treating it has not been shown to improve health status or outcome, and so screening is not recommended.

DIFFERENTIAL DIAGNOSIS

When considering the diagnosis of a UTI, age and anatomy are used as guides. Besides cystitis, the differential diagnosis includes urethritis, vulvitis, vaginitis, cervicitis, prostatitis, and pyelonephritis.

Chlamydial infection of the cervix or urethra, common in young women, can produce a clinical picture similar to that of simple cystitis. A woman with a chlamydial infection and dysuria would have cervical or urethral discharge or a positive culture for chlamydial infec-

> **Differential Diagnosis**
> Cystitis
> Urethritis
> Vulvitis
> Vaginitis
> Cervicitis
> Prostatitis
> Pyelonephritis

tion. Urethritis produces painful urination but usually not urgency and frequency. Vulvitis can cause painful urination as the urine passes over inflamed vulvar tissue; patients describe their pain as external, not internal. Vulvitis can be infectious or can be a dermatitis caused by contact with chemical irritants found in soaps, douches, creams, and spermicides. Vaginitis can present with painful urination, although the patient will often complain of a vaginal discharge in addition to the urinary symptoms. Pyelonephritis, or upper tract infection, can present with similar urinary symptoms as cystitis but is usually accompanied by nausea, back pain, or fever.

The differential diagnosis in elderly women with symptoms of UTI is similar to that in younger women. In addition, postmenopausal women who do not take hormone replacement can suffer from atrophic vaginitis. Symptoms include painful urination, vaginal dryness, and dyspareunia. Many elderly women, especially those with multiple medical problems, have asymptomatic bacteriuria or a positive urine culture in the absence of any urinary symptoms.

Although isolated cystitis does occur in men, bladder infection most commonly results from infection of the nearby prostate gland. Acute prostatitis presents with fever, dysuria, frequency, and abdominal or rectal pain. The prostate is exquisitely tender to examination. Men with chronic prostatitis complain of urinary hesitancy, frequency, dribbling, and vague abdominal or suprapubic pain. The prostate is slightly boggy and enlarged but may not be tender on examination; white blood cells (WBCs) are present in expressed prostatic secretions (EPS). Men who have prostatodynia have symptoms of prostatitis, but repeated workup reveals no microbiologic cause or inflammation. Urethritis can mimic some of these symptoms in men but is usually distinguishable from cystitis or prostatitis on physical examination (urethral discharge) or with a three-glass urine test. Kidney or bladder stones can cause painful urination and frequency; isolated cystitis in an otherwise healthy man may be caused by an infected stone. Symptoms of bladder irritation not caused by infection in an older man could be due to bladder carcinoma.

DIAGNOSIS

Patients who have symptoms of UTI should collect a urine specimen. In a woman, a midstream sample is collected after she wipes her labia from front to back with several moist towelettes; she urinates into the toilet, then (in midstream) into a cup, and then finishes into the toilet. This collection method is an attempt to isolate urine from potential vaginal secretions and skin contaminants during collection.

In men, a three-glass urine test is required to distinguish urethritis, cystitis, and prostatitis. The patient urinates 10 mL of urine into cup 1, the urethral specimen, then collects a midstream sample into cup 2, the bladder specimen. After a prostate examination and massage, prostatic secretions should be expressed onto a slide, and then the third sample, the prostatic sample, is collected.

In a urinary tract infection, bacteria infect the urine and incite an inflammatory reaction in the bladder wall. A urine dipstick will show the presence of leukocyte esterase, an enzyme in WBCs, and sometimes will show the presence of blood or nitrite, a bacterial breakdown product.

In men with prostatitis, the EPS will show more than ten WBCs per high power field. If the prostatitis is causing a cystitis, there may be WBCs in the second cup (midstream bladder), but there should be more in the third cup (prostatic). Isolated cystitis shows a positive dipstick in the second and third cups; urethritis shows the greatest number of WBCs in the first cup.

A urine culture is always positive in a bladder infection (as long as the patient has not taken any antibiotics prior to the specimen collection) and is usually positive from the third specimen in men with bacterial prostatitis. A colony count of greater than 10^2 colonies of a single strain is positive in women; greater than 10^3 is positive in men. Skin flora or multiple strains are usually indicative of a contaminated urine sample. The most common organisms in UTIs in young women are *Escherichia coli, Staphylococcus saprophyticus*, and several species of *Proteus* and *Klebsiella*. These organisms are still the most common in elderly women, but enterococci, pseudomonas, and *Serratia* become more likely. Bacterial prostatitis is usually caused by *E. coli* and other gram-negative organisms. However, nonbacterial prostatitis is more common and can be caused by *Chlamydia, Ureaplasma*, and *Mycoplasma*.

Although culture is the gold standard test for the diagnosis of UTI, it is often not necessary. Because cultures have been shown to add expense to cystitis care but have not been shown to improve outcome, they should be done only in certain cases when a culture might change management, or when the patient is at increased risk of unusual organisms or complications. All men and older women should have cultures, as should women with the risks listed in Table 36-1. The EPS, or the third urine sample, can be sent for culture in men with presumed prostatitis.

TABLE 36-1
COMPLICATING FACTORS IN UTI (NECESSITATING CULTURE)

- Age over 65
- Male sex
- Diabetes
- Pregnancy
- Recent instrumentation of the urinary tract
- Known structural abnormality of the urinary tract
- Recent antibiotic use
- Immunosuppression
- Symptoms for more than 7 days at presentation
- Hospital- or catheter-acquired infection
- Upper tract infection

TREATMENT

Treatment of UTI should maximize the cure rate and minimize side effects. The cure rate is dependent on the length of therapy and the susceptibility pattern of the infecting organism.

Length of treatment for a simple, uncomplicated UTI in a woman should be 3 days of oral antibiotics. Longer courses of therapy increase the side effects but not the cure rate; short-course or single-dose therapy has a higher early recurrence rate. Three-day therapy works best because it treats many cases of subclinical upper tract infection and

> **Simple Cystitis**
> Three days of therapy, no culture necessary

because it is more likely to eradicate the vaginal and urethral reservoirs of bacteria, which can cause relapse and recurrence. Patients with a "complicated" UTI should be treated for 7 days orally; patients with pyelonephritis should be treated for 14 days orally or intravenously.

The first choice for antibiotic therapy for cystitis is trimethoprim-sulfamethoxazole, which is inexpensive and effective (although resistance may be as high as 20% in some geographic locations). An alternative is a member of the fluoroquinolone family; although more expensive, resistance is uncommon. Because of increasing resistance, amoxicillin is no longer recommended for first-line treatment of UTI. Second-line agents include oral cephalosporins, nitrofurantoin, or trimethoprim alone. Pregnant women should be treated with amoxicillin as a first-line agent.

Chronic bacterial prostatitis is difficult to cure, as antibiotics do not penetrate the prostate gland well. Treatment should be with trimethoprim-sulfamethoxazole or a fluoroquinolone for 4–12 weeks. The more common nonbacterial prostatitis should be treated with doxycycline for 2 weeks. Prostatodynia is treated with α-blockers.

Patients who are very uncomfortable with dysuria and frequency may benefit from a medicine that numbs the bladder for the first 2 days of therapy. Phenazopyridine decreases the dysuria and frequency of a UTI within several hours of the first dose (the antibiotics may not help for a day or two) but will turn the patient's urine orange-red and can stain clothing.

Recurrent cystitis is a common outpatient problem in female patients. Women who have recurrent infections (more than two in 1 year) should have the infection documented by culture once and should undergo a complete pelvic examination with cultures to rule out other causes. The majority of women with recurrent UTIs do not need imaging studies to look for abnormalities of the urinary tract because the incidence of treatable abnormalities is very low. The exception is women who have a childhood history of UTIs. These women should have an intravenous pyelogram (IVP) to look for anomalies. If the patient uses a diaphragm, she should be advised to change her method of birth control, since the diaphragm has been shown to increase the incidence of recurrent infection. After this evaluation, the patient can be treated prophylactically. Prophylaxis reduces the rate of recurrence by 95% and is cost-effective.

The options for prophylaxis include *postcoital treatment*. This is most helpful for women who can clearly identify their infections as related to intercourse. The patient takes one tablet (usually double strength trimethoprim-sulfamethoxazole) after intercourse. *Continuous prophylaxis* involves daily or three times weekly treatment with an antibiotic. This strategy is probably the best alternative for women with very frequent infections. *Patient-initiated therapy* works well for patients who identify their problem very early in the course of infection; they take single-dose treatment as soon as symptoms appear. Women in this category have been shown to be good clinicians; they can predict when they have another UTI with 85% accuracy. Postmenopausal women with recurrent infections should first use *estrogen cream*. Vaginal estriol significantly decreases the risk of recurrent UTI in these patients.

No follow-up is needed for patients with a simple UTI whose symptoms resolve. Patients should be told to return to the office if they develop a fever (indicating upper tract infection) or if their symptoms persist for more than 2 days; at that time a repeat evaluation should include a pelvic examination and urine culture. Only pregnant women need a follow-up urine test to document clearance of the infection.

SUGGESTED READING

Nygaard IE, Johnson JM: Urinary tract infections in elderly women. *Am Fam Phys* 53:175–182, 1996.

Stamm WE, Hooton TM: Management of urinary tract infections in adults. *N Engl J Med* 329:1328–1334, 1994.

Wisinger DB: Urinary tract infection. *Postgrad Med* 100:229–236, 1996.

CHAPTER 37
Cellulitis

Robert V. Smith, M.D.

PATIENT

M. White, a 68-year-old woman, comes into the office because she feels "lousy." Today she noticed an area of redness on her right lower leg. Two days ago she was at the beach and sustained several insect bites. She has had a low-grade fever and had a single chill. There is no history of diabetes mellitus. On physical examination, the patient has a temperature of 100°F (37.8°C). An area of erythema about 15 cm in diameter is noted on the leg. The borders of the erythema are indistinct. No erythematous streaks are noted proximal to the area.

CLINICAL PRESENTATION

Cellulitis is an infection that spreads through the subcutaneous tissues. Typically the area is warm, tender, and erythematous. The erythema usually has an indistinct border and is not raised. If lymphangitis is present, streaking erythema can be seen, and proximal lymph nodes may be enlarged and tender. Most cases involve the lower extremities, although the upper extremities can be affected, particularly in women who have had axillary node dissection or radical mastectomy for breast cancer. Systemic symptoms may include malaise, fever, and chills. Sepsis can occur. Immunosuppressed patients are at particularly high risk for sepsis.

ETIOLOGY

The most commonly identified causative organisms are beta-hemolytic streptococci and *Staphylococcus aureus* in that order. Group A *Streptococcus* is the most common pathogen, although groups B, C, and G have also been identified. *Haemophilus influenzae* can be an important cause in children. The organisms may gain entry by way of rashes, abrasions, insect bites, local trauma, or parenteral drug abuse, although often none of these are present.

Streptococcus and *Staphylococcus* are nearly always the causative organisms of cellulitis.

DIFFERENTIAL DIAGNOSIS

Erysipelas is a key alternate diagnosis. The symptoms of erysipelas are virtually identical to cellulitis. Erysipelas involves only the superficial skin layers, and the edema it causes produces a raised, indurated area with a sharply demarcated border. Cellulitis, on the other hand, involves deeper layers of the skin and has an indistinct border. Erysipelas is more likely to involve the face, although the lower extremity is still the most common site. Group A *Streptococcus* is by far the most common causative agent of erysipelas; *Staphylococcus* is a rare cause. Sometimes, at least on initial presentation, it may be impossible to distinguish between cellulitis and erysipelas.

Both cellulitis and erysipelas can usually be distinguished from folliculitis. Folliculitis is a superficial infection characterized by pustules at the openings of hair follicles and is a small, localized infection.

The most feared infections are necrotizing fasciitis and streptococcal toxic shock syndrome. The causative agents of necrotizing fasciitis are the same as for cellulitis, and the clinical presentation, in its early stages, can be similar. Necrotizing fasciitis spreads through the fascia and subcutaneous tissues causing extensive necrosis. Systemic symptoms are much more severe; the patient is very toxic. The affected area is usually very painful and swollen. Bullae may form on the skin. Extensive surgical debridement is essential. Streptococcal toxic shock syndrome is caused by the release of pyogenic exotoxins and cytokines. It is characterized by malaise, fever, chills, nausea, vomiting, and diarrhea. There may be severe pain at the infection site. Shock and organ failure may develop. Necrotizing fasciitis may or may not also be present.

DIAGNOSIS

The diagnosis is established almost entirely on clinical grounds. The white blood cell (WBC) count may reveal a leukocytosis. On the rare occasion when purulent material is present, it should be sent for culture and Gram's stain. In the more severe cases, blood cultures should be obtained. Cultures can also be obtained from the margin of the lesion by injecting and then aspirating a small amount of saline. (Note: Do not use bacteriostatic saline.) However, cultures of blood and aspirate rarely identify an organism.

> It is the history and physical examination that establish the diagnosis. Look for red, warm, and tender.

TREATMENT

Cellulitis is treated with antibiotics, which are chosen empirically to cover both beta-hemolytic streptococci and *Staph. aureus*. The extent, severity, and responsiveness of the disease determine whether oral treatment is sufficient or whether parenteral antibiotics and hospitalization are needed. A penicillinase-resistant penicillin or first-generation cephalosporin is usually chosen. In the penicillin-allergic patient, erythromycin, clarithromycin, or clindamycin will be used most often. Erysipelas is almost always caused by group A streptococci, which may be treated with penicillin. Often, however, the same antibiotics that are used for cellulitis are chosen because *Staphylococcus* may occur (rarely) or because the clinical appearance may not allow clear differentiation between the two entities. Parenteral broad-spectrum antibiotics may be needed for those who are immunosuppressed. Systemic antibiotics are rarely needed for folliculitis; topical antibiotics and local hygiene are usually sufficient.

SUGGESTED READING

Bisno AL, Stevens DL: Streptococcal infections of skin and soft tissues. *N Eng J Med* 334:240–245, 1996.

Hacker SM: Common infections of the skin. *Postgrad Med* 96:43–52, 1994.

Simon MS, Cody RL: Cellulitis after axillary node dissection for carcinoma of the breast. *Am J Med* 93:543–548, 1992.

CHAPTER 38
Asthma

Katherine C. Krause, M.D.

PATIENT

N. Johnson, a 24-year-old man, his wife, and their 2-year-old son went to visit his parents who had just moved to Florida to retire. N. Johnson offered to clean out some old mattresses left in the garage. As a surprise, the grandparents bought a puppy for their grandson who was delighted. After returning home with the dog, N. Johnson experienced a significant flare in his mild asthma symptoms, which were previously well controlled by taking albuterol as needed two or three times a week.

CLINICAL PRESENTATION

Asthma is a reversible obstructive pulmonary disease characterized by narrowed airways, inflammation, and hyperresponsiveness. It can be induced by exposure to an irritant or an allergen. In the latter case, there is an immediate bronchoconstriction lasting 1–2 hours, which results from an antigen binding to immunoglobulin E (IgE) on the surface of mast cells, causing them to degranulate and release chemical mediators (e.g., histamines, leukotrienes, prostaglandins, platelet-activating factor [PAF]). Increased mucus production and capillary leakage occur. The early phase is responsive to treatment with beta agonists. Late-phase bronchoconstriction begins in 1–8 hours and lasts up to 3–4 days following the influx of inflammatory cells, eosinophils, and neutrophils. This response can be prevented and treated with anti-inflammatory drugs such as cromolyn and corticosteroids. Chronic asthma is the persistence of these inflammatory cell infiltrates, which damage the epithelium.

EPIDEMIOLOGY

Onset occurs before the age of 5 in 75%–90% of cases. Peak prevalence is between ages 10 and 12. Asthma affects 4%–7% of the American population and accounts for 4 million office visits, 1 million emergency room visits, 430,000 hospital admissions, and 2 million hospital days annually. The prevalence, severity, and death rate of asthma have increased in the past 15 years, especially in African Americans and Latinos.

Risk factors for asthma include a family history of atopy (e.g., asthma, hay fever, eczema), parental smoking, air pollution, and viral respiratory infections. The recent increases in morbidity and mortality are thought to be due to limited access to care, increase in pollution, and patient and provider underestimation of severity. Depression and previous life-threatening asthma attacks are risks for asthma-related deaths.

DIFFERENTIAL DIAGNOSIS

The diagnosis of asthma is made by establishing episodic airway obstruction and the reversibility of the obstruction. The diagnosis is not made by wheezing alone but by a pattern of shortness of breath, chest tightness, fatigue, cough, and exercise intolerance. On direct exposure to the allergen, the cough, if productive, yields thick, stringy, clear-to-white mucus. The cough can be nonproductive and can occur in spasms that may awaken the patient at night. Attacks tend to occur at night for several reasons: the temperature is cooler, the patient has nasal congestion, the respiratory tree is dry from mouth breathing, and the mucus is viscous. Lying down reduces the size of the chest cavity, causes pooling of secretions, and coincides with the diurnal waning of corticosteroid production in the body and the rise of histamine production.

Acute attacks can be precipitated by multiple *triggers*: exposure to smoke, dust, mites, pollens, grasses, molds, cockroaches, animal dander, or other allergens. Common incitants include cold, exercise, viral respiratory infections, stress, and drugs such as aspirin, nonsteroidal anti-inflammatory drugs (NSAIDs), and beta blockers. Foods are not common asthma triggers.

Findings on *physical examination* include wheezing, prolonged expiratory phase, tachypnea, tachycardia, decreased breath sounds, and the use of accessory muscles for respiration. Other signs of atopy may be noted, such as coryza, rhinorrhea, or postnasal drip. In mild attacks, wheezing may only be elicited on forced expiration. Reduced peak flow alone may signal the beginning of an attack. In severe attacks, the patient may be highly anxious and unable to complete a sentence. As the attack worsens, the patient tires. Wheezing is less audible as the chest gets "tighter" and moves less air. This worsening of respiratory status may be mistaken for improvement. However, the patient may become sleepy and cyanotic, signifying the onset of respiratory failure and the need to intubate.

Not all that wheezes is asthma, and asthma does not always present with wheezes. In an adult presenting with cough and wheezing or dyspnea (shortness of breath), the *differential diagnosis* includes the following: asthma, bronchitis, emphysema, sinusitis, gastroesophageal reflux disease (GERD), foreign body, coronary artery disease (CAD), congestive heart failure (CHF), pulmonary embolus, sarcoid, tuberculosis, or lung cancer. If the origin is infectious, fever and cough productive of purulent sputum would be common. If percussion and auscultation of the chest is asymmetric, a chest x-ray is helpful in localizing a foreign body. In a smoker with constitutional symptoms or a chronic increasing cough, a chest x-ray can identify a tumor or unresolving pneumonia. If the wheezing is cardiac in origin, signs of pump failure will be evident (e.g., rales, peripheral edema, presence of jugular venous distention, and a third heart sound [S_3]). Wheezing with symptoms of regurgitation, esophageal burning, and a cough occurring 1 hour after meals or after lying down at night suggests GERD. In a patient with a recent history of surgery, peripheral vascular disease, cancer, or birth control pill use, poor oxygen saturation and a positive ventilation-perfusion scan are consistent with pulmonary embolus.

DIAGNOSIS

Objective measures of lung function are essential for diagnosing asthma, assessing its severity, and evaluating response to therapy. The history and physical examination correlate poorly with the severity of outflow obstruction. Office spirometry measures forced expiratory volume in 1 second (FEV_1), which can be compared using nomograms to calculate the percent predicted for a person of the same height and age. The peak flow meter is a simple and inexpensive tool available to patients to demonstrate the degree of airway obstruction and the response to bronchodilator treatment. Have the patient stand, place his or her mouth tightly around a tube, and blow out as hard and fast as possible. The gauge measures a peak expiratory flow rate (PEFR), which correlates well with the office spirometry FEV_1. Office oximetry is helpful in determining oxygen saturation. If an arterial blood gas can be obtained, further information will be provided to identify acidosis, a rising PCO_2, and a dropping oxygen level in a patient with compromised respiratory status or a poor response to therapy.

Chest films are useful in selected patients to rule out other diseases. Indications for ordering a chest x-ray include tachypnea, tachycardia, localized rales, localized changes in breath sounds, or cyanosis. The typical asthmatic chest film shows hyperinflation, atelectasis, and rarely, pneumonia.

TREATMENT

The cornerstone of treatment rests on identifying and avoiding asthma triggers, training patients to monitor their respiratory status with a peak flow meter, and stepped therapy. Patients adjust their medications according to written instructions based on peak flow readings and symptoms.

Goals of asthma treatment to improve outcomes include:

- Decreasing symptoms and decreasing the number of episodes
- Decreasing the need for rescue with beta agonists
- Decreasing limitation on activity and exercise
- Decreasing days lost from work or school
- Decreasing emergency room visits or hospitalizations
- Decreasing medication side effects
- Increasing PEFR

Nonpharmacologic Treatment

Nonpharmacologic treatment includes avoiding allergens and trigger agents, especially in the bedroom. Mattresses, springs, foam rubber, and dacron pillows should be covered with plastic. Curtains should be removed and carpets should be replaced with washable cotton throw rugs. Asthma patients should also use wooden furniture with removable foam cushions, and high-efficiency particle arrester (HEPA) portable air filters. Windows in the house and car should be kept closed, and room temperature should be kept lower than 70°F and humidity below 45%.

In addition, smoking should be prohibited inside an asthma patient's house, and furry or feathered pets should be kept outside. Finally, chloride solution or Captan powder should be used to kill molds, and cockroaches should be exterminated.

Pharmacologic Treatment

ANTI-INFLAMMATORY AGENTS

Corticosteroids (Oral or Inhaled)

Regular use of corticosteroids decreases the need for bronchodilators as well as the airway's response to viruses, allergens, and irritants. The long-term side effects of oral steroids are osteoporosis, hypertension, cataracts, Cushing's syndrome, and immunosuppression. This limits the use of corticosteroids to patients who have severe, otherwise unresponsive asthma.

Inhaled steroids have little systemic absorption. Oral candidiasis can be avoided by rinsing the mouth after use or administering steroids with a spacer. Inhaled steroids vary in strength and can be titrated:

- Beclomethasone (42 mcg/puff), 2–4 puffs, two to four times a day
- Triamcinolone (100 mcg/puff), 2–4 puffs, two to four times a day
- Flunisolide (250 mcg/puff), 2–4 puffs, two to four times a day

Systemic steroids are indicated when other modes of therapy fail to control severe asthma. A burst of prednisone is given (1–2 mg/kg/d) for 3–5 days then stopped. If given for longer than 10 days, the dose is gradually reduced over 2–4 weeks. Inhaled steroids are continued during this period. Morning dosing is used to decrease adrenocortical suppression. Every other day dosing is also helpful in this respect.

Cromolyn Sodium

Cromolyn decreases airway hyperresponsiveness, inhibits mast cell degranulation, and inhibits early and late asthmatic responses. It is well tolerated and particularly effective in children and in patients with exercise-induced asthma. A 4–6-week trial is necessary to determine the effective dose of cromolyn. Cromolyn can be administered using a metered dose inhaler (MDI), 1 mg/puff, 2 puffs, two to four times a day.

ANTILEUKOTRIENES

Antileukotrienes are used for prophylaxis and chronic treatment of asthma in adults and children over 6 years of age. They are complementary to anti-inflammatory steroids and bronchodilators. The most common adverse effects are headache, infection, nausea, and diarrhea. The antileukotriene zafirlukast (Accolate) can be used twice a day (20 mg), 1 hour before or 2 hours after meals. Montelukast (Singulaire) is a once a day tablet in a dose of 5 mg for children over 6 and 10 mg for adults. It is best taken at bedtime to avoid headache as a side effect (18%).

BRONCHODILATORS

Beta$_2$ Agonists (albuterol, metaproterenol)

Beta$_2$ agonists are smooth muscle relaxants that may be used intermittently. They improve symptoms not the disease state and are most frequently prescribed in MDIs, 1–2 puffs every 4–6 hours as needed. Albuterol comes in dry powder for inhalation as well as oral syrup and pills. Metaproterenol is available as an inhaler, nebulizer solution, oral syrup, and tablets.

Terbutaline is classified as a B drug and is therefore the recommended choice in pregnant patients with asthma, 2 puffs every 4–6 hours as needed. Patients have difficulty tolerating the accompanying tachycardia.

Pirbuterol and salmeterol MDIs have a longer half-life and are helpful to those with night symptoms, 2 puffs every 8–12 hours. Albuterol can be added for acute exacerbation management if the asthma "breaks through."

Theophylline

Theophylline is a secondary bronchodilator because of its narrow therapeutic index. Serum levels need to be monitored (8–13 µg/mL is a target serum level). Tremors, anxiety, nausea, vomiting, and reflux side effects occur. At higher levels, cardiac dysrhythmias and seizures have been recorded. Certain conditions and many drugs interact with theophylline to raise its level in the bloodstream: high fever, viral infection, heart failure, or liver disease; cimetidine, erythromycin, rifampin, ciprofloxacin, lithium, as well as others. Theophylline is most useful in sustained-release capsules for single-dose nighttime coverage or when other drug management has been inadequate.

GUIDELINES FOR SELF-MANAGEMENT FROM THE NATIONAL ASTHMA EDUCATION EXPERT PANEL RECOMMENDATIONS (TABLE 38-1)

1. Teach each patient proper use of the MDI.
2. Teach each patient proper use of the peak flow meter.
3. Have the patient keep a daily diary during 2 weeks under good control to determine personal best peak flow to be used as the standard for maximum respiratory function.

PROGNOSIS

Onset of the disease predicts neither the length nor the severity of symptoms. The initial severity of asthma and the length of the episodes and hospitalizations are predictors for persistence of asthma into adulthood. Only about 16% of children with asthma are symptom free by early adulthood. There is a second peak of new onset asthma at the age of 40.

SUGGESTED READING

National Asthma Education Program Expert Panel. *Executive Summary: Guidelines for the Diagnosis and Management of Asthma* (DHHS Publication No. 91-3042A). Bethesda, MD: National Heart, Lung, and Blood Institute. 1991.

Rivo ML, Malveaux FJ: Outpatient management of asthma in adults. *Am Fam Physician* 45(5):2105–2112, 1992.

MANAGEMENT OF ASTHMA

		Step Care in Asthma		
Mild	Moderate	Moderate	Severe	Step Down
Beta agonist MDI not greater than three times a week and cromolyn sodium or beta agonist pre-exercise or antigen exposure	Inhaled daily anti-inflammatory: steroid 200–500 µg or cromolyn; may increase inhaled steroid to 400–750 µg; and inhaled beta agonist as needed not more than three to four times a day	Inhaled corticosteroids daily 800–1000 µg; sustained-release theophylline, oral beta agonist, or long-acting inhaled beta agonist, especially for night symptoms; short-acting beta agonist MDI, three to four times a day	Inhaled steroid 800–1000 µg; sustained-release theophylline, long-acting beta agonist, or both; especially for night symptoms, or both; oral steroids every other day or once a day, 40 mg for 7 days then taper over 1 week; short-acting beta agonist MDI three to four times a day	When symptoms are controlled, reduce medication to the minimum needed to maintain control and review signs of worsening; give remedial treatment, and use environmental control

	Clinical Pattern	
Mild	Moderate	Severe
Brief episodes, one to two times a week, night asthma less than one to two times a month, and peak flow greater than 80% as a personal best	Symptoms require beta agonist greater than three times a week, exacerbations greater than once or twice a week or affects activity and sleep, night symptoms greater than twice a month, and PEFR or FEV_1 60%–80% personal best	Frequent exacerbations, symptoms continuous, frequent night symptoms, limited physical activities, and peak flow less than 60% of that predicted

Note: MDI = metered dose inhaler; PEFR = peak expiratory flow rate; FEV_1 = forced expiratory volume in 1 second.
Source: Adapted from National Asthma Education Program Expert Panel. *Executive Summary: Guidelines for the Diagnosis and Management of Asthma* (DHHS Publication No. 91-3042A). Bethesda, MD: National Heart, Lung, and Blood Institute, 1991. Antileukotrienes were not in use at the time of this report.

CHAPTER 39
Chronic Obstructive Pulmonary Disease

Lisa M. Bellini, M.D.

PATIENT

D. Connor, a 50-year-old man, presents to the office complaining of 6 months of progressive dyspnea on exertion. He notes that he has had a cough productive of yellow sputum for years. His exercise tolerance is currently limited to walking one block on level ground. He denies wheezing, hemoptysis, chest pain, orthopnea, and paroxysmal nocturnal dyspnea. He has smoked two packs of cigarettes a day for 30 years and continues to smoke.

CLINICAL PRESENTATION

Chronic obstructive pulmonary disease (COPD) refers to a group of disorders that have in common the presence of persistent airflow limitation. The two frequently overlapping categories of COPD commonly recognized by physicians are chronic bronchitis and emphysema. The spectrum of chronic respiratory disorders is characterized by the following classic symptoms:

- Dyspnea
- Cough
- Sputum production
- Airflow obstruction
- Impaired gas exchange

The classic signs associated with COPD include tachycardia, tachypnea, increased anterior-posterior diameter of the chest, decreased diaphragmatic excursion, and decreased breath sounds. In severe COPD, when the metabolic demands of breathing are much higher than normal, malnutrition can become a significant factor and is manifested as temporal wasting and sunken supraclavicular fossa. Additionally, severe COPD can cause pulmonary hypertension, cor pulmonale, and peripheral edema. Those patients who have received multiple courses of steroids will have symptoms and signs of chronic steroid use including thin skin, cataracts, osteoporosis, and gastritis.

EPIDEMIOLOGY

COPD is a very common disease, estimated to affect at least 15 million Americans. In the United States, the overall prevalence is 4%–6% in men and 1%–3% in women; in adults over age 55 the estimated prevalence is 10%–15%. It is the fourth leading cause of death in the United States, and morbidity and mortality seem to be increasing, especially among women. In the past decade, mortality has risen by 22%, and the mortality rate 10 years after diagnosis is greater than 50%.

Cigarette smoking accounts for more than 90% of cases of COPD. Compared with nonsmokers, smokers have 10 times the relative risk of developing COPD, with the risk being equal for men and women. Given that only 10%–15% of smokers develop clinically significant obstructive lung disease, there is marked individual variation in susceptibility to developing COPD. In susceptible people, smoking causes an acceleration in the progressive decline in respiratory function that accompanies normal aging. The accelerated decline in lung function occurs over many years and is related to the amount of smoking. The large respiratory reserves in healthy lungs cause the disease to go unrecognized until later in life. In addition to smoking, factors modifying the risk of developing the disease include environmental exposures, genetic disorders such as α_1-antitrypsin deficiency, intravenous drug abuse, bronchial hyperreactivity, age, and male gender.

DIAGNOSIS

The development of airflow obstruction in COPD is gradual and insidious, and because of the large reserve in lung function, there is a long latency period before patients develop symptoms. Screening is not currently recommended. As a result, COPD is often identified only when the disease is severe and advanced. Physicians need to have a high index of suspicion for COPD in smokers who present with minor respiratory complaints.

The main feature of COPD necessary for diagnosis is reduced expiratory airflow from increased airway resistance due to airway narrowing. Maximal airflow is best measured with spirometry. It is a safe, reliable, and reproducible test to detect airflow obstruction and stage severity and to follow the course of disease. The hallmark of obstructive lung disease is a reduction in the ratio of forced expiratory volume in 1 second (FEV_1) to the forced vital capacity (FVC)—the FEV_1/FVC ratio. A ratio below 80 indicates airflow obstruction. Once the presence of obstruction is determined, the FEV_1 itself is used to assess disease severity and prognosis. To determine the presence of reversible airflow limitation, spirometry should be performed before and after bronchodilator therapy. Additional lung function studies that can be obtained include a measure of lung volumes and diffusion capacity, which may help to confirm spirometry findings, as emphysema causes a greater increase in lung volumes and a reduced diffusion capacity compared to other obstructive lung diseases. Spirometry should be performed annually to follow changes in lung function.

The use of chest radiographs is limited in the diagnosis of COPD, as they are usually normal in early disease. In advanced emphysema, they may reveal hyperinflation as evidenced by hyperlucency of the lung fields, flattened hemidiaphragms, and increased retrosternal airspace on the lateral view. The main use of chest radiographs in COPD is to eliminate other respiratory and cardiovascular causes of dyspnea.

The relation between the lung function studies and gas exchange is poor, making it important to perform arterial blood gas (ABG) analysis to detect hypoxemia and hypercapnia, especially in patients with advanced disease. It is important to note that hypoxemia can worsen with exercise, sleep, and changes in position. The two classic patterns of patients with COPD—pink puffers and blue bloaters—can be defined by the results of ABG analysis. Pink puffers are characterized by severe dyspnea (resulting in continuous "puffing"), mild hypoxemia (accounting for their pink color), and a lack of hypercapnia. Blue bloaters are characterized by severe hypoxemia (accounting for their blue color or cyanosis), right heart failure (resulting in their bloated appearance), and hypercapnia. In actual practice, most COPD patients fall within these two extremes.

> Those patients who are suspected to have COPD should receive a chest x-ray, spirometry, and an ABG.

TREATMENT

There are five management principles in COPD.

1. **Patient Education.** All patients must become aware of the nature of their disease process and how it will affect their daily functioning, as well as the purpose and value of each aspect of therapy.

2. **Avoid Risk Factors for Disease Progression.** The physician must ensure that the patient is or becomes a nonsmoker. Patients must be told in unequivocal terms that they must quit smoking. Patients must be aware that it may take several attempts before they are able to quit; the average is 3.5 attempts for each successful ex-smoker. Smoking cessation strategies include behavior

modification, counseling, and nicotine replacement therapy in the form of gum or transdermal patches for those who exhibit physical dependence on nicotine. Nicotine replacement therapy should be used cautiously in patients with coronary artery disease, as it can precipitate angina.

3. **Minimize Airflow Limitation.** Secretions and bronchoconstriction are the major factors contributing to airflow limitation. Smoking cessation and avoidance of airway irritants decrease cough and sputum production. The prevention of infection through vaccination for pneumococcus and influenza and the early treatment of recurrent infections with antimicrobial therapy are important.

Bronchodilator therapy is the mainstay of treatment for COPD. Bronchodilators increase airflow and reduce dyspnea in patients with COPD. Patients must be educated in the proper use of metered dose inhalers (MDIs) with a spacer to simplify therapy and improve compliance. The most commonly used bronchodilators are inhaled $beta_2$-adrenoreceptor agonists and inhaled anticholinergic agents. There are many types of $beta_2$ agonists with some having more $beta_2$ selectivity than others and some being long-acting. Isoproterenol and isoetharine have significant $beta_1$ effects and are not frequently used. The most frequently used are albuterol and metaproterenol because of their $beta_2$ selectivity and duration of action of about 4–6 hours. These agents are typically prescribed in doses of 2 puffs, four times a day. Newer agents such as bitolterol and pirbuterol are also $beta_2$ selective and have longer durations of action reducing the frequency of use to twice a day. All have the potential to induce hypokalemia in high doses. Ipratropium bromide is the most commonly used anticholinergic agent. It produces greater bronchodilation than conventional doses of beta agonists. Both classes of medications are equally efficacious in the treatment of acute exacerbations of COPD, and neither potentiates the action of the other. The slower onset and longer duration of action make ipratropium more suitable for use on a regular basis. It is typically prescribed in doses of 2–4 puffs, four times a day. Current recommendations for patients with mild COPD include maintenance therapy with ipratropium with the addition of a $beta_2$ agonist if the response to ipratropium alone is suboptimal. Even if spirometry postbronchodilation reveals no improvement, current recommendations suggest a trial therapy period with the addition of a $beta_2$ agonist. If the addition of a $beta_2$ agonist does not result in symptomatic or objective improvement, as documented by spirometry, it should be discontinued as part of a maintenance regimen. In such patients, $beta_2$ agonists should be reserved for periods of increased dyspnea associated with COPD flares.

The role of theophylline in COPD is controversial. In patients with moderate-to-severe disease, it has been shown to improve symptoms by increasing respiratory muscle function, clearance of secretions, and respiratory drive. In patients who respond suboptimally to bronchodilator therapy, long-acting theophylline can be added to the regimen for a trial period. If there is no symptomatic or objective improvement, as documented by spirometry, it should be discontinued. Theophylline preparations have a narrow therapeutic index, and levels must be monitored during chronic therapy. The target serum drug level is $8-12$ µg/mL.

The role of steroids in treating COPD is also controversial. Short courses of oral steroids are useful in patients with acute exacerbations of COPD to reduce airway inflammation and thus airflow limitation. Acute exacerbations are usually treated with a steroid taper over $1-2$ weeks. Chronic oral steroid therapy should be reserved for those patients with documented improvement in airflow or exercise tolerance and should be prescribed in the lowest possible dose. Unless patients demonstrate a component of asthma in addition to COPD, there is no role for inhaled steroids.

4. **Correct Hypoxemia and Hypercapnia.** In COPD patients with hypoxemia, oxygen therapy has been the only therapy shown to improve survival. The goal of therapy is to maintain oxygen saturation above 90% for a minimum of $12-15$ hours a day. It is important to note that hypoxemia can be exacerbated by activity, sleep, and changes in position, so achieving this goal may require different levels of oxygen therapy with various levels of activity.

Hypercapnia is generally well tolerated. Treatment should focus on decreasing the work of breathing by decreasing secretions and bronchoconstriction and by correcting any metabolic abnormalities.

5. **Optimize Functional Capacity.** It is very important to improve the patient's functional capacity and quality of life in the management of a chronic disease like COPD. Exercise conditioning, including upper extremity training, will improve cardiopulmonary conditioning and promote an improved sense of well-being.

Patients with COPD are at great risk for malnutrition because they have increased energy requirements due to increased work of breathing and recurrent respiratory infections as well as poor nutritional intake due to chronic cough, fatigue, depression, oxyhemoglobin desaturation during eating, and shortness of breath. The goals of nutritional therapy are to supply adequate calories, vitamins, and minerals; provide small frequent meals with nutrient-dense foods like peanut butter; add high-calorie, high-protein nutritional supplements; provide a daily multivitamin; encourage rest before meals; recommend food with little preparation involved like frozen dinners; and time the biggest meal of the day with the period of greatest energy.

> The principles of COPD management are: patient education, avoid risk factors for disease progression, minimize airflow limitation, correct hypoxemia and hypercapnia, and optimize functional capacity including exercise tolerance and nutrition therapy.

SUGGESTED READING

Ries A: Chronic obstructive pulmonary disease. In *Textbook of Internal Medicine*. Edited by Kelly WN. Philadelphia, PA: Lippincott-Raven, 1997, pp 1979–1984.

CHAPTER 40

Human Immunodeficiency Virus Infection

Richard A. Neill, M.D., and David E. Nicklin, M.D.

PATIENT

K. Jones, a 34-year-old man, presents for a health maintenance examination. He has no complaints. His medical history is unremarkable except for an episode of hepatitis B virus (HBV), which resolved 1 year ago. He is a homosexual who admits to having had four partners in a serially monogamous pattern during his lifetime. He has been with his most recent partner for the past 5 years. He denies intravenous drug use or blood transfusions. The remainder of his history and examination are unremarkable. His partner was just diagnosed as human immunodeficiency virus (HIV)-positive. Although the patient has had two negative HIV tests, his most recent test was over 2 years ago. Enzyme-linked immunosorbent assay (ELISA) and Western blot testing confirm that K. Jones is HIV-positive. His CD_4 lymphocyte count is 680 mm^3/μL, and his quantitative viral load is less than 5000 copies/mL of serum. He is diagnosed with asymptomatic HIV infection.

CLINICAL PRESENTATION

Early in the HIV epidemic, the most common initial presenting complaints of HIV or acquired immunodeficiency syndrome (AIDS) patients were due to opportunistic infections arising from immune dysfunction. New skin lesions due to Kaposi's sarcoma, shortness of breath and fever due to *Pneumocystis carinii* pneumonia, and painful swallowing due to oral or esophageal candidiasis were all common presenting complaints.

Fortunately, an expanded knowledge of the risks for and natural course of HIV infection coupled with more effective diagnostic testing have led to earlier diagnosis. As a result, it is now common for patients to present earlier in the course of infection, either at initial exposure or during the long asymptomatic period which follows, as in the case presented above.

EPIDEMIOLOGY

HIV and AIDS are caused by a human retrovirus transmitted through blood and body fluids. In the United States it is more prevalent among intravenous drug users, recipients of blood product transfusions, and men who have sex with men. However, the highest rate of increase is presently occurring in heterosexual men and women, especially African American and Hispanic women in urban areas. As a worldwide epidemic, it disproportionately affects developing countries in Africa and Asia. It is currently the leading cause of death among 25–44-year-old men and women, though declining death rates from AIDS resulting from public education efforts and the advent of highly active antiretroviral therapy (HAART) are likely to lower its ranking in the near future.

DIAGNOSIS

Because use of HAART can prolong life and defer the onset of immune dysfunction in HIV-infected patients, the United States Preventive Services Task Force (USPSTF) recommends that physicians should assess risk factors for HIV infection in all asymptomatic patients by obtaining a careful sexual history and inquiring about drug use. In addition, testing should be considered in any patient manifesting AIDS-indicator conditions (conditions which in the presence of HIV may constitute a diagnosis of AIDS).

Serum ELISA testing is 99.7% sensitive, but its lower specificity requires confirmatory testing by Western blot testing, which detects specific HIV antigens. Results of Western blot testing can be positive, negative, or indeterminate depending on the number and type of antigen bands demonstrated on the blot. Over-the-counter serum testing kits are available (Home Access), and at least one rapid serum test is available for use in health care offices (SUDS). Testing of oral mucosal transudate (Orasure) obviates the need for blood drawing or fingersticks and has similar sensitivity and specificity to serum testing.

Pretest and post-test counseling play a crucial role in helping patients comprehend the implications of testing. This also represents an important window of opportunity to provide counseling regarding high-risk behaviors and methods to reduce the risk of transmission.

Patients Who Should Receive Treatment

- All patients who are high risk by risk assessment
- Pregnant women in communities where seroprevalence in newborns is greater than or equal to 1%
- All children born to HIV-positive mothers
- All patients with active tuberculosis
- Patients with potential AIDS-defining conditions

Common AIDS-Defining Conditions

- *P. carinii* pneumonia
- Esophageal candidiasis
- Wasting syndrome
- Kaposi's sarcoma
- Extrapulmonary tuberculosis
- Persistent (> 1 mo) mucocutaneous herpes simplex
- Cytomegalovirus (CMV), retinitis, or disseminated CMV
- Cerebral toxoplasmosis
- Disseminated *Mycobacterium avium* infection
- Chronic intestinal cryptosporidiosis (> 1 mo)

TREATMENT

Medical treatment of HIV is guided by the patient's clinical condition combined with HIV viral load testing and CD_4 lymphocyte counts (Table 40-1). Treatment should be offered to any patient with a viral load over 5000–10,000 copies/mL of serum regardless of CD_4 lymphocyte count. Treatment should be considered for patients with lower viral loads if their CD_4 lymphocyte count is below 500 $mm^3/\mu L$. Patients at low risk of progression (i.e., those with low viral loads, high CD_4 lymphocyte counts, especially if not already exposed to antiretroviral therapy) may be safely deferred. These latter patients should be reevaluated in 3–6 months.

Optimal initial treatment consists of a combination of three antiretroviral agents, including two nucleoside reverse transcriptase inhibitors (NRTIs) and a protease inhibitor (PI) or a nonnucleoside reverse transcriptase inhibitor (NNRTI). Because of the large number of virions produced, viral resistance develops quickly in less than full-strength regimens or when patient compliance or drug interactions lower drug levels. Patient education regarding compliance and medication interactions is essential to ensure optimal treatment. PIs in particular are subject to development of rapid resistance, with substantial cross-resistance exhibited between PIs. For this reason PIs should be used only at full strength and in combination with other antiretroviral agents.

TABLE 40-1
TREATMENT OPTIONS FOR PATIENTS WITH HIV

Class of Medication	Members of Class	Typical Dosage
Nucleoside reverse transcriptase inhibitors	Zidovudine (AZT, Retrovir)	200 mg PO tid
	Dideoxycytidine (ddC, Zalcitabine)	0.75 mg PO tid
	Lamivudine (3TC, Epivir)	150 mg PO bid
	Stavudine (d4T, Zerit)	20 mg PO bid
	Didanosine (ddl, Videx)	200 mg PO bid

TABLE 40-1 (CONTINUED)

Class of Medication	Members of Class	Typical Dosage
Protease inhibitors	Indinavir (Crixivan)	800 mg PO q8h
	Ritonavir (Norvir)	600 mg PO bid
	Nelfinavir (Viracept)	750 mg PO tid
	Saquinavir (Invirase)	600 mg PO tid
Non-nucleoside reverse transcriptase inhibitors	Nevaripine (Viramune)	200 mg PO qid/bid (200 mg/qid × 14 days followed by 200 mg/bid thereafter)
	Delavaradine (Rescriptor)	200 mg PO tid

Note. PO = orally; tid = three times a day; bid = twice a day; qid = four times a day; q8h = every 8 hours.

The sociopolitical nature of HIV and AIDS also raises difficult treatment issues regarding legal and financial matters. Patients should receive advice regarding their rights to privacy, non-discrimination, and accommodation. Physicians should also encourage review of health or life insurance policies, attention to advance directives (including designation of power of attorney if appropriate), and creation of a will.

Support for the patient's psychosocial well-being should be provided in a nonjudgmental manner. Recruitment of community health resources such as AIDS patient support groups can be invaluable in minimizing the isolating effects of carrying a diagnosis of HIV or AIDS.

Ongoing monitoring for medication compliance and side effects, immune status, and signs or symptoms of opportunistic infection should occur side-by-side with age-and-gender-appropriate health maintenance for HIV or AIDS patients. However, several alterations and additions to health maintenance practices are necessary. Immunizations are more effective when given to immunocompetent patients, however, live virus vaccines (oral polio vaccine in particular) are contraindicated in patients with HIV. Pneumococcal and yearly influenza vaccines are recommended, despite evidence that the latter may transiently increase viral load. Skin testing for tuberculosis should be performed yearly, with some experts promoting isoniazide (INH) prophylaxis for patients in high-risk groups (intravenous drug users, migrant farm workers, homeless people) regardless of purified protein derivative (PPD) status. Papanicolaou (Pap) smears should be performed yearly in HIV-infected women, with aggressive follow-up of dysplastic lesions.

Patients also require specific counseling regarding avoidance of possible exposure to opportunistic infections. Inadvertent exposures from environmental or occupational settings (tuberculosis from health-related facilities or homeless shelters, diarrheal illness in child care facilities, coccidioidomycosis from gardening), pet-related exposures (feline toxoplasmosis, salmonellosis from reptiles), food or water exposures (unpasteurized foods, raw eggs, *Listeria* infection from undercooked meats and soft cheeses), and persistent high-risk behavior all warrant counseling and surveillance.

PROGNOSIS

HIV infection is a chronic illness that follows a predictable course. Acute phase symptoms follow 1–10 weeks after initial exposure and range in severity from no symptoms to a mononucleosis-type syndrome including pharyngitis, low-grade fever, lymphadenopathy, and myalgias. Less frequently seen are gastrointestinal or neurologic symptoms such as are seen in aseptic meningitis. A dramatic viremia during the acute phase induces a host immune response, which usually quells acute phase symptoms and heralds the onset of the second, chronic phase of HIV infection. During the second phase, patients generally remain asymptomatic for 1–10 years without treatment. Plasma viral titers are low during this phase, but virus replication in lymphoid tissue remains abundantly active. Viral production is often in the range of billions of copies daily. Eventually host immune mechanisms yield to relentless viral replication, causing characteristic declines in CD_4 count and rising viral plasma titers. These findings portend the onset of the third stage of infection, which is characterized by immune dysfunction and consequent overwhelming opportunistic infections resulting in death.

Questions to Assess Risk in Asymptomatic Adults

- Have you shared needles or syringes to inject drugs or steroids?
- If questioning a man: Have you had sex with other men?
- Have you had sex with someone who you believe may have been infected with HIV?
- Have you had a sexually transmitted disease (STD)?
- Did you receive a blood transfusion or blood products between 1978 and 1985?
- Have you had unprotected sex with someone who would answer yes to any of the above questions?

PREVENTION

The USPSTF recommends that all adolescent and adult patients be advised about risk factors for STDs and counseled appropriately about effective measures to reduce risk of infection, with counseling tailored to the individual risk factors, needs, and abilities of each patient. Effective measures in reducing sexual transmission include abstaining from sex, maintaining a mutually faithful monogamous sexual relationship with a partner known to be uninfected, regular use of latex condoms, and avoiding sexual contact with casual partners and high-risk individuals (e.g., intravenous drug users, prostitutes, persons with numerous sex partners). Patients should be counseled to avoid alcohol and other drugs that lower inhibitions against high-risk behaviors. Intravenous drug users should be counseled regarding the need to avoid sharing equipment and, when available, referred to sources for uncontaminated injection equipment and condoms. Patients at risk for STDs should be offered testing and treatment in accordance with current Centers for Disease Control recommendations on screening for syphilis, gonorrhea, HIV infection, and chlamydial infection.

Prevention of opportunistic infection in the immunocompromised patient relies heavily on exposure avoidance and prophylactic measures. Because risk for opportunistic infections is related to immune status, prophylactic measures are typically instituted based on a patient's CD_4 lymphocyte count. Asymptomatic patients with CD_4 lymphocyte counts above 200 mm³/μL require no prophylaxis. Symptomatic patients or those with CD_4 lymphocyte counts below 200 mm³/μL should receive trimethoprim-sulfamethoxazole for prophylaxis against *P. carinii*. Patients with CD_4 lymphocyte counts below 50–75 mm³/μL should receive clarithromycin or azithromycin for prevention of *M. avium* infection. Although CD_4 lymphocyte counts may rise dramatically with institution of HAART, current data neither support nor discredit continuation of prophylactic therapy. Most experts recommend continuation of prophylaxis once started, regardless of CD_4 lymphocyte count.

SUGGESTED READING

Carpenter CC, Fishel MA, Hammer SM: Antiretroviral therapy of HIV infection in 1997: updated recommendations of the International AIDS Society—USA panel. *JAMA* 277(24):1962–1969, 1997.

Centers for Disease Control: National AIDS Clearinghouse on the

World Wide Web. URL, http://www.cdcnac.gov/. September, 1997.

Goldschmidt RH, Dong BJ: Treatment of AIDS and HIV-related conditions—1997. *J Am Board Fam Pract* 10(2):144–167, 1997.

The Body: A Multimedia AIDS and HIV Information Resource. URL, http://www.thebody.com/. September, 1997.

CHAPTER 41
Migraine Headache

Kevin M. Fosnocht, M.D.

PATIENT

R. Roberts, a 21-year-old woman, complains of recurrent headaches. She gets several each year, ever since her menstrual period began. She describes them as severe and throbbing. The headaches usually occur on one side of her head. They sometimes last for up to 2 days, during which time she experiences profound nausea and light sensitivity. She feels the need to lie still because moving around makes the pain worse. Just before the headache, she says she sees "flashing lights, like lightning," move across her field of vision, which then disappear. When asked, she says the headaches seem to occur when she is "stressed."

CLINICAL PRESENTATION

Migraine attacks often occur with a characteristic pattern including up to five phases. Approximately 60% of migraine sufferers experience a *prodrome*, often hours to days before the onset of headache. This prodrome phase can include psychological symptoms like depression, irritability, and restlessness or constitutional symptoms like fatigue, anorexia, or "a cold feeling." Some patients describe a nonspecific sensation that they say lets them "know" a migraine is coming.

About 20% of migraine patients then experience an *aura*, which consists of focal neurologic symptoms characterized by visual, sensory, or motor phenomena. The most common of these are visual disturbances, typically consisting of an arc of scintillating lights that gradually expands to encompass a visual field, a loss of vision in a visual field (scotoma), or both. Unilateral numbness in the face and ipsilateral hand or arm is the most common somatosensory aura. Most auras develop over 5–20 minutes and last less than 1 hour. They usually precede but may occur concurrently with the next phase of the migraine attack, the *headache*.

The headache is characteristically episodic, gradual in onset, usually unilateral (though may be bilateral), and reported most commonly in the temporal area. It is usually throbbing or pulsating in quality and is moderate to severe in intensity, limiting daily activities. The headache is worsened with even small amounts of

> A migraine headache is often unilateral, pulsating, moderate to severe in intensity, and exacerbated by physical activity. It can be associated with nausea, vomiting, photophobia, and phonophobia. It may be preceded by an "aura."

physical activity. It is often associated with photophobia, phonophobia, nausea, and occasionally vomiting. As a result, the typical migraine sufferer seeks a quiet, dark room and lies still. The headache usually lasts between 4 and 72 hours in adults, and subsides gradually (*termination phase*). This phase is often followed by a *postdrome phase*, characterized by a feeling of being "washed out," moodiness, or fatigue. On occasion, a patient may feel unusually refreshed or euphoric after the headache has resolved. An important subgroup of migraine patients includes patients who do not experience the headache phase. This is known simply as "migraine aura without headache."

Many patients can identify certain triggers for their attacks, especially when asked, and these should be elicited by the physician. These commonly include stress, menstruation, lack of sleep, certain foods, and alcohol. Caffeine or other substance withdrawal can precipitate a migraine attack.

There are no specific signs of a migraine headache. A complete physical examination is warranted to exclude other causes of headache such as trauma, sinus disease, dental disease, ophthalmologic disease, and more serious conditions like brain tumor and temporal arteritis (see Chap. 1). Features that would lead one *away* from the diagnosis of migraine are fever, stiff neck, altered sensorium, or sinus or scalp tenderness. Patients may demonstrate a temporary focal neurologic deficit during the aura phase of the migraine attack, but it should resolve. Stroke is a possible complication of migraine, and a persistent neurologic deficit needs to be evaluated as such.

EPIDEMIOLOGY

A migraine headache is the second most common cause of primary headache (the most common being tension-type headache in the United States). In the United States, an estimated 17% of women and 6% of men are affected by this disorder. This prevalence translates to approximately 23 million Americans who currently suffer from migraine headaches. Migraine headaches usually begin in childhood or young adulthood and decrease in frequency with advancing age. A family history of migraine headaches is present in about two-thirds of patients. About 10%–15% of women who have migraines experience attacks only in the first few days of menses. Another 15% of women migraine sufferers do not develop attacks until menopause. For many women, pregnancy tends to make the condition better, though oral contraceptives or hormone replacement therapy (HRT) can precipitate a migraine headache. The cause of migraine headaches is unknown but seems to involve changes in cerebral blood flow and serotonergic pathways.

DIAGNOSIS

There is no good diagnostic test for migraine headaches. The diagnosis is made by a characteristic history and the exclusion of other causes of headache, which may require specific testing such as computed tomography (CT) of the head, especially when the history and physical examination have features suggesting sinus disease, trauma, stroke, or intracerebral hemorrhage. A headache with a duration of more than 3–4 days should call the diagnosis of migraine into question and might also prompt CT evaluation if the history and physical examination do not point toward another diagnosis.

Migraine headache is most easily confused with tension-type headache, and it is important to remember that the two may coexist. Depending on the history, a diagnosis of "migraine with aura" or "migraine without aura" is made.

TREATMENT

Treatment for migraine headaches is of two types: *abortive* therapy, designed to ameliorate the symptoms at the time of an attack, and *prophylactic* therapy, designed to prevent migraine attacks from occurring, or at least decrease their frequency. *Nonpharmacologic prophylactic measures* can be very effective in decreasing the frequency of attacks. A "headache diary," in which the patient records his or her migraine attacks, noting their timing and the patient's diet and emotional state, can be useful in identifying precipitants, so that these might later be avoided. Adopting a regular sleep schedule, engaging in regular exercise, and routine performance of relaxation techniques can be helpful in those whose attacks seem to be precipitated by stress.

Medications used to treat a migraine headache include analgesics, anti-inflammatory medications, and medications that affect brain physiology, particularly those which directly or indirectly affect serotonin pathways. Pharmacologic *prophylactic therapy* is generally warranted when a patient experiences migraine attacks that interfere with work or daily activities more than once a week. A variety of agents have been shown to be beneficial. A widely used and extensively studied class of drugs is the *beta-blockers* (e.g., propranolol, atenolol, metoprolol). With beta-blockers most migraine sufferers experience at least a 50% reduction in the frequency of attacks. Their use is often limited by side effects, which include drowsiness, exercise intolerance, and depression. They should not be used in patients with congestive heart failure (CHF), asthma, or peripheral vascular disease. It may take 2–3 months of daily therapy before a benefit is noted. A second class of drugs is the *tricyclic antidepressants* (e.g., amitriptyline, imipramine, doxepin), used in low-to-moderate doses. Their effect on migraine headaches is independent of their antidepressive effect. Side effects include drowsiness, orthostatic hypotension, and urinary retention. Other antidepressants may also be effective.

The calcium channel blocker *verapamil* is the most effective drug for migraine headaches in its class available in the United States. It may be more effective for migraine headaches with aura than for migraine headaches without aura. Side effects of verapamil include hypotension, bradycardia, heart block, and constipation.

Nonsteroidal anti-inflammatory drugs (NSAIDs), particularly naproxen, have also been useful, especially in migraine attacks associated with menstruation, when taken around the time of menses. Side effects include gastrointestinal upset, ulcers, and renal dysfunction.

Anticonvulsants, such as valproic acid and phenytoin, and *serotonin antagonists*, such as methysergide, are also used as prophylactic therapies. Their usefulness is limited by their side effects.

> **Prophylactic Therapies**
> Nonpharmacologic
> - Regular sleep schedule
> - Regular exercise
> - Relaxation techniques
> - Avoidance of precipitating foods
>
> Pharmacologic
> - Beta-blockers (e.g., propranolol)
> - Tricyclic antidepressants (e.g., amitriptyline)
> - Calcium channel blockers (e.g., verapamil)
> - NSAIDs (e.g., naproxen)
> - Anticonvulsants (e.g., valproic acid)
> - Serotonin antagonists (e.g., methysergide)

Several treatment options are available for *abortive therapy*. Their efficacy is maximized with administration early in the migraine attack. *NSAIDs* alone can be effective for acute treatment of a migraine headache. Many patients have used these medications prior to seeking the help of a physician. Aspirin or acetaminophen have been combined with caffeine and butalbital, a short-acting barbiturate. Though these latter preparations are effective, they should not be used frequently because of their addictive potential, especially in a chronic, recurring condition like a migraine headache. They also have a propensity to induce a "rebound" headache on discontinuation of the drug. *Narcotics*, with or without NSAIDs, are also effective, but again, have addictive potential, can induce rebound headache, and should be used only for patients with infrequent migraine attacks.

Ergotamine, and its derivative *dihydroergotamine*, are effective abortive therapies. The former is available in oral form in combination with caffeine and is most effective when given in the prodromal phase of the attack. This combination also can induce nausea and is usually given in conjunction with an antiemetic agent. Both agents are vasoconstrictors and should not be used in patients with known coronary artery disease (CAD) or peripheral vascular disease.

A relatively new agent, and possibly the most effective, is *sumatriptan*, which is a selective serotonin agonist. A single 6-mg subcutaneous injection can lead to a significant response in over 80% of patients within 2 hours. An oral preparation may be equally effective, though time to pain relief is longer owing to the mode of absorption. Because this agent acts as a vasoconstrictor, it should not be used in patients with uncontrolled hypertension or CAD. Side effects include a burning sensation at the site of the injection, flushing, and tingling of the extremities. Chest tightness has been reported.

A newly developed therapy is *transnasal butorphanol*, a synthetically derived opioid analgesic that is rapidly absorbed by the nasal mucosa. Its analgesic effect is rapid, occurring within 15 minutes of administration. It also has a sedative effect, which may be an aid in helping to resolve the attack.

> **Abortive Therapies**
> - NSAIDs
> - Sumatriptan
> - Ergotamine
> - Dihydroergotamine
> - Transnasal butorphanol
> - Narcotics
> - Aspirin or acetaminophen, caffeine, butalbital combination

SUGGESTED READING

Baumel B: Migraine: a pharmacologic review with newer options and delivery modalities. *Neurology* 44(Suppl 3):S13–S17, 1994.

Silberstein SD, Lipton RB: Overview of diagnosis and treatment of migraine. *Neurology* 44(Suppl 7):S6–S16, 1994.

Welch KMA: Drug therapy of migraine. *N Eng J Med* 329:1476–1483, 1993.

CHAPTER 42
Hypertension

Kevin A. Pearce, M.D., M.P.H.

PATIENT

T. Black, a 48-year-old man, comes to the physician's office for a checkup. He has no specific complaints but feels it is time to get a "physical." The following blood pressure readings are obtained: 156/94 mm Hg, 150/92 mm Hg. He says that he has never been treated for high blood pressure but recalls that the nurse at work told him his blood pressure was "up a bit" last month. Chart review shows only two other visits (for minor problems), with blood pressure readings 148/90 mm Hg and 150/94 mm Hg about 2 years ago. He takes no medications and has no chronic health problems to his knowledge.

CLINICAL PRESENTATION

Hypertension is usually asymptomatic. It is most often detected via routine blood pressure measurements taken during a medical visit for another reason. Some people do get symptoms from their hypertension. The most common ones are headache, fatigue, and decreased exercise tolerance. Hypertension may also present with signs and symptoms of a *major complication*, such as: angina or myocardial infarction (MI), transient ischemic attack (TIA) or stroke, congestive heart failure (CHF), and severe headache from subarachnoid hemorrhage.

DEFINITION AND CLASSIFICATION OF HYPERTENSION

Hypertension in adults is defined as: resting systolic blood pressure greater than or equal to 140 mm Hg or diastolic blood pressure greater than or equal to 90 mm Hg, based on the average of several readings taken during at least three office visits. Classification of hypertension is based on the severity of either systolic blood pressure or diastolic blood pressure, according to whichever falls into the higher stage:

Stage 1 = systolic blood pressure 140–159 mm Hg or diastolic blood pressure 90–99 mm Hg

Stage 2 = systolic blood pressure 160–179 mm Hg or diastolic blood pressure 100–109 mm Hg

Stage 3 = systolic blood pressure >180 mm Hg or diastolic blood pressure >110 mm Hg

EPIDEMIOLOGY

An estimated 25% of American adults have hypertension. Its prevalence rises steadily with age, with approximately 60% of people over the age of 65 having hypertension. Although blood pressure rises with age in the United States adult population, this is *not* normal and poses a health risk. Hypertension is more common among African Americans than whites, and it runs in families. It is also more common among people with obesity or type 2 diabetes mellitus (type 2 DM). Hypertension is a major risk factor for stroke, MI, CHF, chronic renal insufficiency (progressing to renal failure), and retinopathy. Cardiovascular complications are much more common than renal failure or retinopathy from high blood pressure. Treatment of hypertension has been *proven* to be effective for preventing stroke, MI, and CHF; it is *probably* effective in the prevention of renal insufficiency and retinopathy.

SCREENING

All adults should be screened at least every 2 years for hypertension. If the average of two blood pressure readings taken at one visit show systolic blood pressure greater than or equal to 140 mm Hg or diastolic blood pressure greater than or equal to 90 mm Hg, subsequent visits and readings should be performed to confirm the diagnosis of hypertension.

DIAGNOSIS

Diagnosis depends on accurate blood pressure readings that reflect the patient's usual resting blood pressure. Readings taken during an acute illness or pain should not be used to diagnose hypertension. Blood pressure measurements are best done with the patient seated, after at least 5 minutes of rest, and with the arm supported at the level of the heart. Supine readings are an acceptable alternative. At least two readings should be taken at each office visit, and the readings from at least three visits should be averaged to estimate the usual resting blood pressure. Systolic blood pressure is recorded at the onset of sounds and diastolic blood pressure at their disappearance. If sounds do not disappear despite complete cuff deflation, diastolic blood pressure is recorded when a muffling is first heard. False readings may occur if the blood pressure cuff is too small, too large, or if the patient has severe atherosclerosis. Home blood pressure levels tend to be 5–10 mm Hg lower than those taken in a medical office. Home blood pressure readings are of limited diagnostic value. A consistently large discrepancy between home and office blood pressure levels may warrant 24-hour automatic ambulatory blood pressure monitoring.

HISTORY AND PHYSICAL EXAMINATION

During the initial evaluation of the hypertensive patient, the history and physical examination should answer the following questions:

- What does the patient know about hypertension?
- Has the patient ever been treated for hypertension? If so, find out the type or types of treatment, plus the patient's feelings about and responses to prior treatments.
- Has the patient had any complications or *target organ damage* from hypertension? Keep in mind that hypertension harms the heart, brain, kidneys, eyes, and large arteries.
- What are the patient's other cardiovascular risk factors?
- What might be exacerbating the hypertension (e.g., alcohol abuse, stress, obesity, or medications)?
- Is there a family history of hypertension and any of its complications?
- Is this essential hypertension or secondary hypertension?

In addition to blood pressure measurement, the physical examination should include:

- A *cardiovascular examination* to look for signs of atherosclerosis (bruits, diminished pulses), CHF (gallop, rales, peripheral edema, jugular venous distention), and left ventricular hypertrophy (displaced point of maximal precordial impulse)
- A *neurologic examination* to look for signs of a prior stroke
- A *funduscopic eye examination* to look for signs of atherosclerosis (arteriolar narrowing) and retinal hemorrhages or exudates

LABORATORY TESTS

Except for the measurement of blood pressure, there is not a diagnostic test for hypertension. However, the following tests should be done to screen for causes, complications, and associated conditions that may affect treatment choices:

- *Serum creatinine level and urinalysis* to assess renal function
- *Serum electrolytes* at baseline prior to starting any diuretic therapy
- *Fasting lipid profile* to assess further cardiovascular risk
- *Resting electrocardiogram* (ECG) to look for baseline abnormalities including left ventricular hypertrophy and conduction abnormalities

ESSENTIAL HYPERTENSION VERSUS SECONDARY HYPERTENSION

Most hypertension (90%–95%) is said to be "essential," which is another way of saying idiopathic. Essential hypertension is considered to be nonreversible but treatable. The term "secondary" refers to hypertension that has a potentially reversible cause. Exacerbation of essential hypertension by obesity, sedentary life style, or alcohol abuse is conceptually distinct from secondary hypertension. However, essential hypertension is occasionally reversed by attention to these life-style factors. With that caveat in mind, causes of secondary (reversible) hypertension to consider in the primary care setting are: renal artery stenosis, hyperaldosteronism, primary renal disease, pregnancy, oral contraceptive use, hypothyroidism, hyperthyroidism, sleep apnea, generalized anxiety disorder, drug abuse (anabolic steroids, amphetamines, appetite suppressants), and pheochromocytoma (very rare). History, physical examination, and the limited laboratory evaluation described above serve as the basic screening tools for ruling out secondary hypertension. If a secondary cause is still suspected, it can be ruled in or out through a few well-chosen tests performed in the outpatient setting. Specific tests used to make the diagnosis of each type of secondary hypertension are described in the book by Kaplan listed in *Suggested Reading*.

TREATMENT

General Considerations

Prescribing a treatment for hypertension is relatively easy; but motivating a patient to stick with it can be quite challenging. Most patients cannot sense their blood pressure level, and they feel no immediate symptoms from high blood pressure. Usually, the "complaint" of hypertension has been introduced by a physician, not by the patient. Difficulty in maintaining prescribed antihypertensive treatments is the most common reason for treatment failures. The key to success is a proactive partnership with the patient, demonstrated by a supportive attitude, an interest in patient education, and good communication skills.

Nonpharmacologic Treatment

Nonpharmacologic treatment should be included in the management of all hypertensive patients. Most patients also require antihypertensive medication. However if blood pressure can be kept under 145/95 mm Hg with nondrug treatment, it can suffice as the sole therapy for asymptomatic patients with stage 1 hypertension who have no evidence of complications and are not diabetic. Most patients with target organ damage or diabetes should have blood pressure kept below 130/85 mm Hg. The recommended life-style therapies are:

- Weight loss if overweight
- Low-sodium diet (no more than 2 g of sodium a day)
- Moderation of alcohol (no more than two alcoholic drinks a day)
- Regular aerobic activity (at least 20 minutes a day, 5 or more days a week)

If these life-style changes do not control blood pressure after 3–6 months, drug therapy should be added.

Pharmacologic Treatment

At least 65 different antihypertensive drugs are now available in the United States with new ones appearing on the market each year. The key to understanding and keeping track of these drugs is to group them into major classes and subclasses, as shown in Table 42-1. Knowing the class in which any given drug belongs is very important for the effective treatment of hypertension. Because of their proven efficacy, diuretics and beta-receptor blockers (beta-blockers) are recommended as first-choice drugs for patients without contraindications to their use. Based on their hemodynamic effects and tolerability, drugs from five other major classes (see Table 42-1) are recommended as alternative first-line antihypertensive medications. Treatment is usually started with one first-line drug. If the blood pressure does not fall enough in the ensuing 4–6 weeks, the dose may be gradually increased up to the maximum recommended over the next 8 weeks. If this does not work and if compliance with the regimen is believed to be good, then it is best to pursue one of the following strategies: (1) *switch* to a drug in a *different* class, (2) *add* a second drug from a different class, or (3) *combine* two other drugs from separate classes at low-to-moderate doses (stopping the original drug). When combining drugs, include a diuretic if possible.

If the blood pressure is *still* not controlled 4–8 weeks later, despite good compliance, the patient will probably require a combination of two or three antihypertensive medications. Second-line drugs can be considered in this situation. The patient's other conditions may help guide drug selection. Avoid combining drugs from the same class, with one *exception*: it is acceptable to combine a potassium-sparing diuretic with a thiazide or loop diuretic. Combinations of two drugs in one pill are available. Hypertension that is difficult to control should raise suspicion that a secondary

TABLE 42-1
ANTIHYPERTENSIVE DRUG CLASSES

Diuretics[a]
　Thiazide: hydrocholorothiazide
　Potassium-sparing: spironolactone
　Loop: furosemide
Beta-blockers[a]
　Without ISA: atenolol
　With ISA: pindolol
Alpha₁-blocker:[a] doxazosin
Alpha-beta blocker:[a] labetalol
Angiotensin-converting enzyme inhibitor:[a] enalapril
Calcium channel blockers[a]
　Dihydropyridine: amlodipine
　Diltiazem
　Verapamil
Angiotensin-receptor blocker:[a] losartan
Central alpha agonist: methyldopa
Peripheral antiadrenergic: reserpine
Direct vasodilator: hydralazine

Note. ISA = intrinsic sympathomimetic activity.
[a] First-line drug.

cause is present, and further diagnostic investigation may be warranted.

Choosing the Best Starting Drug Regimen

First, remember that the main goal of antihypertensive treatment is to reduce cardiovascular risk through the least noxious means possible. Effectiveness, side effects, cost, and dosing schedule should all be considered. Next, think about whether you are trying to prevent a patient's first major complication from hypertension (*primary prevention*) versus trying to prevent a subsequent major complication (*secondary prevention*) in a patient who has already suffered a stroke or MI or who has CHF or nephropathy.

For *primary prevention, thiazide diuretics* and *beta-blockers* are good first choices, provided the patient has no contraindications to their use and has not already failed treatment with both drugs. Only these two classes of antihypertensive drugs have been *proven* effective at preventing a hypertensive patient's first MI or stroke. The others have not yet been tested in terms of their effectiveness for primary prevention. However, an alternative must be chosen for patients who cannot tolerate diuretics or beta-blockers or who have contraindications to their use. The choice should be based on the patient's other medical conditions, potential drug interactions, dosing schedule, and cost. Table 42-2 shows common medical

TABLE 42-2
GUIDELINES FOR FIRST-LINE DRUG TREATMENT OF
ESSENTIAL HYPERTENSION

Drug Class	Coexisting Medical Condition						
	CAD	CHF	↓ HR	DM	COPD	Gout	CRI
Diuretics							
Thiazide	...	Yes	...	...	...	No	No
Loop	...	Yes	...	...	...	No	Yes
Potassium-sparing	...	...	...	...	...	...	No
Beta-blockers[a]							
Without ISA	Yes	...[b]	No	...[b]	No	...	...
With ISA	...	...[b]		...[b]	No	...	...
Labetalol	...	...[b]	No	...[b]	No	...	...
Alpha₁-blockers	...	...	Yes	...	...	...	...
ACE inhibitors	Yes	Yes	...	Yes	...	...	Yes[c]
Calcium channel blockers[a]							
Diltiazem	...	No	No	Yes	...	...	Yes
Verapamil	...	No	No	Yes	...	...	Yes
Dihydropyridines[d]	...	No	...	Yes	...	...	Yes
Angiotensin-receptor blockers	...	...	...	...	...	...	...

Note. Either a thiazide diuretic or a beta-blocker is recommended if coexisting conditions do not suggest otherwise. Monitor for and correct any diuretic-associated hypokalemia. Yes = drug is preferred; No = drug is relatively contra-indicated; ... = drug acceptable; CAD = coronary artery disease; CHF = con-gestive heart failure; ↓ HR = bradycardia; DM = diabetes mellitus; COPD = chronic obstructive pulmonary disease; CRI = chronic renal insufficiency; ISA = intrinsic sympathomimetic activity; ACE = angiotensin-converting enzyme.
[a] Long-acting formulations are recommended.
[b] Use with caution in presence of CHF. Avoid in diabetics taking insulin.
[c] ACE inhibitors are contraindicated in bilateral renal artery stenosis.
[d] Avoid immediately after MI.

conditions in terms of relative indications and contraindications for first-line antihypertensive drugs.

Certain drugs are preferred for the *secondary prevention* of selected hypertensive complications. Angiotensin-converting enzyme (ACE) inhibitors are indicated in patients with CHF, diabetic nephropathy, and some cases of hypertensive nephropathy. Beta-blockers have proven efficacy in the prevention of recurrent MI, and loop diuretics are especially useful in patients with chronic renal insufficiency.

Follow-up

Patients with uncontrolled stage 1 or stage 2 hypertension should be seen at 4–12-week intervals until their blood pressure is controlled; those with uncontrolled stage 3 hypertension should be seen every 2 weeks. Medication adjustments should be made at each of these visits if the blood pressure is not responding. Once the blood pressure is controlled, patients should be seen at least annually. Often, other chronic medical conditions bring the patient back more frequently. Follow-up laboratory tests depend on baseline values, treatment type, and other conditions. Patients treated with a diuretic should have serum potassium and creatinine checked at least twice a year.

HYPERTENSION IN PREGNANCY

There are three types of hypertension associated with pregnancy. *Preeclampsia* is hypertension accompanied by proteinuria and edema with onset after 20 weeks gestation; *transient hypertension of pregnancy* develops after the twentieth week without proteinuria or edema and resolves after delivery; and *chronic hypertension* is present before the twentieth week without edema or proteinuria and persists postpartum. Preeclampsia is the most serious type. It can be superimposed on chronic hypertension. Antihypertensive drugs have no proven benefit for the mother or fetus in preeclampsia and should be used only if the blood pressure level is felt to threaten the mother before the problem is cured by delivery (systolic blood pressure greater than 160 mm Hg or diastolic blood pressure greater than 110 mm Hg are reasonable treatment thresholds). Chronic hypertension can often be controlled without drugs during pregnancy; however, medication should be started for systolic blood pressure greater than 150 mm Hg or diastolic blood pressure greater than 100 mm Hg. Bed rest is the only nondrug treatment recommended during pregnancy. Transient hypertension should be managed the same as chronic hypertension, but it will resolve after delivery. Methyldopa is the drug of choice during pregnancy because of its long history of use (Food and Drug Administration [FDA] pregnancy category B). Intravenous hydralazine is the most well-established treatment for severe hypertension during labor and delivery; intravenous labetolol is a good alternative. Magnesium sulfate may lower blood pressure in preeclampsia, but its blood pressure effects are not reliable. *ACE inhibitors and angiotensin-receptor blockers are contraindicated in pregnancy.* All other antihypertensive drugs are FDA category B or C for use in pregnancy.

SUGGESTED READING

Editor: Drugs for hypertension. *The Medical Letter* 37(949):45–50, 1995.

Joint National Committee on Detection, Evaluation, and Treatment of High Blood Pressure: The Fifth Report of the Joint National Committee on Detection, Evaluation, and Treatment of High Blood Pressure (JNC-VI). *Arch Intern Med* 157:2413, 1997.

Kaplan NM: *Clinical Hypertension*, 6th ed. Baltimore, MD: Williams & Wilkins, 1994.

National High Blood Pressure Education Program Working Group: Report on high blood pressure in pregnancy. *Am J Obstet Gynecol* 163:1689, 1990.

Price DW: The hypertensive patient in family practice. *J Am Board Fam Pract* 7:403, 1994.

CHAPTER 43
Obesity

Marilyn V. Howarth, M.D., and Amy J. Behrman, M.D.

PATIENT

T. Brown, a 45-year-old woman, comes to the office requesting prescription medication to help her lose weight. She describes following multiple different popular diets over nearly 30 years and discusses those diets in detail. Although she has managed to lose weight repeatedly, she has never attained "normal weight" and has always regained at least as much as she had lost with each diet cycle. On further questioning, she describes frequently skipping meals. She consumes most of her daily calories at an evening meal, which she eats alone while watching television. She works as a telephone operator, lives alone, and has little physical activity. Her workplace offers an exercise program, but she has never tried it. She denies frank binge eating, induced vomiting, and laxative abuse. She complains of mild dyspnea on exertion and occasional knee pain when climbing stairs. Her medical history is notable for cholecystectomy at age 40. She is on no medications. Her family history is notable for type 2 diabetes mellitus (type 2 DM) in her mother, who is also chronically overweight. On physical examination she is 5′4″ tall, weighs 180 lbs, and has a blood pressure of 160/100 mm Hg.

CLINICAL PRESENTATION

Obesity, the pathologic accumulation of fat tissue, is generally due to the ingestion of more calories than are used in energy expenditure. The diagnosis of obesity is usually obvious, but treatment is difficult. Moderate obesity is generally defined as more than 30% over ideal body weight, and morbid obesity is defined as more than 100% over ideal body weight. Quantification of obesity may be done by using the body mass index (BMI).

$$BMI = \frac{body\ weight\ (kg)}{height\ (m^2)}$$

BMI	
> 27.3 (women)	Mildly obese
> 27.8 (men)	Mildly obese
28–35	Moderately obese
> 35	Morbidly obese

The recognition of key symptoms and findings in obese patients may point to underlying causes and important associated conditions. These, in turn, may help guide effective management.

The *etiology is usually multifactorial*, reflecting behavioral, psychological, sociocultural, occupational, developmental, and genetic factors. Recent research has revealed genetic mutations that may lead to altered appetite and fat metabolism and thereby constitute risk factors for obesity. The initial history and physical examination should include screening for family history, childhood history, symptoms of depression or personality disorder, eating habits, and exercise habits. Rarely, specific genetic syndromes, endocrine abnormalities, or medication reactions may be sufficient by themselves to cause obesity. Endocrine syndromes that may be marked by key symptoms, include hypothyroidism with possible symptoms of fatigue, weakness, decreased alertness, constipation, hair loss, dry skin, and vocal changes; Cushing's syndrome with truncal obesity, "moon" facies, thinning skin, and peripheral muscle weakness; and Stein-Leventhal syndrome in women with hirsutism, amenorrhea, and polycystic ovaries. Medications that may cause new weight gain include beta-blockers, systemic corticosteroids, tricyclic antidepressants, and oral contraceptives.

Obesity is frequently associated with other serious medical conditions. The prognosis is worse when serious medical conditions are present. The clinical presentation may include symptoms and signs of coronary artery disease, diabetes, hypertension, degenerative joint disease, pulmonary dysfunction with decreased exercise tolerance, obstructive sleep apnea, cholecystitis, or depression. Malignancies that are more common in obese patients include cancers of the breast, ovary, colon, prostate, uterus, and gallbladder.

EPIDEMIOLOGY

One of three adults in the United States is now considered overweight. A 1994 survey of adults in this country indicated that at any given time approximately 25% of men and 45% of women are trying to lose weight, but the population seeking weight loss may not be the group that needs it. Despite the dramatic increase in public awareness of healthy diets, the total calorie intake of an average adult has increased 6% since 1979. Although the problem affects all ethnic groups, all ages, and both genders, the prevalence of obesity is higher with advancing age and with decreasing socioeconomic status. Approximately 9% of Americans are moderately obese, and 0.5% (1.7 million people) are morbidly obese.

SCREENING

The American Academy of Family Physicians and the United States Preventive Services Task Force (USPSTF) recommend periodic height and weight measurement. Individuals who are more than 20% above ideal body weight should receive appropriate nutritional and exercise counseling. The American Medical Association recommends that all adolescents should be screened annually for eating disorders and obesity by measuring weight and stature and by asking about body image and dieting patterns.

TREATMENT

Diet, Behavior Modification, and Exercise

Diet, behavior modification, and exercise comprise the primary approach to treatment. More than 30 billion dollars are spent yearly on diet foods, diet products, and programs. Any diet or program that deviates from standard nutritional recommendations may have serious unintended consequences. The goal of the obese patient and the physician should be to alter dysfunctional eating habits to achieve a healthy, nutritionally complete diet compatible with long-term maintenance of a healthier weight. There may be health benefits with even modest weight loss if it is sustained.

There are a variety of *weight reduction programs*, which vary in their level of complexity from simple menu recommendations and food classification with calorie counting to structured programs with physician, dietitian, psychologist, exercise counselor, and other health professionals involved in the planning, monitoring, and reviewing of the patient's progress and status. There is no convincing data to support any one of these programs over another. Behavioral treatment of obesity alone has been shown to result in an average weight loss of 8.5 kg after 21 weeks of treatment. At the 1-year point, however, behavioral treatment of obesity results in an average weight loss of only 5.6 kg. Patients should be counseled that small sustained weight loss is of greater health benefit than cycles of weight loss and weight gain.

Psychotherapy

Obese individuals who present for psychotherapy often identify a problem other than weight. In the course of therapy, it may become apparent that weight plays a significant role in decreased self-esteem and impaired social relationships. Psychotherapy may be appropriate for some patients with emotional difficulties that are caused by obesity or underlying depression, which may be exacerbating the obesity.

Physical Activity

Physical activity is important in any weight reduction program and may offer additional health benefits such as decreasing the incidence of osteoporosis, diabetes mellitus, coronary artery disease, and even breast cancer.

In designing an appropriate *exercise program*, the following factors must be considered:

1. Co-morbid conditions that may restrict or preclude aerobic exercise such as cardiac disease or peripheral vascular disease

2. Patient's life-style preferences that systematically limit physical activities

3. Body appearance concerns, which may limit a patient's willingness to wear a bathing suit or shorts for activities like swimming or jogging

Walking and stationary biking are excellent first activities for obese patients. Although swimming may not lead to weight loss in all patients, it is an effective way to increase cardiovascular fitness in severely overweight or arthritic patients who need minimal impact activities. Isotonic exercise is generally useful in cardiovascular conditioning and weight loss in contrast to isometric strength training. Weight loss is related to the amount of energy expended, which is a factor of the duration of the exercise and the number of exercise sessions a week. (Patients who exercise without restricting their diets may actually experience modest weight gain with conditioning as muscle is 6% heavier than fat.) The key to a successful exercise program is to identify an activity that the patient will actually do. Individuals with a BMI greater than 30 kg/m² should undergo a complete medical evaluation prior to beginning an aerobic exercise regimen.

Medication

The use of medication to treat obesity is not new. In the 1950s and 1960s, amphetamines were widely prescribed for weight loss purposes. No new class of medication for weight loss was approved by the Food and Drug Administration (FDA) until 1996. In 1996, fenfluramine hydrochloride and phentermine resin were approved by the FDA for the treatment of obesity. However, these medications were subsequently taken off the market when they were found to be associated with abnormalities in heart valves. Although comprehensive treatment programs, which include behavior modification techniques to improve diet and increase physical activity, have been shown to achieve weight loss, maintenance of weight loss is most important in enhancing health benefits for obese patients.

Since most individuals who successfully lose weight on a comprehensive treatment program regain their weight, medication has been considered as an adjunct to help sustain weight loss. This effect has yet to be proven; most studies using medication for the treatment of obesity have also shown a pattern of weight gain after treatment cessation.

Drugs that Promote Weight Loss

1. Catecholaminergic system effectors (amphetamines, phentermine, phenylpropanolamine). Amphetamines are not recommended for the treatment of obesity because of their high potential for abuse. The other medications in this category except phentermine are currently approved in the United States for weight control, but there are no data to show their long-term efficacy.

2. Serotonergic system effectors (fenfluramine, dexfenfluramine, fluoxetine and other selective serotonin-reuptake inhibitors (SSRIs). SSRIs are not recommended for the treatment of obesity in most cases, but may have a role in patients who are obese and clinically depressed.

3. Medications that increase energy expenditure and affect thermogenesis and metabolism. These include ephedrine, caffeine, and some experimental agents. No medications in this group are currently approved by the FDA for weight control.

No single drug has been proven to provide efficacy in achieving or sustaining weight loss. However, the combination of fenfluramine-phentermine has been shown in a controlled study to provide for greater weight loss when compared to placebo. Long-term therapy beyond 1 year has not been prospectively studied.

Serious Adverse Effects of Pharmacotherapy

Primary pulmonary hypertension is a rare but frequently fatal condition that occurs in one to two people per million in the general population each year. In patients taking fenfluramine and phentermine for more than 3 months, there is a 3–5-fold increased incidence of primary pulmonary hypertension equivalent to 1 in 22,000–44,000 patients a year. Valvular heart disease may also be increased in patients taking these drugs. Although rare, the seriousness of these diagnoses led the FDA to remove these medications from the market.

The decision to treat patients with medication is based on several factors. The North American Association for the Study of Obesity has recommended a BMI greater than 27 kg/m² before pharmacotherapy is considered for obesity treatment. In addition to the minimum consideration of the BMI, the presence of obesity-related co-morbidities must be considered.

Although the average weight loss shown in studies using pharmacologic agents has not been large, there is significant variability in the response of the individual patient. Several studies have found that weight loss within the first several weeks of treatment often predicts the efficacy of the drug. When medication is used, it is reasonable to start with a 1-month trial and to reassess the efficacy after 1 month.

Minor Adverse Effects of Pharmacotherapy

Catecholaminergic medications can cause insomnia, nervousness, euphoria, increased blood pressure, and tachycardia. Amphetamines have great potential for abuse or dependence.

Serotonergic medications (fenfluramine and dexfenfluramine) can cause sleep disturbance, somnolence, diarrhea, dry mouth, depression, and polyuria. Medications in this class have not frequently been associated with abuse or dependence although there are case reports published that suggest dependence as a possibility. Caution should be used whenever prescribing these medications to patients with a history of substance abuse. Fluoxetine and other SSRIs may occasionally cause insomnia, nausea, sweating, nervousness, diarrhea, dyspepsia, tremor, and sexual dysfunction.

Depression can also be seen on withdrawal of any anorexiant drug. Short-term memory loss, which is reversible, has been shown in up to 13% of patients taking the fenfluramine-phentermine combination.

Contraindications to Pharmacotherapy

Relative contraindications for treatment with obesity medications are patients with cardiac arrhythmias, symptomatic cardiovascular disease, or severe systemic disease such as hepatic or renal failure. *Absolute contraindications* for all obesity medications are concurrent administration with monoamine oxidase inhibitors and glaucoma.

Since drowsiness is a common side effect, concurrent administration of serotonergic medications with central nervous system (CNS) depressants is not advised. Similarly if general anesthesia is planned, obesity medication should be discontinued prior to surgery whenever possible since there may be synergy of CNS effects.

Surgery

Only patients whose BMI is over 40 kg/m² and who have repeatedly failed conservative weight reduction programs including behavior modification, exercise, pharmacotherapy, and psychotherapy should be considered for surgical management. Most surgical procedures for weight reduction produce a greatly decreased gastric volume (*banded gastroplasty, gastric stapling, gastric bubble pro-*

cedure). Other surgical procedures that are still performed include *gastric bypass* and *jaw wiring*.

On average, there is a 1% mortality rate with surgical procedures and a 15% morbidity rate (some of which is very serious). The efficacy of these techniques has not been well described in controlled studies, but many patients achieve long-term weight loss, improved quality of life, and risk reduction for obesity-related medical conditions. The significant morbidity associated with these procedures must be weighed against the morbidity of untreated obesity.

SUGGESTED READING

Carek PJ, Sherer JT, Carson DS: Management of obesity: medical treatment options. *Am Fam Phys* 55(2):551–558, 1997.

Crimmins-Hintlian C: Evaluation of excessive weight gain and obesity. In *Primary Care Medicine: Office Evaluation and Management of the Adult Patient*, 3rd ed. Philadelphia, PA: J. B. Lippincott, 1995, pp 42–48.

Crimmins-Hintlian C: Management of obesity. In *Primary Care Medicine: Office Evaluation and Management of the Adult Patient*, 3rd ed. Philadelphia, PA: J. B. Lippincott, 1995, pp 1066–1072.

Cummings S, Goodrick K, Foreyt J: Position of The American Dietetic Association: weight management. *J Am Dietetic Assoc* 97(1):71–74, 1997.

Pharmacotherapy for Obesity—National Task Force on Obesity: long-term pharmacotherapy in the management of obesity. *JAMA* 276(23):1907–1915, 1996.

U. S. Department of Health and Human Services: *Clinician's Handbook of Preventive Services*. Washington, DC: Government Printing Office, 1994.

CHAPTER 44
Diabetes Mellitus

Robert K. Cato, M.D.

PATIENT

A. Banks, a 57-year-old administrator, complains of a several-weeks history of "urinating all the time," "always feeling thirsty," blurred vision, and fatigue. She denies fever, abdominal pain, light-headedness, and shortness of breath. She has no medical history except obesity. Her older brother and mother are taking medication for diabetes. Physical examination reveals an obese woman in no acute distress with a blood pressure of 158/90 mm Hg, and a heart rate of 84 beats/min; the remainder of the examination is normal.

CLINICAL PRESENTATION

The clinical presentation of diabetes mellitus varies from patient to patient. A large percentage of patients with type 2 diabetes mellitus (type 2 DM) [non–insulin-dependent diabetes mellitus] are asymptomatic, are found through an abnormal blood glucose level that was drawn for another reason, or have vague symptoms such as fatigue. Any symptoms are usually present for weeks to months and are related to hyperglycemia with resultant polyuria, polydipsia, blurred vision, and excessive thirst. Patients with type 1 diabetes mellitus (type 1 DM) [insulin-dependent diabetes mellitus, juvenile diabetes, or ketosis-prone diabetes], are usually symptomatic for a relatively short period of time, with weight loss, poly-phagia, and symptoms of hyperglycemia. These patients may present to medical attention very ill and in diabetic ketoacidosis. In both types, an acute stressor (e.g., infection) may coincide with a marked worsening in what had been mild symptoms. Uncommonly, a patient with type 2 DM will first come to medical attention with a complication of diabetes mellitus such as neuropathy and will not have any other symptoms even though the symptoms may have been present for years.

EPIDEMIOLOGY

Diabetes mellitus is a very common disease, affecting 1%–3% of all Americans. The diagnosis of diabetes mellitus is established when a fasting plasma glucose level is greater than 126 mg/dL or when repeated nonfasting values are greater than 200 mg/dL. This is somewhat arbitrary, and patients that are close to these criteria are considered "insulin-resistant" and at increased risk for developing frank diabetes mellitus. The epidemiology of type 1 and type 2 DM is very different. Type 2 DM, which is 5–10 times more common than type 1 DM, tends to occur in obese patients over the age of 40. In fact, moderate-to-severe obesity is the strongest risk factor for type 2 DM, and roughly three-fourths of type 2 DM patients are obese. The genetic links in type 2 DM are very strong, with almost 100% concordance in identical twins. Type 2 DM (and obesity) is much more common in African Americans and Hispanics. In the Pima Native American tribe, almost half of the people have type 2 DM. Type 1 DM, on the other hand, has a peak incidence in the teen years, and it occurs almost exclusively in patients under the age of 40 years. Genetic links to type 1 DM are present but are not as strong as type 2 DM and appear to be mediated through certain human leukocyte antigen (HLA) types and a predisposition to autoimmune diseases in general.

> Patients at risk for developing diabetes mellitus (family history, obesity) are often screened with fasting glucose levels or glycosylated hemoglobin levels so that treatment can be initiated at an early stage.

DIFFERENTIAL DIAGNOSIS

Diabetes mellitus is usually an obvious diagnosis, but other causes of hyperglycemia must be excluded. States of glucocorticoid excess (steroid therapy, Cushing's syndrome), severe metabolic stress (e.g., burns), hormone-secreting tumors (growth hormone, catecholamines from pheochromocytoma), and artificial feeding can cause hyperglycemia that resolves with correction of the underlying problem. Pancreatic damage, such as that which occurs after surgical removal of the organ or from alcohol-induced chronic pancreatitis, is different pathophysiologically but requires similar treatment to diabetes mellitus. Pregnancy-induced (gestational) diabetes mellitus is a common problem, and although the patient usually returns to a nondiabetic state postpartum, there is an increased risk of diabetes in later years.

PATHOPHYSIOLOGY

Though they have common complications and share some principles of treatment, type 1 and type 2 DM are quite different pathophysiologically. Type 2 DM is believed to start as an insulin-resistant state with a period of hyperinsulinemia that over time develops into a state of relative insulin deficiency (i.e., inappropriate insulin response given the hyperglycemic state). The insulin-resistant state is at least partly related to obesity in most patients. Importantly, patients with type 2 DM have residual pancreatic beta cell function and therefore have enough insulin to prevent the development of ketoacidosis. In many cases, this allows therapy to be directed towards increasing endogenous insulin secretion, improving the activity of the insulin that is present, or decreasing the need for insulin. In contrast, type 1 DM is believed to be related to a combination of genetic (HLA-related), environmental (viral infection), and autoimmune phenomena that result in destruction of pancreatic beta cells. These mechanisms leave the patient with little or no intrinsic insulin secretion and therefore ketoacidosis prone. Therapy for type 1 DM must include exogenous insulin.

TREATMENT

Goals

Treatment of diabetes mellitus is directed first at eliminating the acute hyperglycemic state and the associated symptoms. Once this is achieved, the focus is to maintain serum glucose levels as near normal as possible to prevent long-term complications. There are two techniques used to monitor glucose control. First, on a day-to-day basis, determination of whole blood glucose values is possible by a small drop of blood obtained by pricking a finger (a "fingerstick"). This is collected onto a reagent strip, which is then inserted into a machine (glucometer) that reads the result. Patients may do this prior to meals 1–6 times a day, depending on how tightly they are being controlled and what medicines are being used. Second, a glycosylated hemoglobin (HbA_{1c}) level is obtained every few months, which is a measurement of the percent of hemoglobin amino acids that are glycosylated (normal being 4%–6%). This value is known to vary directly with glucose levels and reflects roughly 3 months of glycemic control (given the turnover of red blood cells). In combination, one can adjust treatment to keep fingerstick values near the normal range (70–130 mg/dL) and HbA_{1c} values near that seen in nondiabetics.

Diet

Most type 2 DM patients are obese, which plays a large role in their insulin resistance and hyperglycemic state. Exercise and weight loss improve insulin sensitivity. Though difficult, *weight loss should be the cornerstone of therapy in most patients with type 2 DM*. Type 1 DM patients are rarely obese and in fact are usually thin. For any diabetic, avoidance of excessive amounts of concentrated simple sugars, such as candy, cakes, and fruit juices, is generally recommended. A regular pattern of meals is useful, especially in patients on insulin so that dosing is consistent day-to-day. A low-fat, low-salt, well-balanced diet is recommended for all diabetics as a way to minimize other medical problems and to maximize overall health.

Exercise

Exercise decreases blood sugar and improves glycemic control. It is recommended for all diabetics. In type 2 DM patients who are asymptomatic, life-style and diet changes should be tried initially without any medication. Exercise and dietary changes may be successful in delaying or preventing the need for pharmacologic treatment.

Medication

If a patient with type 2 DM requires medication because they are symptomatic or life-style modifications have failed, oral agents are generally attempted first. A significant percentage of patients will never achieve adequate control of their glucose despite maximal doses of oral agents (primary failure), and a large percentage of patients who initially achieve adequate control will worsen with time and eventually require insulin therapy (secondary failure). Most patients would like to avoid or delay insulin therapy and its attendant difficulties (self-injections). For patients with type 1 DM, oral agents are not useful, and insulin therapy is necessary.

Sulfonylureas (e.g., glipizide, glyburide) are well tested and have been used for long periods of time. Sulfonylureas work primarily by increasing pancreatic secretion of insulin; they are relatively well tolerated. Side effects include mild gastrointestinal (GI) disturbances, and the relatively rare but dangerous hypoglycemia (especially in the elderly or in a patient who is not eating well). Sulfonylureas are titrated upward in dose until adequate control is achieved or when the maximal beneficial dose is reached.

Metformin is a biguanide agent that has been in use for several years, though only recently in the United States. Its primary mechanism of action is decreasing hepatic gluconeogenesis possibly by enhancing peripheral glucose uptake. It does *not* increase insulin levels, is not associated with hypoglycemia, and has a favorable effect on body weight and lipids. The most concerning side effect is production of a life-threatening lactic acidosis, which is extremely rare except in patients with chronic renal failure, liver dysfunction, or congestive heart failure (CHF). It is therefore contraindicated in these patients. More commonly, metformin causes nausea and diarrhea, which is greatly minimized if the dose is slowly increased over several weeks. Like sulfonylureas, there is a maximal effective dose (for metformin, 850 mg three times a day). Sulfonylureas and metformin are roughly equal in efficacy and are commonly used together with additive effects. Metformin may also be used in combination with insulin in type 2 DM or as primary therapy (especially in obese patients).

Acarbose is a new agent that slows absorption of carbohydrates, thereby attenuating the rapid postprandial glucose peak. It does this by inducing a relative state of malabsorption and therefore is poorly tolerated as a result of significant GI side effects of nausea, cramping, diarrhea, and flatulence. It is usually used as adjunct therapy in the treatment of type 2 DM, if at all.

Troglitazone is a new agent that works by improving insulin sensitivity in peripheral tissues, and like metformin, does not increase insulin levels. It is relatively well tolerated. Further data are needed, though early results are promising, especially in decreasing insulin doses in severe type 2 DM. Hepatic damage has been seen in a small percentage of patients, and liver enzymes should be closely monitored.

Using Insulin

All type 1 DM patients require insulin injections, and over half of type 2 DM patients will eventually require insulin to obtain tight glycemic control. There are many different schedules by which to dose insulin, but the underlying theme is to attempt to mimic normal physiologic insulin action, thereby maintaining blood glucose values within normal range at all times. It is not possible to duplicate exactly the precise control of the pancreas, but the goal remains. It is crucial to individualize insulin therapy for each patient. For example, an elderly patient with type 2 DM who has a short life expectancy would not benefit from strict control of blood glucose with insulin. However, an otherwise healthy 45-year-old patient would benefit from excellent glycemic control to minimize future complications. The difficulty in obtaining excellent glycemic control rests partly with patient compliance, given that several insulin injections and fingerstick determinations may be needed daily. Also, when one attempts to maintain glucose in the normal range, given the imprecise nature of subcutaneous insulin injections, the risk of dangerous and potentially life-threatening hypoglycemia increases.

> It is necessary to individualize insulin therapy. Often, one must accept poor or fair control of diabetes because of compliance issues, social situations, lifestyle choices, and co-morbid illnesses.

There are different types of insulin. Most insulin used now is recombinant human insulin, though some patients still use bovine or porcine insulin. Short-acting (regular) insulin has onset of action in 30-60 minutes, peaks at 2-4 hours, and lasts about 6-8 hours. Intermediate-acting insulin (NPH or Lente) starts working at 2-4 hours, peaks at 6-12 hours, and lasts up to 24 hours. Long-acting insulin (Ultralente) lasts nearly 24 hours but is not commonly used. There are also premixed preparations of intermediate- and short-acting insulin, for example 70/30 has 70% NPH and 30% regular insulin. The pharmacodynamic and pharmacokinetic principles of insulin can vary widely with different patients, injection sites, and exercise, which must be considered as therapy is tailored. Most type 2 DM patients on insulin begin with one or two daily injections of an intermediate insulin, though many will require two daily injections of an intermediate and regular combination. The doses of insulin are then adjusted by fingerstick values. Some insulin-dependent diabetics are also on two daily combination injections, though often they are on a more aggressive regimen. One protocol for "tight" control calls for injecting short-acting insulin prior to each meal and snack, with adjustments in the dose based on the fingerstick obtained and the number of calories anticipated. A dose of intermediate-acting or long-acting insulin is given at night to offer a low basal level of insulin overnight and through most of the day. Another option in type 1 DM is a subcutaneous insulin pump, which injects a programmed dose of insulin subcutaneously at a steady rate, which can be adjusted by the patient. Some of these regimens are quite sophisticated and require extensive education and adequate resources and abilities in the patient.

COMPLICATIONS

The long-term complications of diabetes are most dreaded and of much more concern than the acute symptoms of hyperglycemia. In fact, it is rather easy to control a patient's glucose enough to prevent acute symptoms (polyuria, polydipsia). However, years of hyperglycemia lead to multiple complications, most of them vascular in nature. Diabetic retinopathy is the leading cause of blindness, diabetic nephropathy is the leading cause of chronic renal failure requiring hemodialysis, and diabetic foot infections are the most common cause of nontraumatic lower extremity amputations. Diabetes is one of the few major risk factors for coronary artery disease, peripheral vascular disease, and strokes. Diabetes mellitus also may lead to various neuropathic states, which can cause chronic pain, numbness, or limb weakness. Diabetic gastroparesis is caused by neuropathy of the enteric nervous system, leading to poor gastric motility and associated postprandial vomiting. Diabetics also have increased risk of CHF, cataracts, pneumonia, gram-negative infections, fungal infections, and overall mortality.

The likelihood of these various complications varies from patient to patient, but the evidence is overwhelming that the risk of these complications are strongly related to degree of glycemic control (as measured by HbA_{1c} values). There are likely other factors as well, including genetic differences. These complications are seen in type 1 DM and type 2 DM, and it appears that the benefits of aggressive control are seen in both types of diabetes.

FOLLOW-UP CARE

Diabetes is a chronic disease that needs very close follow-up. Continuous reaffirmation of important educational topics is paramount, and early intervention can prevent complications.

- Patients should record fingerstick values for analysis by a physician or nurse.
- HbA_{1c} values should be obtained 3–4 times yearly to assess the success of the regimen, and changes should be made as needed.
- A *foot examination at each visit* will detect early signs of infections, toenail problems, and neuropathy.
- Patients should be asked about and re-educated about hypoglycemic symptoms (diaphoresis, tachycardia, lightheadedness, weakness) and be reminded that exercise speeds insulin absorption and increases glucose utilization and can precipitate hypoglycemia.
- Lipid abnormalities and other cardiac risk factors such as tobacco use and hypertension need to be aggressively managed to minimize vascular complications.
- *Yearly urinalysis* for the presence of albuminuria should be obtained, since angiotensin-converting enzyme inhibitors have been shown to slow the rate of progression of diabetic neuropathy when started early (at the stage of microalbuminuria).
- *Yearly ophthalmologic consultation* is mandatory, since early diabetic retinopathy can be treated by laser therapy to prevent vision loss.
- Podiatric and nutrition consultation can be helpful in many patients.
- Physician/patient partnerships with well-informed patients actively participating in their own disease management can improve outcomes.

SUGGESTED READING

Diabetes Control and Complications Trial Group: The effect of intensive treatment of diabetes on the development and progression of long-term complications in insulin-dependent diabetes mellitus. *N Engl J Med* 329:977, 1993.

Gerich JE: Oral hypoglycemic agents. *N Engl J Med* 321:1231, 1989.

Laine C, Caro JF: Preventing complications in diabetes mellitus: the role of the primary care physician. *Med Clin N Am* 80(2):457–474, 1995.

CHAPTER 45
Hypercholesterolemia

Eileen E. Reynolds, M.D.

PATIENT

B. Milton, a 59-year-old man, presents to the office for primary care. He feels well and has not seen a physician for several years. He does not smoke or drink but also does not exercise or watch his diet. As a businessman, he travels frequently and eats fast food while "on the road." His younger brother recently had a heart attack. On examination, he is mildly overweight and has a normal blood pressure. His laboratory tests show a total cholesterol of 289 mg/dL; a second, repeated fasting specimen shows a total cholesterol of 270 mg/dL, a high-density lipoprotein (HDL) of 40 mg/dL, triglycerides of 100 mg/dL, and a low-density lipoprotein (LDL) of 210 mg/dL.

CLINICAL PRESENTATION

Hypercholesterolemia is usually asymptomatic and is most often discovered with laboratory work done for health care maintenance. High blood cholesterol is a major risk factor for coronary artery disease (CAD) and vascular disease and is occasionally discovered when a patient who has previously been out of contact with the medical system presents with symptoms of atherosclerosis. Some forms of high cholesterol run in families. In rare cases, lipid levels are so high that patients present with eruptive or tendinous xanthomas or with pancreatitis.

EPIDEMIOLOGY

CAD, the leading cause of death in the United States, accounts for almost 500,000 deaths each year; half of which are among women. The total yearly cost of care for CAD in the United States is more than 60 billion dollars. Hypercholesterolemia is one of the modifiable major risk factors for CAD.

High blood cholesterol is very common. Levels above 200 mg/dL are considered mildly increased; greater than 240 mg/dL are moderately increased. Cholesterol rises throughout life and is higher in women than in men. Lipid is deposited into the walls of blood vessels beginning in childhood, appearing first as fatty streaks and later as atheromatous plaques. A 1% increase in total cholesterol increases a middle-aged man's risk of CAD by about 3%; the increase in risk probably begins with a cholesterol level as low as 160 mg/dL. High cholesterol predicts CAD mortality as early as age 20 in men, and at least to age 75 in men and women. The relationship between high cholesterol and CAD is stronger for men than for women and weakens with increasing age.

LDL ("bad" cholesterol) is the major constituent of total cholesterol and increasing levels of LDL parallel the rise in risk of CAD. In addition, low levels of HDL ("good" cholesterol) also increase the risk of CAD. This is true especially in women even when the LDL and total cholesterol are normal. Triglycerides and other lipids and lipoproteins may represent risk factors for CAD, but the area is controversial.

Efforts of the United States Public Health Service to lower national cholesterol levels have resulted in a decline in the cholesterol level since the 1980s. Currently, 49% of United States adults aged 20–74 have total cholesterol levels below 200 mg/dL. Thirty-one percent of United States adults have "mildly" elevated levels, 201–239 mg/dL, and 20% are elevated over 240 mg/dL.

Using the current treatment guidelines (see Treatment), approximately 29% of Americans qualify for diet therapy for hypercholesterolemia, and as many as 7% qualify for drug treatment.

SCREENING

Screening for high blood cholesterol for the primary prevention of CAD is recommended for some patients by the United States Preventive Services Task Force (USPSTF), although the recommendations have been somewhat controversial. Epidemiologic studies show that the higher the cholesterol the greater the risk of CAD, but some older treatment studies showed that even though treatment may reduce mortality from CAD, it does not change total mortality and may even increase total mortality. Those studies were done using diet and older drugs for the treatment of high blood cholesterol. Several more recent studies have shown that treating patients at moderate-to-high risk for CAD with hydroxymethylglutaryl coenzyme A (HMG-CoA) reductase inhibitors decreases both CAD and total mortality. The majority of patients in these recent studies were middle-aged men.

Evidence clearly shows that screening for and treating hypercholesterolemia in patients with known CAD reduces total mortality (secondary or tertiary prevention). All patients with cardiovascular disease should have a lipid evaluation.

In addition, in the more controversial area of primary prevention, the USPSTF currently recommends:

- Periodic screening for all men ages 35–65 and all women ages 45–65
- Screening for all older persons with major CAD risk factors (smoking, diabetes, family history of premature CAD, hypertension)
- Screening for asymptomatic persons ages 65–75 at the physician's discretion
- Periodic screening of adolescents and young adults with risk factors for CAD
- No routine screening for children

DIAGNOSIS

The total cholesterol level is an inexpensive blood test that can be performed on patients who are not fasting. The level can vary by about 10% in any individual and can vary more with stress, intercurrent illness, and weight change. HDL, also subject to some natural variability, can also be measured fasting or random. Triglycerides (TG) are very sensitive to recent meals and must be measured after an 8–12-hour fast. LDL is not directly measured in most laboratories; rather, it is calculated from the other values according to the following equation:

$$\text{Total cholesterol} = \text{LDL} + \text{HDL} + \text{TG}/5$$

Some experts recommend an initial screening total cholesterol, and then moving on to confirmatory fasting lipid analysis for patients with levels greater than 240 mg/dL. Others suggest starting with a total cholesterol and HDL (both performed randomly), using a confirmatory fasting panel if levels are abnormal. The latter strategy allows the identification of patients with normal total cholesterol levels but low HDL levels who might be at risk for CAD.

The USPSTF does not make a firm recommendation about what tests to use for screening; they do recommend basing treatment decisions on at least two measures plus an assessment of cardiac risk. A reasonable approach for those at low cardiac risk is to test for total cholesterol as an initial measure; for those at higher risk or with known cardiovascular disease, measuring total cholesterol and HDL is recommended as an initial screening.

The interval for testing has not been firmly established. Repeating the test every 5 years for those at low risk or with low values and repeating more frequently in those with borderline levels or those at risk of more rapid rise (middle age, perimenopausal, weight gain) is one common approach.

DIFFERENTIAL DIAGNOSIS

While most patients with high cholesterol levels will not have the problem as the result of another medical illness, there are several common diseases that can cause hypercholesterolemia. Uncontrolled diabetes can cause an elevation in total cholesterol and triglycerides, as can hypothyroidism and renal insufficiency. Nephrotic syndrome can cause an increase in total cholesterol, and alcohol use can increase triglycerides and HDL. If patients have moderately elevated cholesterol levels and symptoms or signs of any of these diseases, they should be evaluated. Patients with a moderate elevation but no symptoms do not need to have additional tests, but patients with a very high cholesterol (> 300 mg/dL) should be evaluated for these fairly common illnesses, even if asymptomatic.

TREATMENT

First, the physician must decide which patients should be treated for hypercholesterolemia. The benefits of dietary and drug therapy should be balanced against the risks of therapy. The goal should be to identify patients at the highest risk for CAD based on their cholesterol levels and their other cardiac risk factors. Those with the most potential benefit from drug therapy are middle-aged men and postmenopausal women with several risks; those with the least potential benefit are young women and men.

Current guidelines from the National Cholesterol Education Panel (NCEP) suggest adding up a patient's risk factors. Risk factors for this calculation include: age greater than 45 for men, age greater than 55 for women; diabetes; smoking; hypertension; HDL level less than 35 mg/dL; and family history of premature CAD. One risk may be subtracted if the patient has an HDL level greater than 60 mg/dL.

Below are the current threshold levels for instituting diet and drug therapy based on the number of risk factors. The LDL level at which diet therapy is begun is the same as the "goal" LDL level. Diet therapy is the first-line therapy for all patients in the setting of primary prevention and should be combined with exercise and, if appropriate, weight loss in an attempt to lower LDL and raise HDL. A step I diet requires that total fat be limited to 30% of total daily calories and that cholesterol intake be less than 300 mg/d. If the LDL level is still above the threshold level after several months of a step I diet, the patient should move on to a step II diet. This diet, which limits cholesterol to 200 mg/d and saturated fat to 7% of total calories a day, is difficult to adhere to and usually requires the assistance of a dietitian.

Dietary therapy for primary prevention should be tried for at least 6 months. (In patients with known CAD, the clinician may move on to drug therapy more rapidly.) If after 6 months the patient is above the threshold for drug therapy (see below), the patient should be started on a cholesterol-lowering drug. The threshold for drug therapy is higher than that for diet therapy. While the goal LDL level for patients with multiple cardiac risk factors is 130 mg/dL, the recommendation is that the patient not be subjected to the costs and side effects of a potentially lifelong drug unless the LDL level is significantly higher than the goal. (See table below for treatment thresholds, based on the patient's cardiac risks.)

TABLE 45-1
LDL TREATMENT THRESHOLDS: NCEP GUIDELINES

Patient	LDL Threshold Level (mg/dL)	
	Goal on Diet	Goal on Drug
Known CAD ,DM, PVD	100	130
≥ 2 risk factors	130	160
< 2 risk factors	160	190
< 2 risk factors, young	160	220

The drugs of first choice in most patients are the HMG-CoA reductase inhibitors or statins. These drugs inhibit the rate-limiting step of cholesterol synthesis and lower serum LDL levels by 20%–40%, depending on the drug and dose. They are the only class of drugs shown in randomized controlled trials to lower total mortality in the setting of primary prevention. They can be expensive, costing at least $60 a month and often more than $100 a month, depending on drug and dose.

The statins (lovastatin, fluvastatin, pravastatin, simvastatin, and atorvastatin) are well tolerated. They should be taken after dinner or at bedtime; the body manufactures cholesterol at night, and the drug will not work well if taken in the morning. An asymptomatic rise in liver function tests (LFTs) is reported in 1%–2% of patients, but symptomatic hepatitis is quite rare. Patients with baseline liver abnormalities should have baseline and occasional follow-up LFTs. Myositis is the most concerning potential adverse effect with muscle pain, weakness, and 10-fold elevations in serum creatine phosphokinase (CPK) concentration. Patients should be educated about the symptoms of myositis and should stop the medication and seek evaluation should weakness or muscle pain develop. Because the timing of the myositis is unpredictable and because the CPK rise does not occur significantly before the onset of symptoms, most physicians do not order routine CPK levels.

The first-choice drug for postmenopausal women may be hormone-replacement therapy (HRT). HRT lowers the LDL by 20%–25%, raises the HDL by 10%, and has other cardioprotective effects in addition to its lipid-lowering properties. In observational studies, it has been found to decrease the risk of CAD by 40%–50%. Side effects include vaginal bleeding, bloating, and breast tenderness. Questions remain about the potential for breast cancer. HRT with estrogen and progesterone costs about $40 a month.

Niacin is the least expensive drug for the treatment of hyperlipidemia at about $10 a month or less. Its mechanism of action is not well understood, but it significantly lowers LDL and raises HDL more than any other drug. Difficult to take because of side effects, it can cause itching and flushing, which can sometimes be aborted by pretreatment with aspirin.

Other classes of cholesterol-lowering drugs include bile acid-binding resins (cholestyramine and colestipol). They lower LDL levels by about 20% and should be second-line agents for patients who do not tolerate the other drugs or who need to have a second drug added. Gemfibrozil, a fibric acid derivative, is the first choice for patients with very high triglycerides (> 1000 mg/dL). Clofibrate, another fibric acid derivative, may increase the risk of gastrointestinal malignancy and should not be used routinely.

Hypercholesterolemia, once diagnosed, is usually a lifelong condition that requires continuous treatment unless the patient has a dramatic change in weight or life style.

SUGGESTED READING

Editor: Choice of lipid-lowering drugs. *The Medical Letter*. 38:67–70, 1996.

Expert Panel on Detection, Evaluation, and Treatment of High Blood Cholesterol in Adults: Summary of the Second Report of the National Cholesterol Education Panel on Detection, Evaluation, and Treatment of High Blood Cholesterol in Adults. *JAMA* 269:3015–3023, 1993.

Garber AM, Browner WS, Hulley SB: Cholesterol screening in asymptomatic adults, revisited. *Ann Intern Med* 124:518–531, 1996.

CHAPTER 46
Coronary Artery Disease

Mark D. Andrews, M.D.

PATIENT

M. Bolin, a 61-year-old man, is brought in for evaluation of intermittent substernal chest pain with radiation to his left shoulder. The pain has been noted for the past 6 months and is generally fairly sporadic in nature. Episodes are described as mild in intensity, pressure-like in quality, and often associated with physical activity such as walking up steps or an incline. One or two episodes are noted a week lasting 2–4 minutes and relieved by rest. He gives a history of smoking cigarettes, two packs per day for more than 40 years. He is overweight and currently taking hydrochlorothiazide 25 mg/d for control of mild essential hypertension. There is a strong family history of coronary artery disease (CAD) and myocardial infarction (MI) [one brother had a MI at age 48].

CLINICAL PRESENTATION

The primary symptoms of CAD are chest pain and arm pain (usually the left arm) associated with physical activity. The pain is described variably as a heaviness, pressure, or aching sensation but may also be depicted as burning in nature. Symptoms are usually mild, short in duration (lasting a few minutes), and relieved with rest, suggesting anginal ischemia. Angina is the pain syndrome that derives from myocardial stress related to oxygen demand that is outstripping its supply. When the pain is more intense; protracted for one-half hour or more; and associated with systemic symptoms such as nausea, shortness of breath, and diaphoresis; cardiac muscle damage (MI) is likely. The elderly and diabetic patients, for multiple reasons, may have a more atypical or asymptomatic presentation of CAD. Congestive heart failure (CHF) with symptoms of shortness of breath and wheezing with exertion also may be the initial presentation of CAD symptoms. Other provocateurs of anginal chest pain are anemia, a heavy meal, cold exposure, intense emotions, and sexual intercourse.

Recurrent exertional chest pain, arm pain, or both with the appropriate clinical risk factors are highly correlated with significant obstructive CAD. This has been traditionally approached with medical therapy to decrease myocardial oxygen demand, revascularization procedures (i.e., coronary artery bypass grafting [CABG], percutaneous transluminal coronary angioplasty [PTCA]), or both that improve blood flow beyond fixed obstructions. Recent data have suggested a more complex relationship between coronary lesions and clinical events. Thrombotic events may be more likely to occur at sites of less than critical hemodynamically significant lesions (less than 70% and often less than 50%). These types of lesions represent sites that would not be approached by invasive techniques such as CABG or PTCA. Thus, high-risk lesions may not be only those that contribute to symptoms or abnormalities on noninvasive testing but may include a large number of ulcerated, irregular, or complex plaques that are dynamic in terms of vessel function and are a potential for local thrombus formation.

EPIDEMIOLOGY

CAD is the major cause of death and disability in the United States with approximately 500,000 people dying each year of a MI or stroke and greater than 60 billion dollars in resources anticipated to be spent for patient care. Risk factors for CAD include the uncontrollable factors of advanced age, male sex, and genetic predisposition. Additional risk factors that are potentially modifiable include smoking, hypertension, hyperlipidemia, diabetes, obesity, left ventricular hypertrophy, the postmenopausal state, and sedentary life style.

> CAD is the major cause of death and disability in the United States.

SCREENING

Recently there has been increasing recognition of the value of screening. Currently, the United States Public Health Service (USPHS) recommends screening for several risk factors that significantly contribute to the development of CAD. These include blood pressure measurements and total blood cholesterol levels in the 25–64-year-old age group. In addition, the USPHS recommends counseling interventions for tobacco use cessation, limiting fat and cholesterol intake, and regular physical activity in the same age group.

> Screening for a healthy heart.

DIFFERENTIAL DIAGNOSIS

The key diagnoses to consider would encompass noncoronary sources of pain mimicking angina, and these might include the following causes.

- Noncoronary artery disorders (mitral valve prolapse, aortic stenosis, hypertensive cardiomyopathy)

- Pulmonary diseases (pulmonary embolism, pleurisy, pneumothorax, pneumonia)
- Gastrointestinal (GI) disorders (peptic ulcer disease, pancreatitis, esophageal spasm, gastroesophageal reflux, cholecystitis, cholelithiasis)
- Musculoskeletal conditions (costochondritis, chest wall trauma, cervical arthritis with radiculopathy, muscle strain)
- Acute aortic dissection
- Herpes zoster
- Anxiety and panic disorder

The history and physical examination findings often help differentiate GI disorders and pulmonary disease from a true cardiac source. The physical examination findings of reproducible chest wall tenderness or pain suggest musculoskeletal conditions mimicking angina. A radicular pattern of pain even prior to the appearance of the classic zoster eruption is often a clue to this cause of noncardiac chest pain. Acute aortic dissection chest pain may be associated with asymmetric femoral pulses.

DIAGNOSIS

The most essential diagnostic factor in assessment of chest pain remains a *detailed history*. A *physical examination* often plays a secondary role and in many patients is totally normal. Listening for heart murmurs may yield a clue to underlying valvular abnormalities as an etiology for atypical chest pain.

The electrocardiogram (ECG) may show evidence of old myocardial damage (Q waves), transient T-wave inversion, ST-segment depression, or elevation of ischemia, but some patients with CAD have a normal tracing. The chest x-ray, while low yield in the workup of chest pain, may show cardiomegaly or changes associated with CHF that may be seen in CAD with complications. An echocardiogram can find valvular abnormalities that cause chest pain as well as provide information in the form of the calculated ejection fraction, which correlates with left ventricular pump function. In addition, wall motion abnormalities can be identified, which can suggest the possibility of underlying CAD. The routine stress ECG remains an important tool in the diagnostic armamentarium of the physician in evaluating the etiology of chest pain. Even in the classical exertional angina presentation (such as the case at the beginning of the chapter), this test can provide valuable information to allow accurate risk stratification for further management and treatment decision-making. The patient with CAD who can achieve at least a 10 mets workload (equivalent of jogging at a 10 min/mile pace) during study performance has been shown to have as good an outcome with medical therapy as with more invasive strategies, such as CABG. Coronary angiography allows for more exact anatomic definition of obstructive atherosclerotic changes in the setting of patients with jeopardized myocardium (those with single or multivessel disease with persistent symptoms on medical therapy or those with noninvasive testing suggesting proximal left main CAD). These are patients who are actively being considered for CABG or angioplasty procedures.

Functional myocardial circulatory assessment can also be undertaken using two noninvasive imaging approaches, stress echocardiography or thallium stress testing. Both study techniques have augmented formats using dobutamine or dipyridamole, respectively, to allow test application with patients unable to exercise. These modalities allow application of stress testing to patients with baseline abnormal ECGs and other contraindications to routine stress testing. These approaches along with a new imaging agent cardiolyte increase slightly the overall sensitivity of stress electrocardiography for detecting CAD.

TREATMENT

The value of an aggressive approach to life-style changes and medical therapy for the management of stable CAD have been born out by several recent large randomized clinical trials. Aggressive risk factor modification and basic medical intervention have significantly extended overall survival, improved quality of life, decreased the need for interventional procedures (CABG, PTCA), and reduced the incidence of subsequent MIs.

Risk Reduction Strategies

- Smoking cessation (counseling, nicotine-replacement therapy, and more formalized programs)
- Lipid management (primary goal to achieve a LDL level less than 100 mg/dL, a HDL level, greater than 45 mg/dL, and a triglyceride level less than 200 mg/dL. Consider therapy with hydroxymethylglutaryl coenzyme A (HMG-CoA) reductase inhibitors, niacin, cholesterol-binding resins, or clofibrate, depending on the lipid pattern. Follow-up is recommended at 3–6-month intervals depending on the level of control and the need for medication adjustment. Fasting lipid values and liver function tests should be monitored. All patients should be on a healthy heart diet.
- Physical activity (minimal goal 30 minutes, 3–4 times a week of moderate intensity)
- Weight management (consider in patients greater than 120% in excess of ideal bodyweight)

- Antiplatelet agents (aspirin 80–325 mg/d to be considered in all patients)
- Angiotensin-converting enzyme (ACE) inhibitors (post-MI for 2–3 months; should be considered as long-term therapy in patients with ejection fractions less than or equal to 40%)
- Beta-blockers (post-MI, angina management, high blood pressure management, heart rhythm management)
- Nitrates (long-acting, particularly oral sustained-release preparations for managing angina)
- Estrogen (consider in all postmenopausal women)
- Blood pressure control (intensify if above interventions used in risk factor management are not adequate for control)

A treated patient with stable angina pectoris with markedly improved symptom control and a low-risk stress ECG result can safely proceed with comprehensive modifiable risk reduction strategies with close follow-up on a 1–3 month basis. Patients with intermediate stress ECG findings or less than adequate medical treatment response in terms of symptom control warrant either noninvasive imaging studies for assessment of residual ischemic burden (stress echocardiography, stress thallium studies) or coronary catheterization and assessment for invasive therapies (CABG, PTCA).

SUGGESTED READING

Ferre FF: *Practical Guide to the Care of the Medical Patient*, 3rd ed. St. Louis, MO: C. V. Mosby, pp 165–182.

Smith CS: The challenge of risk reduction therapy for cardiovascular disease. *AFP* 55(2):491–492, 1997.

U. S. Preventive Services Task Force: *Guide to Clinical Preventive Services: Report of the U.S. Preventive Services Task Force*, 2nd ed. Baltimore, MD: William & Wilkins, 1996.

CHAPTER 47
Atrial Fibrillation and Flutter

Victor Caraballo, M.D.

PATIENT

S. Robertson, a 52-year-old woman with a history of rheumatic heart disease, presents with chest palpitations and shortness of breath. The patient has a known enlarged heart secondary to rheumatic valvular disease.

CLINICAL PRESENTATION

Atrial fibrillation and atrial flutter are tachydysrhythmias caused by abnormal atrial activity. In atrial fibrillation the atrial tissues lose their normal synchronized sequence of depolarization. Instead, multiple foci depolarize and contract in a chaotic fashion. These depolarizations are transmitted to the atrioventricular (AV) node through which a variable number are transmitted to the ventricles. This variable transmission results in an irregularly irregular, often fast, ventricular rate. In atrial fibrillation, there is a loss of atrial kick, which normally contributes to ventricular filling. In atrial fibrillation, a rapid ventricular rate, the lack of atrial kick, or both can lead to decreased cardiac output and congestive heart failure (CHF). Atrial flutter is a result of an accelerated atrial rate, often between 250–350 beats/min. These rapid atrial depolarizations are also transmitted to the AV node where they are also partially blocked or dampened. This usually occurs in a ratio of a 2:1 or 4:1 block and results in a rapid, regular ventricular rate. Atrial fibrillation may occur in paroxysmal events or may persist as a chronic dysrhythmia. Atrial flutter most often occurs in paroxysmal episodes and either degenerates into atrial fibrillation or reverts to a sinus rhythm; it is basically an unstable rhythm. The clinical symptoms of atrial fibrillation and flutter are a result of the abnormal atrial activity and the rapid ventricular response. They are:

- Chest palpitations
- Chest pain, which is often secondary to rate-related ischemia
- Shortness of breath
- Hypotension
- Syncope or weakness secondary to hypotension caused by rapid ventricular rates
- Thromboembolic events, more common when atrial fibrillation has been present for longer than 3 days

Atrial fibrillation is a common cause of strokes or reversible ischemic neurologic syndrome.

EPIDEMIOLOGY

The prevalence of atrial fibrillation increases with age; from 2%–5% in patients older than 60 years of age have atrial fibrillation. The most common causes of atrial fibrillation include ischemic heart disease, valvular disease (especially secondary to rheumatic heart disease), hyperthyroidism, and hypertensive heart disease. Other causes of atrial fibrillation include pulmonary embolism, chronic obstructive pulmonary disease (COPD), pericarditis, sick sinus syndrome, pheochromocytoma, CHF, cardiac surgery, Wolff-Parkinson-White (WPW) syndrome, and ethanol abuse (otherwise known as the "holiday heart" syndrome).

Atrial flutter most often occurs in patients with heart disease and is most commonly seen in patients with ischemic heart disease or myocardial infarction (MI). Atrial flutter is also associated with CHF, pulmonary embolism, cardiac contusion, myocarditis, and rarely digoxin toxicity. Atrial flutter often degenerates into atrial fibrillation or reverts to a sinus rhythm.

DIAGNOSIS

Atrial fibrillation and atrial flutter are often identified by a 12-lead electrocardiogram (ECG). Atrial fibrillation is characterized on ECG by fibrillatory waves best seen in leads V_1–V_3 and the inferior leads II, III, and aVF. The ventricular response is irregular and rapid but can be in the normal range. The ventricular complex is normally narrow unless associated with bundle branch block or a bypass tract. Atrial flutter is characterized on ECG by a regular atrial rate between 250–350 beats/min; sawtooth flutter waves are most visible in leads II, III, aVF, and V_1; and AV block usually 2:1 or 4:1. Echocardiography may be used to evaluate left atrial size and detect valvular disease or mural thrombus. Other underlying etiologies can be pursued as appropriate (e.g., thyroid function tests).

TREATMENT

In the stable patient, the treatment of acute atrial fibrillation is directed at control of the ventricular rate. Calcium channel blockers (diltiazem or verapamil) or beta-adrenergic blockers (esmolol or propranolol) are useful for this purpose as both drugs slow conduction through the AV node. Digoxin may also be used to achieve rate control but may take several hours to become effective.

After rate control, chemical cardioversion can sometimes be achieved with the use of procainamide or quinidine. When drugs do not result in sinus rhythm, electrical cardioversion is usually attempted. If atrial fibrillation has been present for longer than 2–3-days duration, systemic anticoagulation for 1–3 weeks is indicated prior to cardioversion. Patients with atrial fibrillation, flutter, or both who are hypotensive, in CHF, or who are experiencing myocardial ischemia are considered unstable and should be treated with immediate electrical cardioversion. Electrical cardioversion is also an option when patients are refractory or unable to take standard medical therapy. For patients with chronic atrial fibrillation, long-term anticoagulation with warfarin should be considered; aspirin is a less effective alternative. Low-dose amiodarone is also increasingly used to prevent recurrence of atrial fibrillation.

Atrial flutter is treated very much the same as atrial fibrillation with low-energy cardioversion (25–50 joules) proving effective in over 90% of cases. Adenosine is sometimes used when the heart rate is too fast to determine whether the rhythm is atrial flutter or atrial fibrillation; when the rate slows, the characteristic flutter or fibrillation pattern may be seen. Pharmacologic control of the ventricular rate can be achieved with digoxin, diltiazem, verapamil, esmolol, and propranolol. After rate control, chemical cardioversion can be achieved with procainamide or quinidine. Esmolol and verapamil may convert atrial flutter to sinus rhythm in up to 60% and 30%, respectively, of all cases.

SUGGESTED READING

Anderson JL: Acute treatment of atrial fibrillation and flutter. *Am J Cardiol* 78(8A):17–21, 1996.

Camm AJ, Obel OA: Epidemiology and mechanism of atrial fibrillation and atrial flutter. *Am J Cardiol* 78(8A):3–11, 1996.

Golzari H, Cebul RD, Bahler RC: Atrial fibrillation: restoration and maintenance of sinus rhythm and indications for anticoagulation therapy. *Ann Intern Med* 125(4):311–323, 1996.

Viskin S, Barron HV, Heller K, et al: The treatment of atrial fibrillation: pharmacologic and nonpharmacologic strategies. *Curr Prob Cardiol* 22(2):37–108, 1997.

CHAPTER 48

Congestive Heart Failure

Robert K. Cato, M.D.

PATIENT

B. Barr, a 65-year-old electrician, has a 3-month history of feeling "tired all the time" and "short-winded," and he has noted some swelling in his feet. The symptoms have been worsening. He now has trouble climbing the one flight of stairs in his house. B. Barr states that he feels "like I'm drowning" when lying flat and must prop himself up with two pillows to fall asleep. Review of systems is positive for a mild dry cough and negative for chest pain or palpitations. He has a history of hypertension but stopped taking medicine 6 years ago because it made him impotent. Physical examination reveals an ill-appearing man with a blood pressure of 168/98 mm Hg, a pulse of 104 beats/min and regular, and a respiratory rate of 18 breaths/min. He has bibasilar crackles, a laterally displaced and diffuse point of maximal impulse, a positive third heart sound (S_3), and 1+ edema in the ankles.

CLINICAL PRESENTATION

Patients with congestive heart failure (CHF) can present to medical attention with acute onset of respiratory distress that requires urgent admission to the hospital. More often, they have a multitude of subacute or chronic complaints such as:

- Fatigue, weakness, lack of energy
- Dyspnea on exertion or wheezing
- Orthopnea, paroxysmal nocturnal dyspnea, or both
- Lower extremity edema
- Dry, nonproductive cough
- Nocturia
- Unexplained weight gain
- Decreased exercise tolerance

Patients may have all of these symptoms, though often only the less specific symptoms predominate. Physical examination findings may include tachypnea, tachycardia, lung crackles, a diffuse and displaced point of maximal impulse (PMI), S_3 heart sound, elevated jugular venous pressure, lower extremity edema, and a swollen, tender liver. New-onset wheezing in the elderly is often CHF. Chest x-ray may reveal cardiomegaly, small pleural effusions, or interstitial infiltrates. All or only a few of these objective findings may be present, and the absence of any does *not* exclude the diagnosis of CHF.

EPIDEMIOLOGY

CHF is usually a disease of the elderly, as many of the disease processes that cause CHF take years to affect the heart adversely. The most common causes are hypertension, coronary artery disease (CAD), myocardial infarction (MI), alcohol abuse, and valvular diseases. Many other disease states lead to CHF much less frequently, including severe hypothyroidism or hyperthyroidism, viral myocarditis, hemochromatosis, postpartum cardiomyopathy, congenital heart diseases, restrictive cardiomyopathy, pericardial diseases, cocaine abuse, street drug use, and chronic pulmonary diseases. Hyperthyroidism, thyrotoxicosis, beriberi (severe thiamine deficiency), and severe anemia are causes of "high-output" CHF.

PATHOPHYSIOLOGY

The underlying pathophysiology of CHF is complicated and varies depending on the underlying cause. However, elevated cardiac filling pressures are common to all forms of CHF, resulting in pulmonary vascular congestion, elevated systemic venous pressures, or both. This may be from failure of systolic function (with a resultant depressed stroke volume), failure of diastolic function (preventing the ventricle from properly relaxing and filling), or a combination of the two. Also, the failure of one ventricle may predominate with resultant symptoms of "right heart failure" (edema, congested liver, elevated jugular venous pressure) or "left heart failure" (pulmonary congestion, left ventricular S_3). For CHF in general, the heart is unable to maintain adequate nutrient delivery to body tissues, causing fatigue and decreased exercise tolerance. As a result of these changes, physiologic compensatory mechanisms are activated, such as increases in sympathetic nervous system output, antidiuretic hormone secretion, and the renin–angiotensin–aldosterone axis. These are initially useful, but over time become maladaptive and lead to many of the signs and symptoms of CHF, especially fluid retention and edema.

DIAGNOSIS

History and physical examination are usually enough to make the diagnosis of CHF, but further testing is required to investigate the underlying cause and nature of the disease. Chest x-ray can reveal cardiomegaly, vascular redistribution of pulmonary vessels, pulmonary edema, and pleural effusions, all of which may be confirmatory in the diagnosis of CHF. Chest x-ray may also appear normal. Rarely, findings on x-ray can give a hint as to the underlying cause of CHF, for example, certain congenital heart diseases. Echocardiography is the most used and usually the best test to investigate the cause of CHF. It allows assessment of many cardiac parameters such as systolic function, valvular abnormalities, diastolic function, chamber size, and pericardium. It is noninvasive and easily performed but can be expensive and in some people the study is limited secondary to body habitus (usually obesity). Radionuclide ventriculography uses intravenous radioactive markers, which can be counted over several cardiac cycles to give a numeric indication of ventricular performance. Unlike echocardiography, however, it does not visualize valvular lesions well and requires intravenous injections. Cardiac angiography is considered the gold standard to investigate CAD, which is an important cause of CHF. Cardiac angiography also can assess ventricular function and valvular lesions. It is highly invasive, however, and is used only when necessary. Other avenues of investigation may be needed to elicit the cause of cardiac dysfunction, such as thyroid function tests, stress testing, and cardiac biopsy.

TREATMENT

The first step in the treatment of CHF is to identify the underlying cause or causes, and treat any modifiable conditions. Aggressive control of hypertension is crucial to prevent further cardiac damage. Alcoholic cardiomyopathy may partially reverse with abstinence. Hypothyroidism, hyperthyroidism, beriberi, and severe anemia are all reversible, and cardiac function should return to normal after therapy. Underlying CAD must be identified and treated. Surgical repair of valvular lesions or congenital defects can improve cardiac function and eliminate CHF.

Once all reversible causes of CHF are addressed, treatment involves life-style changes and pharmacologic therapy.

Life-style Changes

- A no-added salt diet, which amounts to approximately 4 g of sodium daily, is a cornerstone in minimizing fluid retention symptoms. For more severe CHF patients, limiting sodium to 2–3 g daily can be very helpful but is difficult to achieve in most Americans accustomed to a high-sodium diet.
- Physician-supervised exercise programs, formal cardiac rehabilitation, or both can improve exercise capacity assuming there are no contraindications.
- Patient education is crucial. This includes understanding medications and understanding the importance of adhering to a healthy diet.

- Recording their weight changes daily or biweekly may help patients catch increases in body volume prior to pedal edema or pulmonary congestion.

Pharmacologic Therapy

Vasodilators are the most important pharmacologic intervention in patients with CHF resulting from systolic dysfunction. Multiple studies have shown decreased morbidity, decreased mortality, and better quality of life for patients on vasodilators (which decrease preload, afterload, or both). The most widely used and best studied are angiotensin-converting enzyme (ACE) inhibitors, which are well tolerated and can be given once or twice daily. If the patient does not tolerate ACE inhibitors, a combination of hydralazine and nitrates has been shown to be nearly as efficacious, though this often requires taking medication three to four times daily, thereby decreasing compliance. For patients that develop a cough with ACE inhibitors, which is the most common side effect and affects up to 10% of patients, early evidence suggests that a new class of drugs (angiotensin II receptor antagonists) are equal to ACE inhibitors in efficacy and convenience (once daily dose).

Diuretics (furosemide) are almost always used in the initial treatment of CHF to remove excess volume. Some patients require diuretics indefinitely. These drugs should be minimized for patient comfort and to avoid side effects, which include: polyuria, hypokalemia, excessive thirst, hyperglycemia, hyperuricemia, and prerenal azotemia. Diuretics are *not* proven to decrease morbidity and mortality and are used when other measures (dietary, vasodilators) do not maintain a euvolemic state. Careful follow-up of renal function and electrolytes is necessary for cardioprotection. Serum potassium levels should be maintained at a level of 4 mg/dL.

Digoxin has been used for decades in the management of CHF as a positive inotropic agent. Despite multiple studies, the data are inconclusive as to whether patients benefit from the use of digoxin. However, the drug is commonly used and seems to help some patients. It is used when patients are having symptoms despite maximal management with other medications and life-style interventions, and it can be helpful in controlling the ventricular rate in patients who have atrial fibrillation.

Avoidance of other drugs that are negative inotropic agents such as verapamil and beta-blockers is generally recommended. However, one of the physiologic manifestations of CHF is an overstimulated sympathetic nervous system, which can be cardiotoxic in the long term. Recent studies suggest that low doses of beta-blockers may be helpful in CHF, though further study is needed.

Patients who have purely diastolic dysfunction with intact left ventricular ejection fraction may have identical symptoms to other patients with CHF. They usually have left ventricular hypertrophy from hypertension or a restrictive cardiomyopathy. Beta-blockers and cardiac calcium channel antagonists (e.g., verapamil) may have a role in these patients, whereas digoxin has no role at all and may be deleterious.

Patients with severely depressed left ventricular function, areas of akinesis from previous infarcts, or both may benefit from chronic anticoagulation, as there is a significant risk of thromboembolic stroke from ventricular clots. Critical risk/benefit assessment is necessary, as long-term warfarin therapy is expensive, inconvenient, and carries significant risk of bleeding.

Patients with atrial fibrillation and CHF can benefit from reversion to normal sinus rhythm.

Many agents are being tried on an experimental basis, such as inotropic agents like milrinone, though the data have been disappointing to date. Further trials are ongoing. When all else fails patients may be considered for cardiac transplantation depending on their underlying health, age, and many other factors.

FOLLOW-UP AND PROGNOSIS

Patients with CHF need close follow-up. Careful attention must be paid to weight gain, and appropriate changes in management should be instituted promptly, prior to the onset of symptoms. Patients on diuretics must have their serum potassium levels and renal function closely monitored. Digoxin can reach toxic levels and cause fatal dysrhythmias in the setting of worsening renal failure and hypokalemia. If patients have an exacerbation of chronic CHF that was previously well controlled, a precipitating factor such as dietary indiscretion, infection (e.g., pneumonia), decreased oxygen saturation, arrhythmia, anemia, or MI must be sought. Prognosis in CHF is partly dependent on the underlying cause of CHF and co-morbid conditions. Patients who have treatable causes of CHF do much better. The patient's functional status correlates quite well with prognosis. Patients who are dyspneic with minimal exertion or at rest have mortality that approaches 50% at 1 year.

SUGGESTED READING

Cohn JN: The management of chronic heart failure. *N Engl J Med* 335:490–498, 1996.

Karon BL: Diagnosis and outpatient management of congestive heart failure. *Mayo Clinic Proceedings* 70(11):1080–1085, 1995.

Sorrentino MJ: Drug therapy for congestive heart failure. Appropriate choices can prolong life. *Postgrad Med* 101(1):83–94, 1997.

CHAPTER 49
Peripheral Vascular Disease

Victor Caraballo, M.D.

PATIENT

C. Jordan, a 68-year-old man, with a history of atrial fibrillation presents with acute severe left leg pain. On physical examination the left leg and foot are cool, pale, and mottled. Dorsalis pedis and posterior tibialis pulses are absent.

CLINICAL PRESENTATION

Peripheral vascular disease is a group of disorders that result in insufficient delivery of oxygenated arterial blood to tissues or poor drainage of venous blood. Peripheral arteriovascular disease occurs secondary to eight pathophysiologic mechanisms: atherosclerosis, embolism, thrombosis, inflammation, aneurysm, vasospasm, trauma, and arteriovenous fistulas. Of these, atherosclerosis and thrombosis are most common. *Claudication* is the most common symptom of peripheral arteriovascular disease and is defined as a crampy pain, ache, or numbness in the muscles. Claudication normally occurs with exercise and is relieved by rest. Tissue loss in the form of *ulcers* or *gangrene* is another common manifestation of peripheral vascular disease. Patients may experience swelling or discoloration. Ulcers occurring secondary to arterial insufficiency should be differentiated from venous stasis ulcers. Ninety percent of lower extremity ulcers are caused by venous stasis. These ulcers are moderate in size and occur proximal to or at the ankle. They have a weeping base, extensive granulation tissue, and are only mildly painful. They are associated with stasis dermatitis. *Arterial insufficiency ulcers* account for approximately 5% of ulcers and are small shallow ulcers that occur distal to the ankle, typically at the distal portions of the toes. They are small, shallow, dry, and extremely painful.

Patients with acute arterial occlusion usually present with one or more of the "five Ps," pain, pallor, paresthesia, pulselessness, and paralysis. Acute arterial occlusion is due to one of two mechanisms: embolism (50%) or in situ thrombus (50%). It may be difficult to differentiate in situ thrombus from embolism. If there is any doubt, angiography is indicated.

Atheroemboli are small emboli composed of cholesterol, calcium, and platelet aggregates, which break off from proximal atherosclerotic plaques and can cause transient ischemic attacks (TIAs) or "blue toe syndrome."

EPIDEMIOLOGY

Risk factors for atherosclerosis, the leading cause of peripheral arteriovascular disease include: smoking, hypertension, diabetes, family history, and hypercholesterolemia. The result of atherosclerosis is insufficient blood flow to the extremities, causing chronic arterial insufficiency. Patients with atherosclerosis are generally older than 40 years of age, while patients with autoimmune causes of vascular disease can present with symptoms at a younger age.

DIAGNOSIS

While arteriography and venography remain the gold standards, Doppler ultrasonography is the most popular modality in assessing vascular disease. It is a noninvasive test, which can evaluate the arterial and venous systems. Magnetic resonance imaging (MRI), angiography (MRA), and MRI venography (MRV) are highly sensitive and specific tests, which are also becoming options at tertiary care centers. Impedance plethysmography (IPG), another modality used for the diagnosis of deep venous thrombosis (DVT), is usually less sensitive and specific depending on the institution. Serum markers for autoimmune disease may be useful.

DIFFERENTIAL DIAGNOSIS

The various disorders that cause peripheral vascular disease are given in Table 49-1.

TABLE 49-1
DISORDERS CAUSING PERIPHERAL VASCULAR DISEASE

Symptoms	Signs	Diagnosis
Thigh, hip, buttock, or leg claudication; may progress to rest pain in severe cases	Diminished or absent pulses, loss of hair growth on dorsum of toes and feet, shiny skin, deformity of nails, and small painful ulcers	Chronic arterial insufficiency
Sudden onset of extremity pain; rare history of claudication; and history of atrial fibrillation, mitral valve disease, myocardial infarction, or congestive heart failure (all sources of cardiac thrombus)	Few findings of chronic arterial insufficiency, contralateral and proximal limb pulses normal, well-defined demarcation of limb ischemia, pallor progressing to cyanosis, tenderness progressing to numbness, and paresthesia and paralysis indicate late ischemia	Embolus

TABLE 49-1 (CONTINUED)

Symptoms	Signs	Diagnosis
Gradual onset of extremity pain, common history of claudication and chronic arterial insufficiency, and source of embolism less commonly present	Physical findings of chronic arterial insufficiency commonly present, contralateral and proximal pulses frequently diminished, and demarcation of limb ischemia is less well defined	Thrombosis
Foot or hand claudication and claudication in a *smoker* with no other risk factors for atherosclerosis	Foot pulses may be absent in spite of normal femoral and popliteal pulses; +/− ulcers and Raynaud-type triphasic color changes in 50% of patients	Buerger's disease (thromboangiitis obliterans)
Sudden onset of small painful area on foot, typically in the toe; patient has risk factors or presence of atherosclerosis	Blue tender area of involved toe; dorsalis pedis and posterior tibialis pulses intact	Blue toe syndrome
Triphasic color response to cold or emotional stress: fingers become white then blue then red; patients typically experience cold then painful fingers; tobacco can also be a trigger; female predominance; no underlying cause; and usually symmetric	Triphasic color response	Raynaud's disease
Triphasic color response; equal male-female incidence; secondary to underlying often autoimmune cause; more often asymmetric; and systemic symptoms of underlying disease	Ischemic ulcers more common	Raynaud's phenomenon
Fever, weight loss, weakness, malaise, joint pains, rash, abdominal pain, headache, numbness, and symptoms of end organ ischemia	Raised nonblanching purple red lesions (palpable purpura) and ischemic ulcers	Vasculitis

TABLE 49-1 (CONTINUED)

Symptoms	Signs	Diagnosis
May be congenital or acquired; symptoms depend on location and size but may include pain, edema, and ischemia	Palpable pulsatile mass, thrill, or bruit; peripheral edema; and stasis dermatitis	Arteriovenous fistula
Symptoms depend on size and location but may include pain and compression of surrounding structures; mural thrombi may form and embolize; and aneurysms may also leak or rupture	Pulsatile mass	Aneurysm

TREATMENT

The treatment of peripheral vascular disease varies with the underlying disorder. Patients with atherosclerosis are initially treated with modification of risk factors and antiplatelet drugs such as aspirin, ticlopidine, and dipyridamole. Eventually, surgical treatment may be required in the form of one of several bypass procedures. Thromboembolic disease is treated with heparin, warfarin, control of atrial fibrillation, or surgical embolectomy. Vascular disease as a result of autoimmune disease is treated as above and by optimizing the treatment of the underlying disorder.

SUGGESTED READING

Cooke E: Current thinking on peripheral vascular disease. *Practitioner* 239(1547):120–124, 1995.

Creager MA, Dzau VJ: Vascular diseases of the extremities. In *Harrison's Principles of Internal Medicine*, 13th ed. Edited by Braunwald E, et al. New York, NY: McGraw-Hill, 1994, pp 1135–1143.

Gerwertz BL, Graham A, Lawrence PF, et al: Diseases of the vascular system. In *Essentials of General Surgery*, 2nd ed. Edited by Lawrence PF, Bell RM, Dayton MT. Baltimore, MD: Williams & Wilkins, 1992, pp 328–347.

Green RM, Ouriel K: Peripheral arterial disease. In *Principles of Surgery*, 6th ed. Edited by Schwartz SI, Shires FC, Cowles HW. New York, NY: McGraw-Hill, 1994, pp 903–924.

Spittel JA Jr: Peripheral arterial disease. *Disease-A-Month* 40(12):641–700, 1994.

CHAPTER 50
Thrombophlebitis

Judith A. Fisher, M.D.

PATIENT

J. Peters, a 25-year-old woman recently discharged from the hospital after childbirth, reports a painful and swollen right lower leg. It is difficult for her to walk because of the pain in this leg. On examination, her physician finds a firm and swollen right calf. On measurement, the diameter of the calf is 2 in larger than that of her left calf. There is no redness or lymph node swelling to her right leg and groin. Palpation of the right calf and dorsiflexion of her right foot elicit the report of extreme pain. An ultrasound of her right leg shows a blockage of her deep calf and thigh venous system. The patient is diagnosed with deep venous thrombophlebitis (DVT).

> Thrombophlebitis is superficial or deep, proximal or distal, and associated with the upper or lower extremity. These distinctions are important when considering the possible morbidity, mortality, and treatment.

Thrombophlebitis is an inflammation of a vein with a blood clot at the site of the inflammation. Thrombophlebitis is classified as superficial or deep, proximal or distal. The morbidity, mortality, and treatment vary according to the classification of this disease.

CLINICAL PRESENTATION

Superficial thrombophlebitis is painful, easily treated with oral anti-inflammatory agents and heat, and generally without significant complications. Deep thrombophlebitis is often less painful but more worrisome as it can lead to pulmonary emboli. Thirty percent of individuals with proximal DVT of a lower extremity go on to have pulmonary emboli. Pulmonary emboli are a significant cause of morbidity and mortality. Pulmonary emboli are the number one cause of preventable in-hospital deaths. Some DVTs (usually those of the upper extremity or neck) are most often secondary to intravenous line placement and become a source of sepsis. The remainder of this chapter will primarily deal with DVT of the lower extremity.

While many patients with DVT have no signs or symptoms, the classic signs and symptoms of DVT are:

- Swelling
- Pain or tenderness
- Increased local temperature
- Dilatation of the superficial veins in the area
- Positive Homan's sign (pain with dorsiflexion of the foot on the affected side)
- Erythema

Only DVTs of the proximal lower extremity, abdomen, and pelvis are thought to cause pulmonary embolism.

ETIOLOGY

With present knowledge, it is felt that many individuals with a DVT have an underlying coagulation disorder:

> Eliciting a positive personal or family history is the most accurate and cost-effective way of screening for the potential of a DVT.

- Poor anticoagulation response to activated protein C
- Mutation in the protein C gene
- Protein S deficiency
- Antithrombin III deficiency
- Presence of lupus anticoagulant
- Increased anticardiolipin antibody
- Homocystinurea
- Excessive plasminogen activator inhibitor
- Increased prothrombin fragment F1.2

These individuals then acquire one or more of the following risk factors.

- Obesity
- Surgery
- Immobilization
- Trauma
- Birth control pill use
- Increased age
- Cancer (may be occult)
- Cerebrovascular accident
- Spinal cord injury
- Congestive heart failure
- Indwelling intravenous catheter

DIAGNOSIS

After a history and physical examination, compression ultrasonography and impedance plethysmography are currently the first and second tools for the diagnosis of DVT. Either of these tools coupled with a moderate-to-high clinical index of suspicion yields a greater than 90% sensitivity and specificity for a positive diagnosis of DVT.

TREATMENT

Many treatment protocols exist. Proximal DVTs of the lower extremity, abdomen, and pelvis are usually treated with unfractionated heparin by the intravenous or subcutaneous routes for 5 days followed by 3–6 months of warfarin therapy. Unfractionated heparin is given in the hospital while carefully monitoring the activated partial thromboplastin time (APTT) to levels between 1.5–2.5 times the control values. Reaching an APTT of greater than or equal to 1.5 within 24 hours of onset of treatment correlates with a smaller recurrence rate. Warfarin is given orally beginning on day 1 or 2 of treatment so that a therapeutic level of 2–3 times the international normalization ratio (INR) for the prothrombin time is reached by the end of day 5 of heparin. Warfarin given for less than 6 months is shown to have a higher recurrence rate for thrombophlebitis. In individuals with a recurrence of thrombophlebitis, warfarin is continued indefinitely. In Europe, a once daily dose of low–molecular-weight heparin (LMWH) has been used in place of the heparin–warfarin regimen that is typical in the United States. Preliminary studies done in the United States show that LMWH can safely treat patients for DVT at home. Despite the fact that LMWH is 10 times as expensive as the unfractionated heparin, LMWH protocols would save the cost of hospitalization and repeated blood tests as LMWH has a long half-life and achieves a consistent steady state rapidly and safely. Some areas in the United States have already changed to this regimen.

Distal DVTs of the lower extremity may be treated to prevent extension into the proximal area. If patients are at an increased risk for internal bleeding or have had recurrent thrombophlebitis despite adequate anticoagulation, a filter device can be inserted in the inferior vena cava to prevent pulmonary emboli.

PREVENTION

Prevention is crucial. Protocols exist in order to decrease the risk of DVT postoperatively and during periods of immobilization. If anticoagulation is contraindicated, alternating compression stockings help to increase venous flow and decrease the incidence of DVT in individuals at risk.

SUGGESTED READING

Dale J.: Deep vein thrombosis. In *The American Journal of Medicine: Continuing Education Series*. Belle Meade, NJ: Cahners Healthcare Communications, 1994, pp 2–27.

Ginsberg JS: Management of venous thromboembolism. *N Engl J Med* 335(24):1816–1828, 1996.

Hirsch J: The optimal duration of anticoagulant therapy for venous thrombosis. *N Engl J Med* 332:1710–1711, 1995.

Koopmen M, Prandoni P, Piovella F, et al.: Treatment of venous thrombosis with intravenous unfractionated heparin administered in the hospital as compared with subcutaneous low-molecular-weight heparin administered at home. *N Engl J Med* 334:682–687, 1996.

Levine M, Gent D, Hirsh J, et al.: Comparison of low–molecular-weight heparin administered primarily at home with unfractionated heparin administered in the hospital for proximal deep-vein thrombosis. *N Engl J Med* 334:676–681, 1996.

Schafer A: Low–molecular-weight heparin—an opportunity for home treatment of venous thrombosis. *N Engl J Med* 334:724–725, 1996.

Schulman S, Rhedin A-S, Lindmarker P, et al.: A comparison of six weeks with six months of oral anticoagulant therapy after a first episode of venous thromboembolism. *N Engl J Med* 332:1661–1665, 1995.

CHAPTER 51
Kidney Stones (Renal Calculi)

Kent K.W. Bream, M.D., and Judith A. Fisher, M.D.

PATIENT

F. Goldsmith, a 35-year-old man, calls his physician at night. He reports that for the last 6 hours he has been having excruciating, intermittent, right-sided back pain and abdominal pain. He reports that it is the worst pain he could imagine. The pain radiates into his groin. The patient has not been able to urinate, and his abdomen is "sticking out." He reports that he is sweating and unable to sit still. He also volunteers that he has had "stones" before and was given "Tylenol with something like oxycodeine in them." The patient tells the physician that he would prefer to get a refill of the pills over the phone, but he promises to strain his urine and bring anything he finds into the office in the morning.

CLINICAL PRESENTATION

Classically, kidney stones or renal calculi present with severe pain. Stones can, however, be asymptomatic and found as an incidental finding on an abdominal x-ray or in a urinalysis. The pain of kidney stones is often described as the worst pain ever felt by the patient. The pain may be located in the affected flank and intermittent in nature. Stone movement causes the pain (renal colic), which frequently radiates downward into the inguinal area and scrotum in men or the labia in women. The pain may be associated with nausea, vomiting, and hematuria. Renal calculi may also present with single or multiple episodes of gross hematuria, which may or may not be associated with pain.

Often the presenting symptom is determined by stone location. Typically, stones become lodged and cause obstruction in four places: the pelvis of the kidney, the ureteropelvic junction (where the ureters leave the kidney), where the ureters cross the iliac vessels, and at the ureterovesical zone (where the ureters enter the bladder wall). The disease involving kidney stones is referred to as nephrolithiasis, ureterolithiasis, or urolithiasis, depending on the location of the stone within the urinary tract. When stones are in the renal calyces, they are often asymptomatic; they may, however, cause hematuria, urinary tract infection, pyelonephritis, or flank pain. In the proximal ureter, classic renal colic predominates (intermittent, sharp pain with nausea and vomiting). In the distal ureter, stones cause pain radiating to the groin or symptoms of bladder irritability. Patients with kidney stones may present with a urinary tract infection, initial or recurrent.

On physical examination, patients with renal colic often writhe on the examination table, unlike patients without kidney stones, who tend to lie or sit very still. Patients with renal colic cannot find a position that relieves the pain. They are often diaphoretic, tachycardic, and tachypneic. Patients with renal colic may have hypertension resulting from either the pain or the obstructing stones. Patients may or may not have a fever. Fever can be caused by pain but may be a sign of infection or impending sepsis. Patients can have tenderness to palpation over their costovertebral angle, a distended abdomen secondary to a reflex ileus, and a distended bladder as a result of urinary retention or bladder outlet obstruction.

Finally, nephrolithiasis may present as an asymptomatic incidental finding on an x-ray, new onset hypertension, or azotemia. The calculus may be seen as either a space-occupying lesion (if the stone is radiolucent) or as a radiopaque object on x-ray. Azotemia is seen with nephrolithiasis secondary to obstruction and renal damage.

EPIDEMIOLOGY

There is an annual incidence of 0.2% for nephrolithiasis. The lifetime risk is approximately 5%–15%. The prognosis for recurrence depends on the stone type but, overall, is about 50%.

Typing a stone is important to understand the etiology and epidemiology as well as to define short- and long-term treatment. Type is defined by the chemical make-up of the stone. The four principal types of kidney stones are: calcium, struvite, uric acid, and cystine. While kidney stones are divided into these specific types, many stones are not purely one type but, when chemically analyzed, are made up of multiple matrices. A struvite stone, for example, may have a calcium component to it. In this chapter, each type is discussed separately.

Calcium stones are the most common. They represent approximately 80% of kidney stones and are radiopaque. There are two types of calcium stones: calcium oxalate, representing approximately 70% of kidney stones, and calcium phosphate, representing 10%. The ratio of male to female for this condition is three to one, and the ratio of white patients to black patients is four to one. Calcium stones are seen more frequently in people with a sedentary life style and individuals with low urine output. As a result of increased urine concentration, there is an increase in calcium stones in the summer months and in individuals who exercise excessively. While environment, diet, fluid intake, and fluid losses (sweating, vomiting, diarrhea) play a part in stone formation, there is also a genetic component for some calcium stone formers. Calcium stone formation is related to inherited diseases such as absorptive hypercalciuria, an autosomal dominant disease seen in some familial recurrent stone formers. Additionally, calcium stone formation can be related to sarcoidosis, Addison's disease, Paget's disease, hyperthyroidism, vitamin D intoxication, milk-alkali syndrome, myeloma, lymphoma, leukemia, renal tubular acidosis type I, hypomagnesemia, renal hypercalciuria, resorptive hypercalciuria, and hypocitruria.

Calcium also forms stones in the presence of high uric acid and cystine levels. Excessive levels of oxalate can cause the formation of calcium oxalate stones. Therefore, patients with hyperoxaluria as a result of excessive vitamin C intake, ethylene glycol ingestion, methoxyflurane anesthesia, inflammatory bowel disease, intestinal bypass surgery, or genetic predispositions are at increased risk for calcium stone formation.

The second most common type of stone is the *struvite stone*. These stones are also known as triple phosphate stones. Struvite stones occur exclusively in patients with renal infections. Most staghorn calculi are struvite stones (staghorn calculi are those calculi lodged in the renal pelvis). Struvite stones occur twice as often in women than in men. They represent approximately 10%–20% of kidney stones. Struvite stones may be associated with a superinfection by *Escherichia coli*.

Uric acid stones represent approximately 5%–10% of kidney stones. Uric acid stones are related to an increased concentration of uric acid in the urine as a result of hyperuricuria. There are four causes of hyperuricuria: (1) idiopathic; (2) hyperuricuria secondary to hyperuricemia, which in turn is secondary to gout, lymphoma, or chemotherapy; (3) hyperuricuria without uricemia (seen in patients on thiazides or salicylates); and (4) chronic dehydration, as seen in patients who have ileostomies or inflammatory bowel disease. Whatever the cause, patients with uric acid stones have an acid pH urine.

Cystine stones are seen least frequently. They make up approximately 1%–5% of kidney stones. Cystine stones form in patients who have an inborn error of metabolism, an autosomal recessive disorder with an early presentation.

DIFFERENTIAL DIAGNOSIS

The differential diagnosis of kidney stones varies with stone presentation. For patients who present acutely in pain, the differential includes abdominal and pelvic pathologies (see Chap. 5). If the presentation is that of hematuria, urinary tract infection and carcinoma must be considered (see Chap. 18). In patients with a distended abdomen caused by a reflex ileus, bowel obstruction is on the differential. For patients in whom a calcification is found incidentally on x-ray, gallstones, calcified lymph node, pelvic phlebolith, intrarenal vascular calcification, pancreatic calcification, foreign body, or calcified rib cartilage are all on the differential list. Finally patients who present with a radiolucent, space-occupying lesion on intravenous pyelogram (IVP) or plain x-ray may have a neoplasm, blood clot, fungus ball, or sloughed renal papillae. Additionally, it must be remembered that a patient with classic renal colic by history may be exhibiting drug-seeking behavior.

DIAGNOSIS

The approach to diagnosis is two pronged. Acutely, one must confirm the diagnosis of renal calculus. Secondarily, one must identify the stone type and pursue the appropriate workup for the underlying pathology.

While crystals on urinalysis or a vague opacity on abdominal x-ray suggest the presence of a renal calculus, these findings are not diagnostic. To diagnose a kidney stone definitively, the stone must be visualized by IVP, urogram, tomogram, ultrasound, or computed tomography (CT) [more specifically "spiral" CT] scan. There is some debate as to which of these modalities is more efficient and cost effective.

In the long run, stone identification is important. A recovered stone should be sent for chemical analysis. Grossly, calcium phosphate stones are classically bipyramidal; uric acid stones are needle-shaped; and cystine stones are flat hexagonal crystals. Further workup is based on stone composition.

The threshold for evaluation varies. Some physicians feel that the first stone should only be worked up in patients with a family history of kidney stones, 20–50-year-old men, children, black women, and patients with struvite stones. Otherwise, these physicians would only do a complete workup for recurrent stone formers. Many physicians work up all first kidney stones. A limited workup includes:

- Serum electrolytes (Table 51-1)
- Creatinine
- Calcium
- Phosphorus
- Uric acid
- Urinalysis
- Urine culture and sensitivities
- Sodium nitroprusside test for cysteine, pH, and volume
- Stone analysis

TABLE 51-1
ABNORMAL URINARY CHEMISTRIES

Presentation	Values
Hypercalciuria	> 200 mg urinary calcium/24 hr
Hyperuricuria	pH < 6 and urinary uric acid > 750 mg/24 hr
Hyperoxaluria	Oxalic acid > 45 mg/d
Hypocitruria[a]	< 320 mg/24 hr
Hypomagnesemia[a]	< 50 mg/24 hr

[a] Citrate and magnesium retard renal stone formation.

A full workup also includes:

- Serum magnesium
- Parathyroid hormone
  1,25 vitamin D
- Two 24-hour urines measuring volume, creatinine, sodium, calcium, magnesium, citrate, oxalate, phosphorus, and uric acid

Additionally, patients with calcium stones should undergo a calcium load test requiring a calcium-restricted diet followed by a measured calcium load and water intake with timed measures of urine calcium and creatinine.

TREATMENT

The first goal of treatment is pain control. Often narcotic analgesia is required. If the patient can tolerate oral therapy, acetaminophen with oxycodone is often effective. Nonsteroidal anti-inflammatory drugs (NSAIDs) can be tried. Stadol is highly effective. After pain control, hydration is important. Hydration can be done orally or intravenously if there is associated nausea and vomiting. Hydration helps push the stone through the ureters to assist in passage. Hydration also helps to prevent further stone formation by decreasing the concentration of the precipitating substances.

It is important to note that stones less than 5 mm in diameter usually pass without further intervention. Only 50% of stones 5–10 mm pass. Intervention is indicated for large stones, obstructing stones, stones causing intractable pain, and infected stones. Modalities for intervention include altering the pH of the urine, direct irrigation with stone dissolution, stone fragmentation with ultrasound, and manual stone removal.

After the acute presentation of the calculus, prevention becomes the goal of treatment. The first mode of prevention in all stones except struvite is to assure adequate urine flow. This prevents super-saturation of the urine. Patients should have a daily urine volume of 2–3 L; this requires drinking 4 L of water in a 24-hour period. It is important to maintain the dilute urine during sleep. Additional intake may be required in hot climates, in patients with chronic diarrhea or other gastrointestinal fluid loss, and in physically active patients.

Next, dietary changes are sometimes effective (Table 51-2). In the past hypercalciuria was treated with a calcium-restricted diet. Several recent studies suggest that a high-calcium diet leads to the formation of fewer calcium stones. It is important to note, however, that compliance with these dietary interventions is difficult.

TABLE 51-2
DIETARY MEASURES FOR THE TREATMENT OF URINARY STONE DISEASE

Abnormality	Change	Affected Foods
Hypercalciuria	Change in calcium intake	Dairy foods
Hypercalciuria	Decrease calcium absorption from intestines	Bran and fiber
Hypercalciuria	Decrease oxalate	Nuts, chocolate, tea, and green leafy vegetables
Hyperuricuria	Decrease purine	Red meats
Hyperoxaluria	Decrease oxalate	Nuts, chocolate, tea, and green leafy vegetables
Hypocitruria[a]	Decrease methionine	Meat, eggs, wheat, and peanuts

[a] Citrate retards renal stone formation.

Alkalinizing the urine with bicarbonate may be effective over the long term with cystine and uric acid stones. Citrate also alkalinizes the urine. As noted in Table 51-1, citrate inhibits stone formation. Dietary supplements of zinc and magnesium also inhibit stone formation. Allopurinol lowers uric acid production in patients forming uric acid stones. Sodium cellulose phosphate binds calcium and provides inhibitory phosphate. Magnesium must be supplemented, then, because the cellulose binds magnesium as well. Thiazide diuretics decrease calcium absorption. Pyridoxine (vitamin B_6) is effective in decreasing oxalate. Phosphate supplementation may help decrease calcium and oxalate. Penicillamine, alpha-mercaptopropionylglycine, and captopril bind cystine. These substances can be used with cystine stones. Captopril is often used in patients with cystine stones and hypertension.

Struvite stones require ablation, treatment with antibiotics (as they are associated with infection), and acidification of the urine. Acutely, direct stone lavage with citrate may be effective. If a struvite stone is completely removed, there is only a 10% recurrence. Patients who retain even small remnants of struvite stones experience an 85% recurrence rate. For this reason it is important to follow up with all patients with struvite stones at increasing intervals for 1 to 2 years. Long-term antibiotic prophylaxis and urease inhibition with acetohydroxamic acid can be helpful over the long term.

> Treatment is directed by stone type. The goal is prevention of stone formation to prevent kidney damage.

SUGGESTED READING

Begun FP, Foley WD, Peterson A, et al: Patient evaluation: laboratory and imaging studies. *Urol Clin North Am* 24:97–116, 1997.

LeRoy AJ: Diagnosis and treatment of nephrolithiasis: current perspectives. *AJR* 163:1309–1313, 1994.

Rutchik SD, Resnick MI: Cystine calculi: diagnosis and management. *Urol Clin North Am* 24:163–171, 1997.

Spirnak JP, Resnick MI: Urinary stones. In *Smith's General Urology*, 13th ed. Edited by Tanagho EA, McAninch JW. Norwalk, CT: Appleton and Lange, 1992, pp 271–291.

Trivedi BK: Nephrolithiasis. *Postgrad Med* 100:63–77, 1996.

Wang LP, Wong HY, Griffith DP: Treatment options in struvite stones. *Urol Clin North Am* 24:149–162, 1997.

CHAPTER 52
Cholelithiasis and Cholecystitis

Steven C. Larson, M.D.

PATIENT

P. Hill, an obese 40-year-old woman, presents to the office complaining of 2 hours of aching pressure localized to her right upper quadrant. The pain is worsened with deep inspiration and is associated with pain in her right shoulder. She denies fevers or chills but notes nausea and several episodes of emesis since the onset of pain. The patient has no medical history but on further questioning, relates a milder, similar episode several months earlier that resolved spontaneously. Her examination is unrevealing except for mild right upper quadrant tenderness on deep palpation with no peritoneal signs or fever.

CLINICAL PRESENTATION

Cholelithiasis refers to the presence of gallstones in the gallbladder. Approximately 10% of the United States population has gallstones, and many of these patients are asymptomatic. When symptoms develop, they are generally related to the development of inflammation from stones, obstruction of the cystic or common bile duct, or both. The inflammatory process is termed cholecystitis and presents in two varieties: acute and chronic. Acute and chronic cholecystitis share many of the same clinical features. Both present with the pain of biliary colic, which is a severe, steady ache or pressure localized to the epigastrum or right upper quadrant. It is often sudden in onset and reaches peak intensity early in its clinical course. The pain frequently radiates to the right scapula or shoulder and is worsened with deep inspiration. It is often associated with nausea and vomiting. It may be precipitated by a fatty or large meal following a fasting state. The pain of chronic cholecystitis persists for 1–4 hours before resolving spontaneously. Acute cholecystitis typically lasts more than 6 hours and is often associated with fevers, rigors, and active infection. On examination, mild right upper quadrant tenderness with an absence of peritoneal signs or fever suggests a diagnosis of chronic cholecystitis. The diagnosis of acute cholecystitis is suspected in the patient with fever, dehydration, hypoactive bowel sounds, and right upper quadrant pain that increases on deep inspiration and palpation (Murphy's sign). Elderly patients frequently have more subtle presentations.

EPIDEMIOLOGY

Cholelithiasis is more common in middle-aged, overweight, and fertile women but is present in both sexes and all adult ages. It has a familial tendency, can develop during pregnancy, and has been associated with certain drugs such as oral contraceptive agents.

DIFFERENTIAL DIAGNOSIS

The complaint of right upper quadrant pain presents the physician with a very broad differential diagnosis, which includes: hepatitis, cholangitis, pyelonephritis, right lower lobe pneumonia, myocardial infarction, pancreatitis, peptic ulcer disease, and appendicitis. A thorough history and physical examination should enable the physician to narrow the list to processes affecting the hepatobiliary system; however, further laboratory data and diagnostic tests are often needed to help delineate the exact pathologic process.

DIAGNOSIS

In acute cholecystitis, a leukocytosis of 10,000–15,000 with a left shift is not uncommon. The white blood count (WBC) is normal in chronic cholecystitis. Liver function tests in either case are usually unrevealing, although a mild elevation in serum aminotransferase, bilirubin, and alkaline phosphatase may be noted in acute cholecystitis. Serum amylase may be elevated, suggesting the diagnosis of gallstone pancreatitis. Plain films of the abdomen may reveal calcified stones but are not recommended given their low yield. Ultrasound is the test usually used to diagnose gallstones. Ultrasound is extremely accurate and, in addition to the presence of stones or sludge, may reveal a thickened gallbladder wall or pericholecystic fluid suggestive of cholecystitis. Nuclear medicine tests such as the iminodiacetic acid (IDA) scans remain the tests of choice for acute cholecystitis. Visualization of the hepatic and common ducts, coupled with the failure to visualize the gallbladder 1 hour after administration of radiolabeled IDA, indicates cystic duct obstruction.

TREATMENT

Cholelithiasis

The treatment of choice for symptomatic patients is surgical removal of the gallbladder, either by laparoscopy or open cholecystectomy. Treatment modalities using gallstone dissolution with ursodeoxycholic acid or lithotripsy are rarely used because of low effectiveness and high rates of recurrence. It should be noted that the risk of developing symptoms or complications in asymptomatic patients with cholelithiasis is very small. This has led to the general consensus that elective cholecystectomy is not recommended for asymptomatic patients. However, some physicians believe that patients with diabetes should have prophylactic cholecystectomy because they experience higher rates of complications from cholecystitis.

Cholecystitis

Patients presenting with acute cholecystitis require hydration, analgesia, observation, and often hospitalization. Emesis is managed with antiemetics and nasogastric suction. Pain is best controlled with meperidine, as morphine may increase spasm in the sphincter of Oddi. A single broad-spectrum antibiotic such as a second- or third-generation cephalosporin provides adequate coverage in uncomplicated cases. Debilitated patients, diabetics, or those patients with gram-negative sepsis require combination antibiotic treatment. Surgical intervention remains the mainstay of therapy in acute cholecystitis. If the patient remains febrile, leukocytosis increases, and abdominal findings worsen, emergent surgery is required to prevent gangrenous cholecystitis and perforation. In uncomplicated cases of acute cholecystitis, early surgery (within 24–72 hours) is indicated in individuals who fail to respond to medical management. Delayed surgical intervention is reserved for patients with underlying medical conditions that present unacceptable risk for early surgery.

SUGGESTED READING

Kadakia SC: Biliary tract emergencies: Acute cholecystitis, acute cholangitis, and acute pancreatitis. *Med Clin North Am* 77(5):1015–1036, 1993.

Mezey E, Bender J: Diseases of the biliary tract. In *Ambulatory Medicine*, 4th ed. Edited by Barker L, Burton J, Zieve P. Baltimore, MD: William & Wilkins, 1995, p 1331.

CHAPTER 53
Acute and Chronic Pancreatitis

Sarah A. Stahmer, M.D.

PATIENT

L. Hartmann, a 50-year-old man, presents complaining of severe abdominal pain, which is localized to his upper abdomen and radiates into his back. He has been unable to keep anything down for 24 hours. He notes that the pain is worse when lying down, and he is only comfortable when he is sitting with his knees drawn up to his chest. He is a chronic alcoholic and describes recent heavy alcohol ingestion. He is diagnosed with acute pancreatitis secondary to alcohol abuse.

> In the patient with severe abdominal or flank pain, vomiting, and an elevated serum amylase level—think pancreatitis, cholecystitis, or perforated peptic ulcer.

CLINICAL PRESENTATION

Pancreatitis is an inflammatory disease that is classified as acute or chronic pancreatitis. In acute pancreatitis, there is restoration of normal pancreatic function following resolution of clinical symptoms; in chronic pancreatitis, there is evidence of residual damage to the pancreas. The clinical presentation of acute pancreatitis is not subtle; patients usually complain of abdominal pain that is often severe and constant rather than intermittent or colicky. It is localized to the epigastrium and usually radiates to the back and flanks. As is often observed with inflammatory processes involving retroperitoneal structures, patients describe worsening pain when lying supine and relief when sitting in a flexed position with knees drawn to the chest. Nausea and vomiting, often severe, are usually present.

Patients may give a history of alcohol dependence, recent binging, or both. A history of elevated triglycerides, cholelithiasis, recent abdominal surgery, or trauma are all relevant clues to the diagnosis. Careful questioning may reveal recent infectious illnesses, specifically viral syndromes. In addition, the patient should be asked about recent medications; a number of commonly prescribed drugs can independently cause pancreatitis. Table 53-1 lists the possible causes of pancreatitis.

TABLE 53-1
CAUSES OF PANCREATITIS

Alcohol ingestion (acute and chronic)	Infectious
Cholelithiasis	Mumps, mononucleosis, viral
Postoperative endoscopic retrograde	hepatitis
cholangiopancreatography (ERCP)	Gram-negative sepsis
Metabolic	Other viral infections
Acute renal failure	(coxsackievirus, echovirus)
Hypertriglyceridemia	Ascariasis
Hypercalcemia	Mycoplasma
Trauma	Vascular
Drug associated	Polyarteritis nodosa
Azathioprine	Systemic lupus erythematosus
Sulfonamides	Atherosclerotic embolization
Thiazide diuretics	Pancreas divisum
Furosemide	Obstruction of the ampulla of Vater
Estrogens	
Tetracycline	
Valproic acid	

Patients with acute pancreatitis often are in distress due to pain, intractable vomiting, and dehydration. Vital signs may reveal tachycardia, varying degrees of hypotension, and low-grade fever. Jaundice is an infrequent but important clinical finding; when present, it suggests edema of the pancreatic head with obstruction of the intrapancreatic portion of the common bile duct. Patients may have bibasilar rales or dullness due to a pleural effusion, usually located on the left. Erythematous skin nodules resulting from subcutaneous fat necrosis are an infrequent finding. The most notable findings are moderate-to-severe epigastric tenderness with guarding. The physical findings are often less impressive than the patient's complaints suggest. Abdominal distention and diminution of bowel sounds are common.

ETIOLOGY

Pancreatitis is usually an adult disease. Gallstones and alcohol abuse account for most cases of acute pancreatitis. Less common causes include trauma, hypertriglyceridemia, infections, drug reactions, pancreas divisum, and sphincter of Oddi dysfunction. Ten percent of cases are idiopathic.

DIFFERENTIAL DIAGNOSIS

Other causes of acute abdominal pain need to be considered, particularly in the patient presenting with acute and severe symptoms. Diseases that would require acute surgical intervention need to be excluded early in the patient's evaluation. These include a perforated viscus, particularly peptic ulcer, cholecystitis, appendicitis, intestinal obstruction, and ischemic bowel. Nonsurgical disorders that can have similar presentations include renal colic, pelvic inflammatory disease, pyelonephritis, gastroenteritis (viral, bacterial), alcoholic ketoacidosis, pneumonia, and myocardial infarction.

DIAGNOSIS

The diagnosis of acute pancreatitis is made by demonstrating an elevation of serum amylase, lipase, or both in a patient presenting with typical clinical symptoms. Amylase is a sensitive but non-specific marker of pancreatic injury and can be elevated in patients with metabolic acidosis, acute bowel ischemia, or perforation. Serum lipase is another enzyme that is released in pancreatic injury, it is as sensitive a marker as amylase and persists in the serum longer than amylase. Serum lipase and trypsin are helpful in identifying those patients with nonpancreatic causes of hyperamylasemia. There is no correlation between the degree of amylase or lipase elevation and the severity of pancreatic injury. A number of pancreas-specific markers have been found to be valuable in distinguishing pancreatic sources of hyperamylasemia in addition to providing prognostic information. These include:

- **Isoamylase.** This is a very sensitive and specific marker for acute pancreatitis, especially when used in combination with phospholipase A_2.
- **Phospholipase A_2.** This is a very specific marker for acute pancreatitis. Markedly elevated levels are seen in patients who develop complications (sepsis, respiratory failure, shock).

C-reactive protein is an acute-phase protein. Higher levels are predictive of poor outcome in patients with acute pancreatitis.

Other laboratory findings that may occur in acute pancreatitis include:

- Leukocytosis
- Hyperglycemia
- Hypocalcemia
- Hyperbilirubinemia
- Hypertriglyceridemia
- Hypoxemia

Factors that predict poor outcome in patients with acute pancreatitis are:

On presentation:

- Age greater than 55 years
- Hypotension
- Abnormal pulmonary findings

- Abdominal mass
- Hemorrhagic peritoneal fluid
- Increased serum lactate dehydrogenase

- Leukocytosis
- Hyperglycemia

At 48 hours:

- Fall in hematocrit greater than 10% with hydration
- Need for massive volume resuscitation

- Hypocalcemia
- Hypoxemia
- Azotemia
- Hypoalbuminemia

While some patients require hospitalization for acute symptoms, those with a clear diagnosis of pancreatitis and mild symptoms may not require admission. Patients with any of the factors predicting a poor outcome should be hospitalized.

Imaging studies can exclude other diagnoses, identify precipitants (e.g., gallstones), and visualize the pancreas to determine the severity of injury (edema vs. necrosis or hemorrhage). A chest x-ray and obstruction series are useful initial studies to exclude a perforated viscus, bowel obstruction, and pneumonia. Ultrasonography and computed tomography (CT) are used most frequently in diagnosing pancreatitis. Ultrasonography is an excellent initial test to evaluate the gallbladder and biliary tree for gallstones (a potential cause of acute pancreatitis) or cholecystitis (an alternative diagnosis). CT is the single best test to screen for alternative diagnoses such as gallstones (which can be missed on initial ultrasound), tumor, or mesenteric ischemia, in addition to gauging disease severity and prognosis. A normal or mildly edematous pancreas generally carries an excellent prognosis with respect to symptom duration and risk of complications. A CT that reveals diffuse pancreatic inflammation extending into the peripancreatic fat or phlegmon suggests a more prolonged and complicated course.

TREATMENT

In most patients, the disease is self-limited and subsides spontaneously within 3–7 days. Indications for hospitalization include intractable pain or vomiting, dehydration, fever, or suspicion of an alternative diagnosis. For patients with mild disease as determined by less than three risk factors and imaging studies that are normal or consistent with mild inflammation, the treatment is:

- Analgesics for pain
- Intravenous fluids to maintain normal intravascular volume

- Nothing by mouth
- Consideration of nasogastric suction for patients with symptomatic ileus (vomiting, diminished bowel sounds)

For patients with moderate-to-severe disease as determined by three or more risk factors and a CT revealing extensive inflammation, phlegmon, or both, the treatment is the same as for mild disease with the following additions:

- Aggressive volume resuscitation with colloid and close monitoring of clients for hypovolemic shock as a result of third spacing
- Close monitoring for pulmonary insufficiency
- Careful screening for complications requiring surgical or radiographic intervention (phlegmon, impacted stone)
- Broad-spectrum antibiotics

Alternative therapies that may be useful adjuncts for selected patients are listed below.

- **ERCP.** This may reduce complications in patients with suspected gallstones.
- **Enzyme Inhibitors.** Aprotinin and gabexate may reduce complications of acute pancreatitis.
- **Cytokine Inhibitors.** Lexipafant is a potent receptor antagonist of platelet-activating factor (PAF) and in experimental trials has reduced the incidence of multiorgan failure in acute pancreatitis.

PATIENT

The patient described earlier now presents 1 year later complaining of diarrhea of several months duration. He is now abstaining from alcohol use and generally feels well except for frequent bowel movements that typically occur after eating. He has noted an approximate 10-lb weight loss but denies abdominal pain, vomiting, fevers, recent travel, or new medications. He has been tested for human immunodeficiency virus, and the results were negative.

CLINICAL PRESENTATION

The classic presentation of chronic pancreatitis is the triad of pancreatic calcification, steatorrhea, and diabetes mellitus. This triad reflects insufficiency of pancreatic exocrine and endocrine function. One-third of patients present with all three. Patients with chronic pancreatitis often complain of abdominal or epigastric

> Steatorrhea, pancreatic calcifications, and hyperglycemia in an alcoholic is likely to be chronic pancreatitis.

pain that is deep-seated, persistent, usually refractory to antacids, and frequently requiring analgesics for relief. Patients may note that the pain is worsened with meals (particularly fatty foods) and alcohol. Symptoms resulting from malabsorption, such as fatty stools (steatorrhea) and weight loss, are common.

Physical findings are usually unremarkable. Of note is the often observed discrepancy between the severity of complaints of abdominal pain (when present) and a relatively benign abdominal examination. Signs of vitamin deficiency such as easy bruising may be present. Stools are usually soft, brown, and often foul smelling. Complications of chronic pancreatitis are steatorrhea; vitamin B_{12} malabsorption; impaired glucose tolerance; pleural, pericardial, and peritoneal effusions with elevated amylase levels; subcutaneous fat necrosis; and bone pain resulting from intramedullary fat necrosis.

EPIDEMIOLOGY

The cause of chronic pancreatitis is frequently unknown. For those patients with an identifiable cause, the etiologies are similar to acute pancreatitis. In developed countries, 60%–70% of patients with chronic pancreatitis have a long history of heavy alcohol consumption. Chronic pancreatitis is seen most commonly in middle-aged male alcoholics (35–45 years of age). In underdeveloped areas, specifically Africa and Asia, chronic pancreatitis is a disease of young people and is thought to be due to either protein malnutrition or ingestion of potentially toxic substances such as cyanogens in the cassava root.

PROGNOSIS

Chronic pancreatic injury is not reversible and is characterized by progressive loss of pancreatic tissue and eventual loss of endocrine and exocrine function. The impact of alcohol cessation on the natural history of alcoholic pancreatitis is not clear. Some investigators believe that cessation halts progression, while others feel that once established, the disease progresses even without further exposure to alcohol. Chronic pancreatitis is associated with a mortality rate that approaches 50% within 20–25 years. Causes of death are variable and include malnutrition, liver failure, infection, and trauma. Most of these reflect the risks inherent to the life style of the chronic alcoholic, rather than the disease itself. Patients with chronic pancreatitis are also at increased risk of developing pancreatic cancer. Approximately 4% of patients go on to develop pancreatic cancer within 20 years of the diagnosis.

DIFFERENTIAL DIAGNOSIS

Alternative diagnoses include all other causes of chronic diarrhea, particularly malabsorptive syndromes, lactose intolerance, malignancy, parasites, and bacterial overgrowth. Other causes of chronic abdominal pain associated with changes in appetite or food intolerance include gastroesophageal reflux disease, hiatal hernia, dyspepsia, peptic ulcer disease, cholelithiasis, and malignancies (specifically those involving the stomach, pancreas, and liver). Pancreatic cancer is particularly difficult to diagnose, and ERCP with brush cytology may be helpful. Gastroparesis is a complication of diabetes that can cause similar symptoms, although pain is usually not as predominant a complaint as it is in chronic pancreatitis.

DIAGNOSIS
- Serum electrolytes, glucose, and hemoglobin A_{1c}
- Complete blood count (CBC), prothrombin time (PT), and partial thromboplastin time (PTT) may be abnormal resulting from vitamin B_{12} deficiency, vitamin K deficiency, or both.
- Liver function tests may be abnormal in the presence of alcoholic liver disease. When there is compression of the intrapancreatic portion of the bile duct, alkaline phosphatase and bilirubin may be elevated.
- Urine for glucose and ketones
- Sudan stain of stool for fat
- Stool for culture, parasites, and *Clostridium difficile* toxin if alternative diagnoses are suspected
- Abdominal radiographs reveal *pancreatic calcifications* in 30% of patients.
- Ultrasound may reveal pancreatic enlargement, ductal dilatation, or pseudocysts.
- CT scan diagnoses chronic pancreatitis with sensitivity of up to 90% and specificity of 85%.
- ERCP is the gold standard for diagnosing chronic pancreatitis and planning treatment.

The gold standard pancreatic function test involves collection of duodenal juice and measurement of its volume, collection of bicarbonate and protein concentrations after a meal, or administration of secretin (+/– cholecystokinin [CCK]). Simpler but somewhat less sensitive tests involve oral administration of pancreatic enzyme substrates and measurement of their products of digestion—the bentiromide and the pancreolauryl tests.

TREATMENT

Treatment is aimed at relieving pain and symptoms resulting from pancreatic exocrine and endocrine insufficiencies. Many patients require chronic analgesics for pain control. Issues pertaining to narcotic dependence and abuse often arise during the chronic management of these patients. Noninvasive approaches include abstinence from alcohol and other triggers, analgesics, and nerve blocks. Recent research efforts have focused on blocking pancreatic secretion via administration of exogenous enzymes such as trypsin, somatostatin, and CCK-receptor antagonists. The results of these trials on pain relief are confounded by a high-placebo response rate, but in certain patients (particularly young women), this may be an effective approach. Alternative treatments for patients with pain that is refractory to medical management are surgical procedures aimed at relieving pancreatic duct stricture. These procedures involve bypassing the primary pancreatic duct or removing a portion of the pancreas. Nonsurgical approaches include endoscopic placement of stents in the pancreatic duct. Preliminary reports suggest that this is a potentially useful approach to the treatment of chronic pancreatitis.

For mild symptoms of pancreatic exocrine insufficiency, a low-fat diet should be the initial approach. The treatment is to restore lipase activity through oral administration of a commercially prepared enzyme replacement. This is taken with or immediately after meals. Large amounts are usually required to control diarrhea. In vivo lipase activity is affected by gastric pH, so the addition of antacids or H_2 blockers can improve response to enzyme replacement. Periodic monitoring of fecal fat is recommended to assess treatment response.

Most patients with pancreatic endocrine insufficiency have impaired glucose tolerance, but diabetic ketoacidosis is rare. Dietary changes can achieve control for most patients.

SUGGESTED READING

Ranson JH: Diagnostic standards for acute pancreatitis. *World J Surg* 21(2):136–142, 1997.

Sidhu S, Tandon RK: Chronic pancreatitis: diagnosis and treatment. *Postgrad Med J* 72(848):327–333, 1996.

Skaife P, Kingsnorth AN: Acute pancreatitis: assessment and management. *Postgrad Med J* 72(847):277–283, 1996.

Steer ML, Waxman I, Freedman S: Medical progress: chronic pancreatitis. *N Engl J Med* 332(22):1482–1490, 1995.

Steinberg W, Tenner S: Acute pancreatitis. *N Engl J Med* 330(17): 1198–1210, 1994.

Stimac D, Rubinic M, Lenac T, et al: Biochemical parameters in the early differentiation of the etiology of acute pancreatitis. *Am J Gastroenterol* 91(11):2355–2359, 1996.

CHAPTER 54
Gastroesophageal Reflux Disease

- -

Robert K. Cato, M.D.

PATIENT

R. Jackson, a 39-year-old lawyer, has noted a "hot, burning feeling in her chest for several years, which shoots upwards," often occurring at night or after meals. She also reports a "sour taste" in her mouth at times. These symptoms are sometimes relieved with Rolaids, but they have been worsening over the past few months and now occur daily. She smokes cigarettes, drinks two glasses of wine with dinner nightly, and tends to eat large, heavy dinners. Examination is notable only for obesity.

CLINICAL PRESENTATION

Patients with gastroesophageal reflux disease (GERD) classically describe a retrosternal "burning" or "heat" sensation that radiates upwards, most often 1 hour after a meal or when supine. Patients also may mention a sour taste, bad breath, or the sensation of a "lump in the throat." Some note only a "dull ache" in the chest. Still others present to the physician with a complication of GERD, presumably after years of asymptomatic disease. Patients commonly have tried various antacid combinations with some success. Physical examination is usually unremarkable but may include mild epigastric tenderness.

EPIDEMIOLOGY

GERD is an extremely common problem, with up to one-third of people reporting symptoms of "heartburn" at least once monthly. It can affect adults at any age. Risk factors include obesity, pregnancy, cigarette smoking, and alcohol abuse.

DIFFERENTIAL DIAGNOSIS

GERD can usually be diagnosed by history alone, but as is true of many diseases, patients may present atypically. It may be difficult to distinguish between myocardial ischemic chest pain and GERD. For example, some patients

> Many patients with acute symptoms of GERD are admitted to the hospital emergently to exclude unstable angina and myocardial infarction. Similarly, some patients who describe "really bad heartburn" for a few hours actually have had a myocardial infarction (MI).

report chest pain or chest pressure that occurs at various times of the day and in various situations, without the classic postprandial or supine GERD description. In this situation further testing may be necessary to rule out the presence of potentially life-threatening coronary artery disease (CAD). Other esophageal disorders such as achalasia, esophageal spasm, esophageal infections, or cancers also can be confused with GERD.

PATHOPHYSIOLOGY

The pathophysiology of GERD involves a combination of decreased basal lower esophageal sphincter (LES) pressure, abnormal peristalsis, and inappropriate periodic relaxation of the LES. This allows acidic gastric contents to contact the esophageal mucosa, which is sensitive to low pH. GERD is more common in people who smoke tobacco and drink alcohol, both of which are known to decrease LES tone.

DIAGNOSIS

The clinical history is often enough to make a tentative diagnosis of GERD, and a therapeutic trial can be initiated. Definitive diagnostic testing is necessary only when the diagnosis is unclear, when symptoms fail to respond to therapy, or when complications of GERD (see below) are suspected. An upper gastrointestinal series, a barium swallow, or both can demonstrate reflux, but false-positive and false-negative results are common. Endoscopy does not demonstrate reflux per se but is the best approach to investigate possible complications of GERD. The most sensitive and specific test to diagnose GERD involves 24-hour esophageal pH monitoring, via a probe passed through the nose. This is uncomfortable, expensive, and only rarely necessary. It is most often used when there is significant concern for CAD, and with this test the physician can verify that a patient's symptoms coincide with acid reflux. Overall, a minority of patients with GERD require diagnostic testing.

TREATMENT

There are several facets to therapy.

- *Avoidance* of factors that alter LES pressure such as *tobacco, alcohol, chocolate, citrus, mints, caffeine*, and *high-fat foods*
- *Eating smaller meals* and *avoiding* eating within 2–3 hours of sleep
- *Weight loss*
- *Elevating* the head of the bed several inches for persistent nocturnal symptoms

- Over-the-counter *antacids* for occasional symptoms or regularly after meals
- *Prescribing* regular medication for persistent symptoms, either *histamine (H_2)-receptor antagonists* (e.g., ranitidine) or proton-pump inhibitors (e.g., omeprazole). *Proton-pump inhibitors* are more potent and increasingly are being used as first-line therapy.
- *Prokinetic agents* such as cisapride may be helpful in severe cases
- Surgical intervention (e.g., laparoscopic fundoplication) is reserved for severe, refractory cases

COMPLICATIONS AND PROGNOSIS

Many patients require lifelong therapy, though some patients will have complete resolution of their symptoms and can be weaned from medications. Chronic GERD can lead to reflux esophagitis, which is an inflammatory condition that leads to the production of columnar-lined epithelium of the esophagus (Barrett's esophagus). This metaplastic change greatly increases the risk for esophageal adenocarcinoma, and patients with Barrett's esophagus must undergo periodic endoscopic surveillance biopsies in an attempt to diagnose carcinoma at an early stage. Chronic GERD can also lead to esophageal strictures, which may require dilating procedures or surgery. Any patient with GERD who has new onset of dysphagia, odynophagia (painful swallowing), hoarseness, or lymphadenopathy should have prompt endoscopic evaluation to exclude the development of a cancer or stricture. Reactive airway disease (asthma, wheezing) is an increasingly recognized result of GERD, presumably related to small aspirations of gastric contents, alterations in parasympathetic cholinergic inputs to bronchial smooth muscle, or both.

SUGGESTED READING

Altorki NK, Skinner DB: Pathophysiology of gastroesophageal reflux. *Am J Med* 86:685, 1989.

Larsen, R: Gastroesophageal reflux disease. *Postgrad Med* 101(2): 181–187, 1997.

CHAPTER 55
Peptic Ulcer Disease

Robert K. Cato, M.D.

PATIENT

J. McCarthy, a 36-year-old man, complains of "stomach pains" for 2 months. The pain is intermittent throughout the day, especially a few hours after dinner, and it occasionally wakes him at 2–3 A.M. Food often relieves the pain. He takes antacids several times a week, which temporarily relieve the pain. He describes the pain as "burning, gnawing, and achy" and localizes it to the middle of his abdomen. He denies fatigue, weight loss, vomiting of blood, black stools, and rectal bleeding. Physical examination is entirely within normal limits and notable for the lack of tenderness on abdominal examination.

CLINICAL PRESENTATION

Peptic ulcer disease (PUD) refers to gastric or duodenal ulceration. Classically, duodenal ulceration is characterized by a dull, burning, epigastric pain, which is intermittent throughout the day, relieved by food and antacids, and most painful 2–3 hours postprandially, and which may awaken the patient from sleep. Gastric ulcers present with similar pain, though food may aggravate the symptoms. There is great overlap between the two, however, and one cannot definitively diagnose either solely on clinical grounds. Many patients are asymptomatic until they present with a complication, for example, weakness secondary to anemia from a chronically bleeding ulcer.

EPIDEMIOLOGY

PUD has a peak incidence between the ages of 40 and 60 but can occur at any age. Men slightly outnumber women. It is a very common disease, affecting 5%–10% of people at some point in their lifetime.

PROGNOSIS

Prognosis for patients with PUD is excellent. Acid-suppression therapy yields complete healing of the ulcer in most patients, and relapses are very uncommon if underlying risk factors (see below) are addressed. Complications such as gastrointestinal (GI) hemorrhage, perforation, and scarring with obstruction are uncommon in patients treated for PUD.

PATHOPHYSIOLOGY AND RISK FACTORS

Recent insights into the role of *H. pylori* in PUD has revolutionized the understanding of the mechanisms and treatment of ulcers. It is believed to be transmitted via fecal-oral routes, and in the Third World, infection rates are well over 50%. Infection also appears to be a risk factor for gastric lymphoma and carcinoma.

Nearly all duodenal ulcers, and over half of gastric ulcers, are associated with chronic gastric infection with the bacteria *Helicobacter pylori*. However, for unknown reasons only a minority of infected people ever develop PUD, and most remain asymptomatic. *Nonsteroidal anti-inflammatory drugs (NSAIDs)* are major risk factors for gastric ulcers (and to a lesser degree duodenal ulcers). They inhibit prostaglandin synthesis, thereby interfering with gastric mucosal defenses. Many patients on NSAIDs have asymptomatic gastric ulceration. *Tobacco use, alcohol, stress and anxiety, caffeine, genetics, glucocorticoid* use, and some *chronic illnesses* may also predispose a patient to PUD, though to much lesser degrees than *H. pylori* and NSAIDs. *Zollinger-Ellison syndrome*, a disease characterized by excess acid production secondary to hypergastrinemia from a gastrin-secreting tumor, is a rare cause of PUD.

DIFFERENTIAL DIAGNOSIS

In patients over 40 years old, new symptoms of PUD warrant investigation to exclude gastric carcinoma.

Many disease states can cause abdominal pain similar to PUD. Biliary colic, pancreatitis, irritable bowel syndrome, gastroesophageal reflux disease, angina, and liver disease can sometimes mimic PUD. Other gastric conditions such as gastritis and nonulcer dyspepsia are also on the list. The most important condition to consider is gastric carcinoma, which can ulcerate and cause symptoms identical to PUD.

DIAGNOSIS

A thorough history and physical examination (including testing for occult fecal blood) is necessary in all patients suspected of having PUD. In a young patient with straightforward symptoms, further diagnostic testing may not be necessary prior to initiating therapy. Testing for *H. pylori* infection should be considered, however, unless empiric antibacterial therapy is initiated. If there are any concerns about malignancy, diagnostic testing is required to exclude that possibility. Signs to look for are weight loss, early satiety, anemia, and lymphadenopathy. Double-contrast upper GI barium studies are noninvasive, well tolerated, relatively inexpensive, and sensitive in identifying PUD. However, if a gastric ulcer is identified, it is not possible to exclude cancer satisfactorily without further testing. Duodenal ulcers can almost always be considered benign. Endoscopy is slightly more sensitive than barium studies, and it allows biopsies to identify malignancy or the

> Several regimens exist that are effective in eradicating *H. pylori*, and they differ primarily in cost and side effect profile. Regimens include 1–3 antibiotics for 2–4 weeks, in addition to acid-suppression therapy.

presence of *H. pylori*. It is the procedure of choice in patients with complications such as acute GI bleeding. However, it is significantly more expensive and invasive. Testing for infection with *H. pylori* can be done in several ways. Gastric tissue obtained on biopsy from upper endoscopy can be tested for *H. pylori*, and this is considered by many to be the "gold standard" for diagnosis. The radioactive carbon-labeled urea breath test is also quite sensitive and specific, and it is noninvasive and safe. *H. pylori* antibody testing is quite sensitive and can be done in the office setting but cannot distinguish active versus prior infection.

TREATMENT

Once PUD is identified or highly suspected, acute treatment involves acid-suppression therapy. High doses of antacids (aluminum-, calcium-, or magnesium-based) are effective and quite inexpensive but are limited by GI side effects and compliance problems (therapy 4–6 times daily). H_2-receptor antagonists (cimetidine, ranitidine) are well tolerated, highly effective, and moderately priced. The most potent acid-suppression therapy is proton-pump inhibitors such as omeprazole. Proton-pump inhibitors are the most effective of all the therapies but are very

> Surgery, with gastric antrectomy, vagotomy, or both, once played a pivotal role in the treatment of PUD. Today, with the advent of *H. pylori* therapy and powerful antacids, it is rarely needed in uncomplicated disease.

expensive. Any of the above therapies promote complete ulcer healing in 4–12 weeks in most patients. However, recurrence rates are
over 50% if the underlying risk factors are not addressed. If at all
possible, NSAIDs, tobacco, and alcohol should be stopped. If *H.
pylori* is identified, antibacterial therapy will speed ulcer healing
and reduce recurrence rates to less than 5%. Along with acid-
suppression therapy, bismuth salicylate, tetracycline, amoxicillin,
metronidazole, and clarithromycin are some of the antibiotics used
in various combinations to eradicate *H. pylori*. Once antibacterial
therapy is complete and acid-suppressing therapy has been in place
for several weeks, all medications can be stopped. No follow-up
testing is needed unless symptoms recur.

SUGGESTED READING

Goodwin CS, Mendall MM, Northfield TC: *Helicobacter pylori* infection. *Lancet* 349:265–269, 1997.

Hebtscgek EM, Brabdstatter G, Dragosics B, et al: Effect of ranitidine and amoxicillin plus metronidazole on the eradication
of *Helicobacter pylori* and the recurrence of duodenal ulcer. *N Engl
J Med* 328:308, 1993.

Soll AH, Weinsten WM, Kurata J, et al: Nonsteroidal anti-inflammatory drugs and peptic ulcer disease. *Ann Intern Med* 114:307,
1991.

CHAPTER 56
Hepatitis

Marc W. McKenna, M.D.

PATIENT

S. Simpson, a 25-year-old woman, presents with fatigue, anorexia, and malaise for the past week. She is now reporting some nausea and vomiting and is quite concerned because she has started passing dark urine.

CLINICAL PRESENTATION

Hepatitis is an inflammatory process of the liver. The typical presentation of acute hepatitis is similar to a flu-like illness. Patients initially develop fatigue followed by anorexia, nausea, and vomiting. The patient can also experience fever, muscle aches, diarrhea, and arthralgias. On physical examination, the patient often has abdominal discomfort, especially in the right upper quadrant. These symptoms all constitute the preicteric phase and often precede the onset of jaundice by up to a week. The icteric phase, when present, is characterized by jaundice. This is commonly manifested in the patient by the conjunctiva and skin turning yellow and more dramatically by the onset of dark tea-colored urine. The latter is easily diagnosed by confirming the presence of bilirubin in the urine with a dipstick.

The severity of the illness can range from mild to fulminant. Mild cases can be subclinical. More severe cases can cause significant and prolonged morbidity and, in rare instances, hepatic necrosis and death.

ETIOLOGY

Viral Hepatitis

Viruses account for most cases of hepatitis. Hepatitis can be part of the systemic manifestation of some common viral infections including infectious mononucleosis and cytomegalovirus. The viruses that more specifically affect the liver are hepatitis A (HAV), hepatitis B (HBV), and hepatitis C (HCV). These are the most frequent causes of viral hepatitis, and they are all very contagious (Table 56-1).

> **Three Most Common Causes of Hepatitis**
> Viruses
> Drugs
> Alcohol

HAV is transmitted through the fecal-oral route and is highly

Table 56-1
Types of Hepatitis Virus

	Hepatitis A	Hepatitis B	Hepatitis C
Common route of transmission	Fecal-oral	Parenteral or sexual contact	Parenteral
Incubation period (days)	15–60	60–180	15–150
Severity of acute illness	Usually mild	More severe	Frequently subclinical
Long-term complications	Rare	Occasional	Frequent
Postexposure prophylaxis	Immune globulin	HBIG	Possibly immune globulin
Immunization	Yes	Yes	No
Marker of acute infection	HAV IgM	HBV surface antigen or core antibody	HCV antibody later in the course

Note. HBIG = hepatitis B immune globulin; IgM = immunoglobulin M.

contagious in areas of poor hygiene. It is commonly spread at day care centers and through contaminated food and water. Symptoms usually last 1–3 months. It is rarely fatal.

HBV is typically spread through percutaneous transmission of contaminated blood, intimate sexual contact, or vertical transmission from mother to infant. HBV can have associated serum sickness-type symptoms, and the transaminase elevation is usually higher than in HAV. The clinical course of HBV is usually 2–6 months, and there is a 1% mortality from acute fulminant hepatitis.

HCV infection is transmitted primarily through exposure to contaminated blood from blood transfusion or intravenous drug use. The initial clinical course is the mildest of the three and is often subclinical. Many patients never become clinically jaundiced.

Drugs

Many prescribed drugs can cause hepatitis. Physicians should warn patients about the typical signs and symptoms of hepatitis before prescribing these medications. Drugs that may cause hepatitis include: acetaminophen, nonsteroidal anti-inflammatory drugs (NSAIDs), phenytoin, niacin, sulfonamides, rifampin, nitrofurantoin, methyldopa, isoniazid, halothane, and antifungal agents. The inflammation can range from subclinical transaminase elevation to full-blown hepatitis. The condition is usually reversible with removal of the offending agent. It is important to note that an overdose of acetaminophen can cause acute liver necrosis, which requires immediate life-saving treatment.

Alcohol

While many toxins can cause hepatitis, the most common by far is alcohol. Alcoholic hepatitis can be caused by either prolonged use of alcohol or heavy intermittent use. The diagnosis is primarily made with a thorough medical history taken from the patient or family members. With good nutritional support and abstinence, alcoholic hepatitis is often reversible. Prolonged intake of alcohol can lead to cirrhosis and liver failure.

DIAGNOSIS

The diagnosis of hepatitis is typically made by the presence of elevated transaminases, alanine aminotransferase (ALT), and aspartate aminotransferase (AST). In viral hepatitis the rise can be 10–100 times normal. The total bilirubin can also rise 2–20 times normal,

> The most common cause of marked elevation of serum transaminases is viral hepatitis.

but it is not always a good marker for the severity of the illness. In alcoholic hepatitis there is a modest elevation of the transaminases of 3–5 times normal, and often the most sensitive marker of alcoholic liver disease is an elevated γ-glutamyltransferase (GGT). In all types of acute hepatitis, an elevation of the prothrombin time (PT) is a sign of serious liver damage and decreased hepatic function (Fig. 56-1).

Specific serum markers differentiate acute HAV, HBV, and HCV. Acute HAV is diagnosed by the presence of IgM antibodies to HAV. IgG antibodies to HAV are associated with previous infection.

Figure 56-1
Clinical Course of Acute Hepatitis B

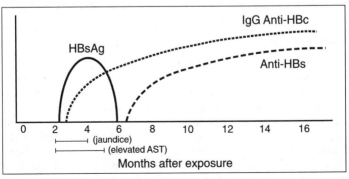

AST = aspartate aminotransferase; HBsAg = hepatitis B surface antigen; anti-HBc = hepatitis B core antibody; anti-HBs = hepatitis B surface antibody.

Acute HBV is diagnosed by the presence of hepatitis B surface antigen (HBsAg) or a positive hepatitis B core antibody (anti-HBc). The presence of antibody to HBV denotes previous infection and, as is in the case with IgG antibodies to HAV, represents immunity from future infection with that virus. Antibodies to HCV are present in acute and chronic HCV infection but may not turn positive until 4 months after the acute infection.

TREATMENT

Treatment for acute hepatitis is supportive. Rest and hydration are the mainstays. Occasionally, the patient needs to be admitted to the hospital for intravenous hydration. Otherwise, only the most severe cases require inpatient management. In the case of drug- or alcohol-related hepatitis, removal of the offending substance is essential. Periodic monitoring of liver function tests every 3–6 months after the acute infection is recommended to identify the development of chronic hepatitis. In 5%–10% of HBV cases, the surface antigen persists, indicating that the patient is still contagious and at high risk for developing chronic active hepatitis.

PROGNOSIS

Most cases of acute hepatitis are self-limited. Acute fulminant hepatitis, which can lead to liver failure and death, is rare, occurring in less than 1% of cases.

Chronic hepatitis occurs in 10% of those with HBV and in almost 50% of those with HCV. A small percentage of those with chronic HBV develop cirrhosis, while an estimated 20% of those with chronic HCV develop cirrhosis. Cirrhosis can lead to liver failure over a period of years. There is also an association between the HBV and HCV viruses and development of hepatocellular carcinoma. Chronic alcoholic hepatitis can also lead to cirrhosis and liver failure.

PREVENTION

Since the isolation and identification of HAV, HBV, and HCV, much progress has been made in the area of prevention. Hand washing and good hygiene are helpful. Public health policies have decreased the spread of HAV from food handlers and have been quick to identify day care centers and schools where an outbreak may have started. Passive immunization with immune globulin is recommended to all close household or intimate contacts of patients with HAV and to those who were exposed to contaminated food or water. Immune globulin can be given for immediate protection to those who are traveling to highly endemic areas. Travelers should receive the HAV vaccine before visiting areas of the world where HAV is endemic. The first in a series of two shots must be given 4 weeks before travel commences (Table 56-2).

Table 56-2
Recommended Groups for the Hepatitis Vaccines

Hepatitis A	Hepatitis B
International travelers to areas of high endemism	All newborn infants
Children in communities with high rates of HAV	All children 11–12 years of age who have not been vaccinated
Homosexual men	Adults with increased risk of HBV:
Intravenous drug users	Intravenous drug users
Patients with chronic liver disease	Those with multiple sexual partners
Individuals with occupational risks (e.g., exposure to nonhuman primates)	Sexual partner or household contact of HBsAg-positive people
Persons with clotting factor disorders	International travelers to areas of high endemism
	Individuals whose occupations expose them to blood or bodily fluids
	Residents or staff of institutionalized disabled persons
	Individuals with chronic renal failure
	Individuals with clotting factor disorders

Note. HBsAg = hepatitis B surface antigen.

Those exposed to HBV through sexual contact or exposure to contaminated blood should be treated with hepatitis B immune globulin (HBIG). Active immunization with HBV vaccine is now recommended for all newborn infants. A series of three shots is given

> Postexposure treatment is recommended and effective for HAV and HBV.

in the first 6 months of life. Those not immunized at birth should receive the HBV vaccine before the onset of puberty. It is also recommended that all adults at high risk for contracting HBV be vaccinated. All pregnant women should be screened for HBsAg during pregnancy because perinatal spread is common and administration of HBIG to the infant at birth can prevent the infant from developing chronic active hepatitis. Universal administration of HBV vaccine will go a long way not only to prevent acute HBV infections but also to prevent the sequelae of chronic infections, namely cirrhosis and hepatocellular carcinoma.

SUGGESTED READING

Lee WM: Medical progress: drug-induced hepatotoxicity. *N Engl J Med* 333:1118–1127, 1995.

Lemon SM, Thomas DL: Vaccines to prevent viral hepatitis. *N Engl J Med* 336:196–204, 1997.

Peter G: Hepatitis. In *1994 Red Book: Report of the Committee on Infectious Diseases* 23rd ed. Edited by Peter G. Elk Grove Village, IL: American Academy of Pediatrics, 1994, pp 221–238.

CHAPTER 57
Inflammatory Bowel Disease

Iris M. Reyes, M.D.

PATIENT

L. Peterson, a 20-year-old college student, complains of abdominal pain intermittently over several months, which is now severe and persistent for 2 days. The pain is generalized, crampy, and associated with anorexia and fatigue. He denies nausea and vomiting. He has had several bouts of bloody diarrhea today and has lost 10 lbs over the previous 6 weeks. His temperature is 100.6°F. He thinks that his grandfather had a "bowel condition."

CLINICAL PRESENTATION

Inflammatory bowel disease (IBD) is divided into two distinct conditions: Crohn's disease and ulcerative colitis. These conditions are characterized by chronic inflammation of a segment of bowel of unclear etiology and generally involve long periods of remission interspersed with episodes of acute inflammation. These conditions also have distinct differences.

Crohn's disease is segmental with normal areas interspersed between diseased bowel. All layers of the bowel wall are involved. It can involve any part of the gastrointestinal (GI) tract from mouth to anus. The terminal ileum is involved in most cases, but Crohn's disease may also be confined to the colon. Patients typically present with abdominal pain, anorexia, weight loss, and nonbloody diarrhea. The clinical course varies, however, with some patients developing only mild symptoms and others developing fistulas, abscesses, bowel obstruction, and perianal disease. Patients who have undergone recurrent bowel resections can develop short-bowel syndrome. Endoscopic and radiologic studies reveal a thickened bowel wall with stricture formation and deep ulcerations. Extra-intestinal manifestations of Crohn's disease include arthritis, uveitis, erythema nodosum, pyoderma gangrenosum, ankylosing spondylitis, cholangitis, hepatitis, and vasculitis.

Ulcerative colitis involves the rectum and colon only. The inflammation begins in the rectum, progresses proximally through the colon, and is localized to the mucosal layer of the bowel. Patients typically present with diarrhea and rectal bleeding. The severity of the disease is dependent on its anatomic distribution in the colon. Those patients with severe disease tend to have a higher incidence of extraintestinal manifestations, which are the same as those in Crohn's disease. Complications of ulcerative colitis include massive GI hemorrhage, bowel obstruction, toxic megacolon, and bowel perforation. There is a substantially increased risk for the development of colon cancer in patients with ulcerative colitis. Endoscopic and radiologic studies reveal a friable, edematous mucosa with bleeding and ulcerations.

EPIDEMIOLOGY

The peak incidence of IBD is in young adulthood with a second peak during middle age. The disease is more common in people of European descent and more common in people of Jewish ancestry. Patients often have a family member with the disease.

DIFFERENTIAL DIAGNOSIS

Diseases that should be considered in the differential diagnosis of IBD include infectious conditions caused by *Giardia, Cryptosporidium, Campylobacter, Shigella, Salmonella*, enterotoxigenic *Escherichia coli*, and *Yersinia* organisms. Diseases that may mimic colitis include gonorrhea, syphilis, and herpes. These can be diagnosed by appropriate cultures. Pseudomembranous colitis (often seen in patients after antibiotic therapy) and ischemic bowel disease should also be considered. Ischemic bowel disease usually presents in the elderly patient with risk factors for atherosclerosis.

DIAGNOSIS

Most patients with IBD present with nonspecific GI symptoms that have generally been present intermittently over months or years preceding the diagnosis. Laboratory tests are nonspecific for diagnosing the disease but can indicate the severity of the patient's presenting condition. For example, patients with Crohn's disease often are anemic and have an elevated sedimentation rate. Radiologic and endoscopic studies remain the mainstay of diagnosing IBD and its severity. An upper GI series with small-bowel followthrough, air-contrast barium enema, and colonoscopy with biopsy can provide a definitive diagnosis in Crohn's disease. Classic radiologic findings include fistulas, segmental narrowing, and an abnormal mucosal pattern.

In ulcerative colitis, presenting symptoms, signs, and laboratory findings may also be nonspecific. It is imperative to rule out parasitic and bacterial pathogens that may cause symptoms that mimic ulcerative colitis. Sigmoidoscopy and rectal biopsy can confirm the presence of disease. Colonoscopy reveals the extent of colon involvement and the severity of the disease.

TREATMENT

The goal of treatment of IBD is not only to treat active disease but also to maintain remission. Although Crohn's disease and ulcerative colitis are different diseases based on their natural history and pathologic findings, the medical therapy used to treat them is similar. The mainstay of therapy for IBD has been the 5-aminosalicylic acid (5-ASA) group of drugs. The original drug developed was sulfasalazine. Now 5-ASA, the active component of this drug, has been found to be effective with fewer side effects. The newer formulations release 5-ASA directly into the affected areas of the bowel. This drug is available in oral and topical preparations especially for ulcerative colitis and Crohn's disease.

Steroid use (systemic and topical) has been reserved for patients not responding to 5-ASA and for those with a severe flare. Because of the side effects, steroids are not routinely used for maintenance therapy.

Use of the antibiotics metronidazole and ciprofloxacin is increasing for IBD. These have been shown to be effective in patients who have Crohn's colitis with perianal disease and for the prevention of postoperative recurrences.

Azathioprine and 6-mercaptopurine are the immunosuppressive agents most commonly used in the treatment of IBD. More recently, cyclosporine and methotrexate have been used for refractory cases.

Surgical intervention in the management of Crohn's disease is not curative; it is used to treat complications such as bowel obstruction, intestinal perforation, abscess formation, hemorrhage, and fistula formation. Recurrence of disease postoperatively is common. Surgery in ulcerative colitis is curative and is generally required for hemorrhage, perforation, presence of colonic dysplasia, and toxic megacolon.

PROGNOSIS

While characterized by episodes of remissions, Crohn's disease is ultimately incurable. Ulcerative colitis can be cured by total colectomy and removal of rectal mucosa. There is an increased incidence of malignancy in patients with ulcerative colitis 10 years after the onset of colitis. Routine screening is essential.

SUGGESTED READING

Hanauer SB: Inflammatory bowel disease. *Drug Therapy* 334(13): 841–848, 1996.

Kornbluth A, Sachar DB: Ulcerative colitis practice guidelines in adults. *Am J Gastroenterol* 92(2):204–211, 1997.

Mascarenhas MR, Altschuler SM: Treatment of inflammatory bowel disease. *Pediatr Rev* 18(3):95–98, 1997.

CHAPTER 58
Irritable Bowel Syndrome

Marjorie A. Bowman, M.D., M.P.A.

PATIENT

E. Conway, a 19-year-old woman, complains of abdominal pain. She cannot easily describe its location. It happens most days and has been worse since she started college 3 months ago. She sometimes has nausea and vomits maybe once a month. She does not feel that she is constipated often, but her stools are often hard, and her bowel movement frequency is irregular. She has episodes where her stools will be loose for a day or two. The pain improves with passing gas or having a bowel movement. There has been no blood in the stool. Her weight is stable. Her examination is benign.

CLINICAL PRESENTATION

Irritable bowel syndrome (IBS) is considered a functional gastro-intestinal (GI) problem. The primary symptom of IBS is abdominal pain, which tends to be diffuse and often crampy. It is relieved by having a bowel movement or the passage of flatus. The pain does not occur while the patient is asleep. IBS is often accompanied by erratic stool patterns, classically alternating constipation and diarrhea, but many variations on this exist. The patient complains of visible abdominal swelling. Nausea and vomiting can occur but are not usually the presenting symptoms. IBS is a common cause of chronic pelvic pain in women.

> Irritable bowel syndrome presents as chronic, nonspecific abdominal pain.

There are thought to be psychological aspects to IBS, but the exact interaction is unclear. Flare-ups of symptoms often occur at times of stress. Patients with severe IBS often have concurrent psychiatric illness, such as panic disorder. IBS patients seem to have sensitive bowels—the same amount of pressure in the bowel that leads to pain in a person with IBS would not do so in someone without the syndrome.

EPIDEMIOLOGY

IBS usually starts in young adults but can start in childhood. It is common (perhaps 15%–20% of adults have it to some degree) and is the most common cause of chronic abdominal pain.

DIFFERENTIAL DIAGNOSIS

In young patients, the key alternate diagnosis to be considered is inflammatory bowel disease. Blood with the stool, anemia, fevers, weight loss, or nocturnal diarrhea are key symptoms that would suggest inflammatory bowel disease rather than IBS. Symptoms also may lead the physician to suspect other differential diagnoses, such as bowel cancer or gallbladder disease. Lactose intolerance, which leads to flatulence and diarrhea with the ingestion of milk products, is sometimes confused and can coexist with IBS.

DIAGNOSIS

There is no specific diagnostic test for IBS. Frequently, tests such as a complete blood count (CBC), erythrocyte sedimentation rate (ESR), and imaging studies of the bowel are done to exclude inflammatory bowel disease. Avoiding lactose for a couple of weeks or tests for lactose intolerance are often helpful. A dietary assessment may help elucidate exacerbating food substances, such as sorbitol or fructose. A patient over 50 years of age or who has a family history of colon cancer should be screened for colon cancer.

TREATMENT

Increasing fiber in the diet can help many individuals with IBS, loose stools, or constipation, but it may make other patients' cramping worse. As this is safe and generally healthy, it is reasonable to try fiber first, starting in low doses and gradually increasing. This can be accomplished through high-fiber foods or by adding psyllium. Patients with moderate or severe symptoms, however, will also often need medications at least intermittently. Medications should be symptom driven. The medications most frequently successful are anticholinergic agents and low-dose antidepressants. Of the antidepressants, the tricyclic antidepressants have been the most frequently used. Antianxiety agents are also sometimes helpful. Newer agents being used are the GI prokinetic agents (such as cisapride) particularly when constipation is a major symptom. Stress management may help with milder cases. If there are significant concurrent psychological problems, therapy, specific medication, or both can help. There are no specific follow-up studies needed, and the frequency of follow-up is dictated by patient circumstances.

PROGNOSIS

The pain tends to be chronic and intermittent. Some patients seem to adjust or have fewer symptoms over the years.

SUGGESTED READING

Bonis PAL, Norton RA: The challenge of irritable bowel syndrome. *Am Fam Phys* 53:1229–1236, 1996.

Dalton CB, Drossman DA: Diagnosis and treatment of irritable bowel syndrome. *Am Fam Phys* 55:875–880, 1997.

Lynn RB, Friedman LS: Irritable bowel syndrome. *N Engl J Med* 329:1940–1945, 1993.

Tolliver BA, Herrera JL, DiPalma JA: Evaluation of patients who meet clinical criteria for irritable bowel syndrome. *Am J Gastroenterol* 89:176–178, 1994.

CHAPTER 59
Lung Cancer

Jason D. Christie, M.D., and Lisa M. Bellini, M.D.

PATIENT

L. Michael, a 59-year-old man with a 100-pack-year history of tobacco use, presents with a 1-month history of cough productive of blood-tinged sputum. Over the past few months, he has noted worsening shortness of breath and a 10-lb weight loss. Physical examination reveals tachypnea, coarse breath sounds with a wheeze over his right middle lung field, and digital clubbing.

CLINICAL PRESENTATION

Lung cancer is divided into *small cell* (or oat cell) *carcinoma* and *non–small cell carcinoma* because of the differences in presentation and treatment. Non–small cell carcinomas (commonly referred to as bronchogenic tumors) include squamous cell carcinoma, large cell carcinoma, and adenocarcinomas. Clinically, they all behave similarly. Non–small cell carcinomas account for 75%–80% of all new lung cancers, while small cell tumors account for 20%–25%. The most common presenting symptoms of lung cancer are cough, dyspnea, hemoptysis, and chest pain. Symptoms and signs can result from systemic effects, local effects, intrathoracic metastases, extrathoracic metastases, and paraneoplastic syndromes.

Systemic symptoms include weight loss, anorexia, and fever. *Local symptoms* include cough, wheezing, stridor, dyspnea, hemoptysis, and recurrent pneumonia. *Intrathoracic metastases* can cause dysphagia, facial swelling from compression of the superior vena cava (SVC syndrome), shortness of breath from pleural or pericardial effusions, hoarseness from laryngeal nerve compression, and Horner's syndrome (sympathetic nerve paralysis with unilateral ptosis, miosis, and dry skin). *Extrathoracic metastases* can cause seizures as a result of brain involvement, pathologic fractures or bone pain, spinal cord compression, and jaundice resulting from extensive liver involvement. *Paraneoplastic syndromes* occur in approximately 10% of lung cancer patients. These syndromes are poorly understood but may result from ectopic hormone production by the tumor.

> The most common presenting symptoms of lung cancer are cough, dyspnea, hemoptysis, and chest pain.

The most clinically significant syndromes include: hypercalcemia, caused by the production of a parathyroid hormone-like substance; Cushing's syndrome from excess adrenocorticotropic hormone (ACTH) production; syndrome of inappropriate antidiuretic hormone (ADH) production; the Lambert-Eaton syndrome, caused by antibody-mediated failure of acetylcholine release from terminal axons; clubbing; and hypertrophic pulmonary osteoarthropathy.

EPIDEMIOLOGY

Lung cancer is the second most common type of cancer to affect men and women, and it is the leading cause of cancer-related death for both sexes. In 1995, 24% of all cancer deaths in women and 33% of all cancer deaths in men were due to lung cancer. There is an increasing rate of lung cancer among women over the age of 30 years, a disturbing trend that reflects new smoking patterns among women. Lung cancer typically presents between the ages of 35 and 54 years; peak cancer deaths are between the ages of 55 and 74 years.

In 1991, an estimated 90% of lung cancer deaths in the United States in men and 78% in women were attributed to smoking. Men and women who smoke have a 17.4% and 10.8% increased risk of lung cancer, respectively, when compared to nonsmokers. The relative risk of developing lung cancer increases with the number of cigarettes smoked a day, ranging from 5.5% for those who smoke one to ten cigarettes a day to greater than 20% for those who smoke one pack a day. Women are at higher risk for lung cancer at any level of smoking. Risk increases with duration of smoking, earlier age at onset of smoking, and smoking unfiltered or high-tar cigarettes.

Only 10% of smokers develop lung cancer, and 10% of lung cancers develop in persons who never smoked. This suggests that factors other than cigarette smoking are important for the development of lung cancer. These include age; preexisting lung disease; passive smoking; and occupational exposures to contaminants such as asbestos, radon, nickel, and chromates. Most occupational exposure risks are multiplied by smoking. Screening for lung cancer with chest radiographs and sputum cytology has not been shown to be cost-effective or to improve survival.

DIAGNOSIS

The above symptoms in the setting of risk factors for lung cancer require a chest radiograph. The chest radiograph has a 70%–89% sensitivity for detecting lung cancer. If a lesion is found, old radiographs should be obtained for comparison. Any abnormality that has been stable for a period of 2 years or has a benign pattern of calcification (central, ring, target, popcorn) represents benign disease. If the chest radiograph does not reveal any lesions but the symptoms are cause for concern, a chest computed tomography (CT) scan should be performed and referral to a pulmonologist for fiberoptic bronchoscopy should be considered to rule out endobronchial lesions.

Establishing a histologic diagnosis is critical because different types of lung cancer are treated differently. An important consideration in deciding where to biopsy is the ease in obtaining a specimen. Sputum cytology is the least invasive method with a 98% sensitivity for five early morning specimens. Easily accessible lymph nodes can be removed, and pleural effusions can be tapped for cytology. Other approaches include mediastinoscopy for bulky mediastinal adenopathy, CT-guided transthoracic needle aspiration for peripheral lesions, and fiberoptic bronchoscopy for central lesions.

Anatomic and Physiologic Staging

Once the diagnosis is established, anatomic and physiologic staging must be performed to determine the extent of tumor spread, to select appropriate treatment, and to estimate prognosis. Anatomic staging for non–small cell tumors is based on the TNM classification system reflecting the size, location, and extent of the primary tumor (T), nodal involvement (N), and presence or absence of distant metastasis (M). Increasing stage portends a poorer prognosis.

Anatomic staging typically includes a chest CT scan with extension through the liver and adrenal glands to evaluate the size and extent of the lesion, local invasion, presence or absence of lymphadenopathy, as well as liver or adrenal metastases. Anatomic staging also includes magnetic resonance imaging (MRI) of the head to rule out brain metastases and a bone scan to rule out bone metastases. Fiberoptic or rigid bronchoscopy may be performed to determine the distance of the lesion from the carina. Anatomic staging for small cell carcinoma also focuses on disease extent but broadly classifies it as limited stage (confined to one hemithorax) or extensive disease.

If surgery is indicated after this evaluation, physiologic staging is performed to assess operative risk and to determine whether postoperative reserve will be adequate to maintain ventilatory and gas exchange needs. Pulmonary function studies and arterial blood gas (ABG) analysis are the most common ways to assess if the patient can tolerate surgery. A forced expiratory volume in one second (FEV_1) is the most reliable predictor of postoperative functional status. If the FEV_1 is greater than 2 L, a pneumonectomy should be well tolerated. If the preoperative or predicted postoperative FEV_1

is less than 800 mL, surgery is contraindicated. If the patient's FEV_1 is borderline, a differential perfusion scan is performed to determine the percentage of blood flow to each lobe of the lung. The sum of the percentages of blood flow to each remaining lobe of the lung multiplied by the preoperative FEV_1 gives an estimate of the postoperative FEV_1. An ABG revealing hypercapnia is a relative contraindication to thoracotomy and is the most reliable predictor of postoperative complications. In addition, patients must have an adequate functional and nutritional status to withstand surgery.

> Once the diagnosis is established, anatomic and physiologic staging must be performed to determine optimal management.

TREATMENT

Treatment depends primarily on the stage and the type of tumor. Patients with stage I, II, and IIIa non-small cell carcinomas are treated with surgery if they can tolerate an operation. Stage IIIb and IV non-small cell carcinomas are treated with chemotherapy. The role of adjuvant chemotherapy for non-small cell carcinoma is being established. Small cell carcinomas are treated primarily with radiation and chemotherapy.

PROGNOSIS

In non-small cell carcinoma, prognosis depends mostly on the stage of the tumor and the patient's ability to tolerate surgery. Table 59-1 illustrates the 5-year survival rates in those patients with non-small cell carcinoma who are surgical candidates as well as the percentage of patients presenting at a given stage.

TABLE 59-1
5-YEAR SURVIVAL RATES FOR PATIENTS WITH NON-SMALL CELL CARCINOMA

Stage	Population at Presentation (%)	5-Year Survival Rate
I	20%–30%	65%–85% (operable)
II	5%–10%	40%–50% (operable)
III	20%–30%	20%–45% (operable)
IV	40%–50%	Mean survival < 1 year

Extensive disease is seen in 60%–70% of small cell cancer patients at presentation. The mean 1-year survival is less than 1 year. In the 30% of patients who present with limited disease, combination chemotherapy can lead to a 30% 5-year survival rate.

Palliative care is an important part of lung cancer treatment, as most patients die of the disease. Pain control, air hunger, psychosocial problems, nutrition, functional status, and other complications of metastatic disease are important issues in the quality of life of the dying patient. When a patient's life expectancy is less than 6 months, referral to a hospice organization may be appropriate. Smoking cessation can improve symptoms and should be strongly encouraged.

SUGGESTED READING

Kern JA, Clamon G: Lung cancer. In *Textbook of Internal Medicine.* Edited by Kelly WN. Philadelphia, PA: Lippincott-Raven, 1997, pp 2047–2057.

Simon H: Lung Cancer. In *Primary Care Medicine: Office Evaluation and Management of the Adult Patient.* Edited by Goroll A, May L, Mulley A. Philadelphia, PA: Lippincott-Raven, 1995, pp 294–299.

CHAPTER 60
Colon Cancer

Iris M. Reyes, M.D.

PATIENT

K. Lorence, a 73-year-old woman, complains of fatigue and a 20-lb weight loss over the previous 3 months. She has a decreased appetite. She has noticed that her stools have been loose and narrower than usual for 1 week. Occasionally she has noticed bloody streaks in the stool. She has had a dull pain in the right upper quadrant (RUQ) of her abdomen for several weeks. The examination is notable for a thin, wasted, elderly woman with fullness in the RUQ and grossly heme-positive stool. Her laboratory tests reveal a microcytic anemia.

CLINICAL PRESENTATION

The diagnosis of colon cancer must be considered in patients presenting with a change in bowel habits, rectal bleeding, iron deficiency anemia, and unexplained abdominal pain. Each of these findings can be explained by other diseases, but colon cancer should be suspected especially in at-risk patients. Patients at increased risk for colon cancer are those with a family history, a prior removal of a malignant lesion in the colon, a history of gynecologic malignancy, a history of ulcerative colitis or familial polyposis, and those who are older than 40 years of age. It is not uncommon for patients to present with symptoms related to metastasis of the tumor. The liver is a common site of metastasis in patients presenting with RUQ pain, but metastases to the lung and bone are also frequent. Local invasion may cause urinary symptoms, bowel obstruction, or periodic release of gas from the vagina.

EPIDEMIOLOGY

The prevalence of colorectal cancer is higher in developed countries than in undeveloped countries. It is a leading cause of death by cancer in the United States. Migrants from low- to high-risk areas assume the higher risk of colon cancer. It is likely that environmental factors, particularly dietary fiber and fat content, play a role in the development of this disease. Also, research suggests that genetic make up can predict a poor prognosis in a subgroup of patients.

DIFFERENTIAL DIAGNOSIS

Rectal bleeding is common in non-neoplastic conditions such as diverticular disease, angiodysplasia of the colon, ischemic colitis, benign tumors (polyps), rectal hemorrhoids, and anal fissures. Changes in stool caliber can also be found in diverticular disease and benign tumors.

DIAGNOSIS

A thorough history and physical examination are essential in generating a suspicion of colon cancer. The history should include a search for markers that may indicate a patient at risk (i.e., family history of colon cancer). The physical examination may reveal findings consistent with familial colon cancer syndromes such as Gardner's and Peutz-Jeghers syndrome. It may also reveal evidence of metastatic disease. The digital rectal examination is used to detect low-lying tumors. Testing for fecal occult blood is a screening technique for detecting colon cancer. However, it has a high false-positive rate in asymptomatic patients and is an inadequate test for a symptomatic patient. Those patients with suspicious signs or symptoms of colon cancer should have a colonoscopy, a double-contrast barium enema, or both.

TREATMENT

Surgical removal as a cure is generally attempted if signs of limited local disease are found. Most patient series have indicated that approximately one-half of patients treated with potentially curative surgical intervention eventually develop and die from recurrent disease. Patients with metastatic disease may require surgery if hemorrhage, perforation, or obstruction develops. Adjuvant chemotherapy has been effective for patients with either Dukes' B or C colon cancer. Fluorouracil is the most effective chemotherapeutic agent for colorectal cancer; it is incorporated into the cancer cell's DNA and RNA. Adjuvant chemotherapy consists of treatment with fluorouracil with either calcium folinate or levamisole for variable periods of time depending on staging of the malignancy. Radiation therapy has been used in both the preoperative and postoperative setting to reduce local recurrence of colorectal cancer. Evidence suggests that radiation therapy combined with chemotherapy significantly improves survivability, particularly in patients with primary resectable rectal cancer.

PROGNOSIS

There is adequate evidence that early detection can prevent and cure colon cancer. However, in those with advanced disease, survival depends on the stage of the disease. The best prognosis is found in cancer confined to the mucosa. Prognosis is poorer in patients with cancer involving all the layers of the bowel wall and lymph nodes.

PREVENTION

Several factors have been linked with increased risk for development of colorectal cancer. These include dietary factors, familial predisposition, inheritable syndromes (e.g., Gardner's, familial adenomatous polyposis), and inflammatory bowel disease, particularly ulcerative colitis. It is clear that the Western diet—high in saturated fat and animal protein and low in fiber, fruit, and vegetables—is associated with increased risk. The exact mechanism by which this occurs is as yet unclear.

Prevention can be divided into primary and secondary prevention. In primary prevention, an adjustment in the diet may, theoretically, reduce the risk for development of colorectal cancer. Secondary prevention involves screening to detect premalignant lesions or malignancy in its earliest and most curative stages. The *United States Preventive Services Task Force*, 2nd ed., currently recommends screening for all persons aged 50 and older by annual fecal occult blood testing, sigmoidoscopy, or both. Data are insufficient to determine which strategy is best, and neither test is ideal; however, recent studies indicate that their use is associated with lower colon cancer mortality. Screening provides detection for removal of premalignant adenomas, thus reducing the development of colon cancers and deaths from colorectal cancer. The use of molecular genetics techniques may help reduce the incidence of colon cancer by identifying individuals at risk and targeting appropriate screening techniques.

SUGGESTED READING

Burt WB: Familial risk and colorectal cancer. *Gastroenterol Clin North Am* 25(4):793–803, 1996.

Labianca R, Pessi MA, Zamparelli G: Drug treatment of colorectal cancer. *Drugs* 53(4):593–607, 1997.

United States Preventive Task Force: *Guide to Clinical Preventive Services*, 2nd ed. Baltimore, MD: Williams & Wilkins, 1996.

Wilmink AB: Overview of the epidemiology of colorectal cancer. *Dis Colon Rectum* 40(4):483–493, 1997.

CHAPTER 61
Breast Cancer

Mark P. Knudson, M.D., M.S.P.H.

PATIENT

K. Sharp, a 42-year-old woman, presents with a palpable breast mass noted on self-examination that has persisted through two menstrual cycles. The patient denies pain, nipple discharge, or skin changes. Her history is unremarkable except for a history of breast cancer in her mother, who was diagnosed at age 56. Physical examination by the physician reveals a single, firm, irregular 1.5-cm mass in the upper outer quadrant of the left breast.

> **Key Symptoms**
> Breast mass
> Pain
> Nipple discharge
> Skin changes

CLINICAL PRESENTATION

The most common presentation of breast cancer is a female patient with a "breast lump." A palpable mass, found either by the patient or the physician, accounts for 80% of detected breast cancers. Only 10% of these breast masses are painful. Approximately 20% of breast cancers are detected by a routine screening mammography. Pain without a detectable mass, nipple discharge, skin changes in the breast, or signs of distant spread are all possible but rare presentations of breast cancer, and reflect a small proportion of all diagnosed breast cancers. With the exception of age, most breast cancers occur in women without risk factors. Likewise, only 5% of breast cancers in women are related to one of the known breast cancer genes (BRCA1, BRCA2).

The diagnosis of breast cancer is important in primary care because of the frequency of the complaint of breast mass, the high level of "breast cancer fear" that exists among women today, the relative frequency of breast cancer in the United States, and the significant morbidity and mortality caused by breast cancer.

EPIDEMIOLOGY

Breast cancer is the most common solid cancer diagnosed in women, representing 25% of all cancers in women. It is a common cause of death from cancer among women in the United States, second only to lung cancer. Since the 1940s, the incidence of breast cancer has been increasing. The incidence of breast cancer increases with age with less than 2% occurring under the age of 30 and 80% occurring after the age of 40. A lifetime incidence of breast cancer is 10%–12% with a 3.6% lifetime incidence of death from breast cancer.

Risk factors for breast cancer include: early menarche; late menopause; nulliparous or late first pregnancy; and significant exposure to radiation, estrogen, or alcohol. The risk increases with age with roughly twice the risk for breast cancer attributed to each 15 years of advanced age. Genetics plays a significant role with almost twice the risk for breast cancer if the patient's mother or sister has breast cancer. Premenopausal or bilateral breast cancer in a family member conveys greater risk. High-fat diet, oral contraceptive use, and tobacco use are less well-proven risk factors for breast cancer.

> **Genetics and prolonged, uninterrupted exposure to estrogen at a young age contribute to the risk of developing breast cancer.**

DIFFERENTIAL DIAGNOSIS

Most palpable masses, especially in younger women, represent normal breast tissue (Table 61-1). In response to hormonal stimulation, thickening, cords, and cysts can form. At the extreme is fibrocystic breast disease, which is characterized by recurrent tender and worrisome masses caused by hormonal proliferation of breast elements. Benign cysts of the breast are common and also present as masses. Mastitis can cause a mass and is associated with redness and tenderness especially in the postpartum period. A swollen axillary lymph node (common with many viral and bacterial infections) may present as a mass in the breast. Infiltrating ductal

TABLE 61-1
DIFFERENTIAL DIAGNOSIS OF A BREAST MASS

Diagnosis	Signs and Symptoms
Normal breast tissue	Irregular fullness felt prior to menses
Lymph node	In or near axilla and associated with infections
Fibrocystic breast	Mix of cystic and noncystic masses with tenderness and increased size prior to menses
Adenoma	Firm, tender, movable mass that persists through menses
Mastitis	Tender mass after pregnancy, with overlying redness, fever, and systemic symptoms
Breast cancer	Hard, fixed, nontender mass that persists through menses

carcinoma, represents 50% of breast cancers. Medullary breast cancer, lobular carcinoma, tubular carcinoma, infiltrating papillary cancer, and Paget's disease represent other types of tumors found; most of these have a better prognosis than the infiltrating ductal type.

SCREENING

Three methods of screening for breast cancer are widely used. Breast self-examination (BSE) is practiced by many women on a monthly basis after each menses. No randomized controlled trials have proved BSE's effectiveness at detecting breast cancer early and reducing morbidity or mortality. Clinical breast examination (CBE) is performed by a physician or health care provider during annual or periodic health maintenance. While studies suggest that BSE and CBE are less effective than mammography in detecting breast cancers, it is a useful screen for the many women who do not get regular mammographic screening. In addition, CBE and SBE can, at times, detect cancers that are not detected on routine mammography.

Mammography is the most effective screening method available. In women between the ages of 50 and 75, annual mammography can reduce the breast cancer mortality rate by 25% or more. There is still debate, however, whether annual mammography in low-risk women under the age of 50 reduces mortality in a cost-effective manner. The denser breast tissue and lower incidence of breast cancer in women under age 50 result in a lower sensitivity and specificity for mammography in women 40–50 years of age. Several ongoing studies are investigating the ability of mammography to reduce morbidity and mortality from breast cancer in women 40–50 years of age. Current recommendations by the American Cancer Society call for a monthly BSE and a CBE every third year for women 20–39 years of age; a monthly BSE, an annual CBE, and mammography every 1–2 years for women 40–50 years of age; and a monthly BSE, an annual CBE, and annual mammography for women over 50 years of age. The United States Preventive Services Task Force (USPSTF) published more stringent guidelines in 1996 based on a comprehensive review of available scientific studies on breast cancer screening. The lack of support for BSE and weaker support for CBE caused them to recommend mammographic screening for women between the ages of 50 and 75. Mammography outside of this age group, BSE, and CBE may be recommended by the physician based on specific patient needs, patient risks, practice patterns, and availability of screening tests. Most physicians offer mammography to women under the age of 50 when there is increased risk such as a history of breast cancer in the patient or a family history of breast cancer in first-degree relatives of the patient.

| **Screening for breast cancer as recommended by the American Cancer Society.** | • Age 20–39: BSE monthly, CBE every 3 years
• Age 40–49: BSE monthly, CBE yearly, mammography every 1–2 years
• Age over 50: BSE monthly, CBE yearly, mammogram yearly |

Screening for breast cancer as Recommended by the USPSTF.

Screen every 1–2 years with mammogram or mammogram and CBE in women aged 50–69. Screening before age 50 and after age 69 is not supported by sufficient evidence; however, it may be recommended for high-risk women or healthy women over the age of 70 on other grounds. There is not sufficient evidence to recommend or advise against BSE.

DIAGNOSIS

Mammography is now often coupled with ultrasound to determine the presence of cysts in the breast. It is an excellent screening tool, but it is not a diagnostic test. Fifteen percent of cancers may not be seen on mammography, and most abnormal findings on mammography are not cancers. For the many patients who present with a suspicious and persistent mass or those with an abnormal lesion on mammogram, the definitive diagnosis is made with tissue biopsy.

Physical Signs of Breast Cancer
A hard, non-tender, fixed mass that persists through several menstrual cycles with overlying skin dimpling, bloody nipple discharge, or palpable lymph nodes in axilla.

For breast lesions that may be cystic, needle aspiration is an informative and often definitive first step and can be performed in the office. Aspiration of clear fluid with resolution of the cyst is diagnostic of a simple benign cyst. Aspiration of bloody fluid should prompt cytologic evaluation of the fluid. Lack of resolution or recurrence of the lesion any time after aspiration should prompt further diagnostic evaluation such as biopsy.

For lesions that persist or recur after needle aspiration or lesions that do not seem cystic and have persisted through more than one menstrual cycle, a mammogram may be helpful. While not diagnostic, the mammogram may help define the location of the lesion and might identify other breast lesions not felt on examination. Presence of microcalcifications and a stellate pattern on the mammogram are associated with an increased likelihood of cancer.

Open biopsy remains the diagnostic method of choice, but use of fine needle or stereotactic-guided needle biopsy is growing. For the patient with a suspicious lesion on examination and an abnormal mammogram, open biopsy is the diagnostic method of choice, as more than 30% of such patients can be misdiagnosed with fine needle biopsy.

In the patient who presents with nipple discharge and no mass to prompt the workup above, a clear approach is needed. Expressed nipple discharge is common and is found in as many as 50% of women. While potentially of social importance, it is not indicative of significant underlying breast disease. Spontaneous discharge is more serious. Milky (thin, white, or cloudy) or opalescent (thicker, white, or colored) fluid is not associated with breast cancer. Serous, bloody, or serosanguineous fluid is worrisome for underlying cancer, especially if it is associated with nipple redness, rawness, or thickening. If it is unilateral and if it originates from one duct, the fluid should be evaluated. Mammography should be followed by either cytology of bloody fluid, cannulation of the duct with galactography, or more appropriately, surgical evaluation. Fortunately, even the more worrisome bloody fluid is associated with breast cancer in only approximately 11% of cases (Table 61-2).

TABLE 61-2
TYPES OF SPONTANEOUS NIPPLE DISCHARGE

Fluid Type	Differential Diagnosis
Milky (clear, cloudy, or white but thin discharge)	Excessive prolactin, mechanical stimulation, drugs, and postlactation
Opalescent (white, yellow, green, or black and thick)	Duct ectasia, epithelial hyperplasia, or enlarged duct cysts
Serous, sanguine, or serosanguine	Pregnancy, duct ectasia, papilloma, or cancer

TREATMENT

This woman was diagnosed with infiltrating ductal carcinoma of the breast. Variations of mastectomy were the treatment of choice for breast cancer in the past. Awareness of the significant emotional burden of breast removal, the major physical complications associated with mastectomy, and the success of a variety of less invasive treatments for breast cancer has led to other treatment options. For locally confined disease, either lumpectomy with radiation or total simple mastectomy are reasonable treatment options. Local disease with positive nodes may be treated with simple mastectomy combined with chemotherapy. Tamoxifen, an estrogen antagonist, may be added to the various therapies to delay tumor recurrence or prolong survival, especially in postmenopausal women or those with estrogen-receptor positive tumors. In more advanced disease, local treatment (surgery, radiation, or both) is coupled with chemotherapy and hormonal therapy. This maximizes survival while minimizing the ill effects of treatment. Finally, new and improved methods of treatment include bone marrow transplant with chemotherapy. This expensive form of therapy is being used more frequently, in spite of a lack of consensus or clear evidence regarding its appropriate use.

PROGNOSIS

Early diagnosis and aggressive treatment have improved survival in patients with breast cancer. Treated in the earliest stage, carcinoma in situ patients may have less than a 5% chance of recurrent cancer. For more advanced local disease with no evidence of lymph node involvement, the 8-year survival rate is roughly 80%. For patients with evidence of lymph node involvement, the 8-year survival rate drops to 60%. Even the most advanced cancers with evidence of distant metastases have a survival rate of more than 2 years for roughly 50% of the patients and more than 10 years for as many as 10%.

SUGGESTED READING

Henderson I: *Breast Cancer.* In *Textbook of Clinical Oncology,* 2nd ed. Atlanta, GA: American Cancer Society, 1995, pp 198–219.

Lindfors KK, Rosenquist CJ: The cost-effectiveness of mammographic screening strategies. *JAMA* 274:881–884, 1995.

Phillips DM, Balducci L: Current management of breast cancer. *Am Fam Physician* 52(2):657–665, 1996.

CHAPTER 62
Prostate Cancer

Robert V. Smith, M.D.

PATIENT

V. Conor, a 70-year-old man, presents for a physical examination. He has been feeling well but does complain of nocturia "times two," some urinary hesitancy, and a decrease in his urinary stream. On physical examination, his prostate is enlarged, and a nodular area is detected in the right lobe.

CLINICAL PRESENTATION

Prostate cancer may be asymptomatic or may present with symptoms suggesting bladder outlet obstruction or metastatic disease. The symptoms of bladder outlet obstruction, including urinary hesitancy, urinary frequency, nocturia, and a diminished stream, are also symptoms of benign prostatic hypertrophy (BPH) and are nonspecific for prostate cancer. The diagnosis is often first suspected when an abnormality is detected on digital rectal examination or a prostate-specific antigen (PSA) level is elevated. At other times, prostate cancer may be an unanticipated finding when a transurethral prostatic resection (TURP) is performed for BPH. Rarely, it is diagnosed when metastatic disease manifests as bone pain, spinal cord compression, or renal failure as a result of urinary obstruction.

> Approximately 50% of palpable prostatic nodules are malignant.

EPIDEMIOLOGY

Only lung cancer causes more cancer deaths in men in the United States than prostate cancer. Each year, there are over 200,000 new cases and 40,000 deaths. It is rare before age 50 and is more common in African-American men than in white American men. A positive family history is a risk factor. As many as 70% of men who die of other causes after age 70 may have occult foci of prostate cancer identified at autopsy.

SCREENING

Screening for prostate cancer has engendered huge debate and disagreement. The American Cancer Society recommends an annual digital rectal examination for all men, starting at age 40. It also

> The recommen-
> dations of
> various national
> organizations
> disagree on the
> issue of screen-
> ing.

recommends that an annual test of the PSA be done on all men age 50 and older and that African-American men and those with a positive family history begin PSA screening at age 40. The American College of Radiology and the American Urological Association support these recommendations. The United States Preventive Services Task Force (USPSTF), on the other hand, does not recommend routine screening with digital rectal examination, PSA, or transrectal ultrasound. The USPSTF cites the lack of evidence regarding screening benefits and the risks of adverse effects. These risks include unnecessary biopsies or surgery with the possible consequences of impotence or incontinence. If a patient requests screening, the USPSTF recommends that the patient be informed about the potential benefits and risks of early detection and treatment and that screening be limited to men with a life expectancy greater than 10 years. The American Academy of Family Physicians (AAFP) recommends that men aged 50 to 65 be counseled about the known risks and uncertain benefits of screening for prostate cancer. Most recently, the American College of Physicians recommended that instead of routinely screening all men, physicians should have a full discussion with patients regarding benefits and risks and individualize medical decisions.

DIAGNOSIS

Often the diagnosis of prostate cancer is first suspected after digital rectal examination. The prostate may be firmer than normal or an indurated or nodular area may be palpated. A large tumor may extend beyond the capsule, rendering the boundaries of the gland indistinct. The serum PSA level should be measured in all individuals with an abnormality on palpation. On the other hand, an elevated PSA level detected by screening may be the only apparent sign. In either event, transrectal ultrasound should be performed. It can help to identify abnormal areas, which can be biopsied via transrectal needle biopsy. If no abnormalities are detected by ultrasound, several "blind" biopsies can be taken. Transrectal ultrasound can also be used to determine local tumor spread. Once prostate cancer has been diagnosed, computerized tomography (CT) or magnetic resonance imaging (MRI) of the pelvis may be useful in trying to assess local or lymph node spread. Other studies such as bone scans, plain x-rays, or intravenous pyelography may be needed to determine the extent of disease. Laboratory assessment should also include serum acid phosphatase, alkaline phosphatase, creatinine, and blood urea nitrogen (BUN).

Almost all prostate cancers are adenocarcinomas. Adenocarcinomas are more common at the periphery of the gland, but if they arise or spread into the periurethral region, urethral obstruction and its associated symptoms may occur.

Accurate staging is essential in determining prognosis and treatment options. Unfortunately, there are several classification systems in use. The traditional staging system, known as the Whitmore System, uses four stages (A to D) with some subdivisions. Another system uses the tumor, node, metastases (TNM) classification (Table 62-1).

TABLE 62-1
MAJOR ASPECTS OF PROSTATE CANCER STAGING SYSTEMS

TNM	Whitmore	Descriptions
T1a	Stage A1	Well-differentiated tumor found in less than 5% of specimens obtained at transurethral resection
T1b	Stage A2	Well-differentiated tumor found in four or more chips or tumor that is not well-differentiated
T2	Stage B	Asymptomatic prostatic nodule
T3	Stage C	Tumor extends locally beyond the prostatic capsule but with no distant metastases
	Stage D0	Metastatic disease as indicated by an elevated acid phosphatase level alone
N+	Stage D1	Metastases to pelvic lymph nodes
M+	Stage D2	Distant metastases

TREATMENT

The choice of treatment is based on the stage of the disease and the medical condition of the patient. *Watchful waiting* may be appropriate for individuals with well-differentiated tumors and a life expectancy of less than 10 years. *Radical prostatectomy*, the removal of the entire prostate and both seminal vesicles, is generally recommended for stages A2, B, and sometimes stage A1. A radical prostatectomy with lymph node dissection and orchiectomy is sometimes recommended for stage D1. *Radiation therapy* can be used for stages A2, B, C, and sometimes D1. For stage B, however, radical prostatectomy has a slightly more favorable outcome. *Hormonal therapy* is based on the fact that androgen deprivation can produce regression of primary and metastatic disease. Androgen deprivation can be accomplished by either surgical or medical castration. Medical castration can be achieved with luteinizing hormone–releasing hormone (LH-RH) analogues or antiandrogens. LH-RH analogues, such as leuprolide, inhibit the release of pituitary gonadotropins. Antiandrogens, such as flutamide, block the action of dihydrotestosterone (DHT) on prostate cancer cells. LH-RH analogues and antiandrogens can be used in combination. Hormonal therapy is usually limited to stage D2 disease. *Chemotherapy* may be used for advanced disease refractory to other treatments, but it is generally of limited benefit. Radiation therapy may also be used in a palliative fashion for the pain of bony metastases, to prevent pathologic fractures in weight-bearing bones, or for the treatment of spinal cord compression.

Periodic digital rectal examination and measurement of PSA levels are commonly used to follow patients with prostate cancer. Other aspects of follow-up are very dependent on the staging and specialized treatments the patient receives.

PROGNOSIS

The natural course of prostate cancer can be extremely variable. The prognosis varies greatly with the extent of disease from a life expectancy close to the general population for small cancers discovered incidentally at TURP to a median survival of a little more than 2 years for disseminated disease.

SUGGESTED READING

American College of Physicians: Screening for prostate cancer. *Ann Intern Med* 126:480–484, 1997.

Garnick MB, Fair W: Prostate cancer: emerging concepts (part I). *Ann Intern Med* 125:118–125, 1996.

Garnick MB, Fair W: Prostate cancer: emerging concepts (part II). *Ann Intern Med* 125:205–212, 1996.

Taub M, Begas A, Leve N: Advanced prostate cancer: endocrine therapies and palliative measures. *Postgrad Med* 100:139–154, 1996.

United States Preventive Services Task Force: *Guide to Clinical Preventive Services*, 2nd ed. Baltimore, MD: Williams & Wilkins, 1996.

Williams TR, Love N: Treatment of localized prostate cancer. *Postgrad Med* 100:105–120, 1996.

CHAPTER 63
Anemia

Richard A. Neill, M.D.

PATIENT

C. Richardson, a 26-year-old woman, complains of the gradual onset of fatigue and headaches over the preceding 6 months. She has a history of heavy menses, occurring regularly every 29 days and lasting 7 days. She denies any skin or hair changes, but she does complain of feeling cool when others are warm.

CLINICAL PRESENTATION

Anemia is defined as an abnormally low hemoglobin concentration. As such it is commonly diagnosed as an abnormal laboratory finding incidental to evaluation of other illnesses. Because of this, the symptoms of anemia vary widely and are usually attributable to the underlying cause of anemia. When the onset is gradual, the symptoms can be minimal or absent even in the face of marked anemia (Hgb, 9 mg/dL). Physical findings of nail-bed pallor, palmar crease pallor, conjunctival pallor, or an absence of nail-bed blanching are found to varying degrees in patients with anemia. In more acute or severe cases, tachycardia, orthostasis, and outright cardiovascular collapse can be seen.

Certain symptoms in association with anemia can provide a clue to diagnosis. Fatigue, headache, cheilitis, and pica—a predilection for chewing ice, dirt, clay, or other unusual substances—are all consistent with iron deficiency anemia, as are the symptoms in the case described above. Symmetric paresthesias, ataxia, mental status changes, and glossitis ("strawberry tongue") suggest vitamin B_{12} deficiency. Thalassemia minor and folate deficiency are often asymptomatic. Sickle cell anemia and glucose-6-phosphate dehydrogenase (G6PD) deficiency often present with dramatic symptoms. Recurring, painful sickle cell crises lasting hours or days are the hallmark symptom of sickle cell disease. G6PD deficiency results in a hemolytic anemia of varying severity in response to stressors such as drugs (sulfonamides specifically), fever, or diet. Joint

> Anemia is a symptom of an underlying illness. Iron deficiency, thalassemia trait, and chronic disease are the most common etiologies.

aches, jaundice, fever, or outright cardiovascular collapse can all occur in severe hemolytic anemia.

EPIDEMIOLOGY

Each of the causes of anemia has its own unique population distribution. The most common causes of anemia in the United States include iron deficiency (most often a result of blood loss), thalassemia minor, and anemia of chronic disease in almost equal proportions. Taken together these account for approximately 75% of all anemias. The remainder of anemias can be attributed to sickle cell anemia, nutritional deficiencies such as vitamin B_{12} or folate deficiency, G6PD deficiency, autoimmune hemolytic anemias, and disorders of red blood cell (RBC) production (aplasia).

Iron deficiency as a result of dietary insufficiency typically occurs only in infants and menstruating women. In infants, an expanding RBC mass creates iron demands that can outstrip supply in the absence of iron-fortified formula or cereals; in menstruating women, monthly blood loss approximately doubles the normally low daily iron need. Over time, this increment, if unreplaced, can result in anemia. In nonmenstruating women and adult men, iron deficiency demands an evaluation for sources of blood loss to rule out conditions such as colon and stomach cancer, peptic ulcer disease, and inflammatory bowel disease.

Vitamin B_{12} deficiency typically occurs in illnesses affecting secretion of intrinsic factors from the stomach or absorption of vitamin B_{12}/intrinsic factor complex in the terminal ileum. Examples include atrophic gastritis, Crohn's disease, postsurgical states, and achlorhydria. Folate deficiencies are commonly seen in alcoholics and other nutritionally challenged patients.

Thalassemia minor occurs most frequently in persons of Mediterranean, African, Southeast Asian, or Southern European descent. Sickle cell anemia is overwhelmingly a disease of African Americans. Underproduction anemias (aplasias) occur most commonly in response to marrow-toxic drugs or infections.

SCREENING

The United States Preventive Services Task Force (USPSTF) recommends screening for iron deficiency anemia using hemoglobin or hematocrit in all pregnant women. There is insufficient evidence to recommend for or against routine screening for anemia in other asymptomatic persons.

DIAGNOSIS

Examination of a *peripheral blood smear* is critical to the diagnosis. Characteristic findings such as sickled cells in sickle cell anemia,

schistocytes (RBC fragments) in hemolytic anemias, hypersegmented polymorphonuclear cells in vitamin B_{12} deficiency, or the small hypochromic cells
of iron deficiency can all confirm a diagnosis.

> Examination of
> the peripheral
> smear is the
> single most im-
> portant diagnos-
> tic test.

Mean corpuscular volume (MCV) has
been used to separate anemias into
three broad, overlapping classes based
on RBC size:

1. **Microcytic anemias**, including iron-deficiency anemia
   and thalassemia
2. **Macrocytic anemias**, including those resulting from alcohol abuse, liver disease, hypothyroidism, and vitamin B_{12}
   and folate deficiencies
3. **Normocytic anemias**, including anemia of chronic diseases such as tuberculosis, rheumatologic diseases, malignancies, or renal disease. Unfortunately many causes of
   anemia produce dimorphic populations of RBCs, which
   when read by an automated counter suggest a normocytic
   process. An increased *red cell distribution width (RDW)* can
   be a clue to this. In the end, nothing substitutes for personal examination of the smear.

Iron deficiency is characterized by decreased *ferritin*, decreased
percent transferrin saturation, and increased *iron-binding capacity*. A
definitive diagnosis requires bone marrow biopsy demonstrating
diminished iron stores on prussian blue staining, although this is
rarely necessary to establish the diagnosis. Thalassemia, while also
microcytic, is differentiated from iron deficiency by the finding of
normal iron studies and an increased to high normal RBC count.

The *reticulocyte count* can establish whether the bone marrow is
responding to an anemia appropriately by releasing newly formed
RBCs into the blood. A low reticulocyte count may imply an anemia
from underproduction, as in iron deficiency or nutritional deficiencies. Remember to use a corrected reticulocyte count (% retic-
ulocytes × patient Hgb/45). An elevated reticulocyte count implies
hemolysis or acute hemorrhage. When hemolysis is suspected, *serum haptoglobin, bilirubin,* and *lactate dehydrogenase (LDH)* can all
confirm the diagnosis. *Direct and indirect Coombs' test, cold agglutinins,*
or *hemoglobin electrophoresis* can separate acquired immune hemolytic anemias resulting from infections (cytomegalovirus [CMV],
Mycoplasma) or drugs (quinidine, methyldopa) from genetic hemolytic anemias (G6PD deficiency, sickle cell anemia).

TREATMENT

Treatment is directed at the underlying cause. Iron sulfate (325 mg) by mouth three times daily suffices to induce a brisk reticulocytosis in iron deficiency anemia. Because iron is better absorbed in an acidic environment, it is frequently given with ascorbic acid (vitamin C).

Intramuscular vitamin B_{12} injections will quickly reverse pernicious anemia, as will oral folate in folate deficiencies. Anemias of chronic disease respond only to treatment of the underlying condition. G6PD deficiency is managed through scrupulous avoidance of inciting factors.

In the absence of continuing blood loss or dramatic symptoms, transfusion is rarely necessary. Treatment of the underlying conditions, where possible, will allow the bone marrow to replace RBC mass normally. Overreliance on transfusion simply to return hemoglobin to normal levels can result in iron overload, with resultant liver and other organ damage, not to mention the risk of transfusion reactions and transfusion-associated hepatitis and human immunodeficiency virus. While the risk of the latter has been greatly reduced through source screening, a small but measurable risk remains. As a result, transfusions of any blood product should occur only when absolutely necessary.

SUGGESTED READING

Beuther E: The common anemias. *JAMA* 259(16):2433–2437, 1988.

Panzer RJ, Black ER, Griner PF (eds): Microcytic anemias. In *Diagnostic Strategies for Common Medical Problems*. Philadelphia, PA: American College of Physicians, 1991, pp 448–457.

CHAPTER 64
Hypothyroidism

Marjorie A. Bowman, M.D., M.P.A.

PATIENT

C. Simms, a 55-year-old woman, says "she just does not feel well." She feels tired all the time in spite of sleeping fine. In the last couple of years she has gained 10 lbs, and her skin is dry. She denies depressive feelings or crying. On further questioning, she has also had increasing constipation.

CLINICAL PRESENTATION

Hypothyroidism is a sneaky disease. The symptoms tend to be mild and progress gradually. The progression of symptoms is so gradual that they may go unrecognized. With increased screening, many cases are diagnosed by laboratory tests, rather than as a result of testing based on specific patient complaints. The classic symptoms are:

- Dry, dull skin and hair
- Intolerance to cold
- Puffiness and swelling
- Diminished sweating in a warm environment
- Weight increase
- Paresthesias
- Constipation
- Deepening voice, hoarseness
- Weakness, malaise, and fatigue
- Menorrhagia
- Mental dullness
- Arthralgias and myalgias
- Slowed movements

> Think "slow" (onset, muscles, heart, bowels, thinking, reflexes) and "swollen" (legs; vocal cords; heart; pericardial, pleural, peritoneal fluid)

Progressive hearing loss has a high specificity for hypothyroidism but is uncommon. Congestive heart failure, psychosis, peripheral edema, myxedema, coma, and death can occur with severe hypothyroidism or long-term hypothyroidism.

The signs most suggestive of hypothyroidism are goiter, slow return of the ankle reflexes, thinning of the outer eyebrows, a thick tongue, and slow movements observed by the physician. Of these, the slow return of the ankle reflexes is the most common. Vital signs may reveal bradycardia and hypothermia. Pleural, pericardial, and peritoneal effusions can occur. Galactorrhea may be found. The dry skin is nonspecific. The most important factor in diagnosis is a high index of suspicion.

EPIDEMIOLOGY

Hypothyroidism is common. There is a gradually increasing prevalence with age. It is more common in patients with other endocrine diseases and in those with family histories of thyroid disease. The most common cause of hypothyroidism is basically thyroid failure, such as from Hashimoto's thyroiditis or multinodular goiter. Hypothyroidism can also result from pituitary failure.

SCREENING

Recently, there has been increasing recognition of the potential value of screening. Currently the United States Public Health Service (USPHS) does not recommend screening with the sensitive thyroid-stimulating hormone (TSH) but suggests that physicians have a low threshold for ordering the test.

DIAGNOSIS

In thyroid gland failure, the TSH level is increased, and the thyroxine (T_4) level is low. Confusion can occur with mild abnormalities, which can happen during acute illnesses. Anemia, hyponatremia, hypercholesterolemia, hyperprolactinemia, and elevated liver enzymes can occur.

TREATMENT

The treatment is basically thyroid replacement hormone, which will need to be taken for the remainder of the patient's life, except in the uncommon cases of transient postpregnancy hypothyroidism. Patients with severe hypothyroidism or who are elderly should be started at low doses (25–50 µg/d). The usual replacement dose is about 0.001 mg per pound of body weight. The patient should have intermittent TSH tests to monitor treatment (every 6–12 months once stable). The goal should be a normal TSH, since too much thyroid hormone can cause iatrogenic problems such as atrial fibrillation or osteoporosis. In general, the patient should receive a set brand of thyroid hormone to limit changes in therapeutic levels.

SUGGESTED READING

Singer PA, Cooper DS, Levy EG, et al: Treatment guidelines for patients with hyperthyroidism and hypothyroidism. *JAMA* 273:808–812, 1995.

Zulewski H, Muller B, Exer P, et al: Estimation of tissue hypo-thyroidism by a new clinical score: evaluation of patients with various grades of hypothyroidism and controls. *J Clin Endocrinol Metabl* 82:771–776, 1997.

CHAPTER 65
Hyperthyroidism

Russell S. Breish, M.D.

PATIENT

K. Wells, a 32-year-old weightlifter, has noticed several months of intermittent rapid heartbeats; weight loss; loose, frequent stools; and an inability to lift as much weight as he had been lifting. Until this point, he has been in excellent health. His social history is unremarkable. His family history is positive for a sister with Graves' disease. On physical examination his eyes look normal, his thyroid gland feels normal, and there is no thyroid bruit. His heart is regular at 120 beats/min. His abdomen is soft. He does have a mild tremor of his hands and 3+–4+ deep tendon reflexes diffusely.

CLINICAL PRESENTATION

Hyperthyroidism presents with a constellation of signs and symptoms that are typical for the condition. The symptoms are caused by an excessive amount of thyroxine (T_4), which drives cell function in all tissue. Common symptoms include nervousness, sweating, heat intolerance, palpitations, dyspnea, fatigue, weight loss, and eye complaints such as eye redness or dryness. Less common symptoms include increased quantity of stool, eyelid retraction, congestive heart failure (CHF), and proximal myopathy. Physical examination frequently reveals an enlarged thyroid gland with a thyroid bruit, muscular tremor, tachycardia, and hyperkinetic muscle activity. In Graves' disease, exophthalmos (a protrusion of the eye caused by deposition of tissue in the orbit) can be quite severe, with ophthalmoplegia, conjunctivitis, and even visual loss. Exophthalmos is diagnosed on physical examination by observing irritated conjunctivae or sclerae, proptosis, lid lag, and a widened palpebral fissure. Also seen in Graves' disease are pretibial myxedema, clubbing, and dermopathy. Hyperthyroidism in the elderly is often a much more

> Common signs and symptoms are nervousness, sweating, heat intolerance, palpitations, dyspnea, fatigue, weight loss, and eye complaints. Less common symptoms are increased quantity of stool, arrhythmia, eyelid retraction, edema, CHF, and proximal muscle weakness.

subtle condition. Frequently symptoms include apathy, weakness, constipation, weight loss, and atrial fibrillation. A high index of suspicion for thyroid disease is important when caring for the elderly.

EPIDEMIOLOGY

Hyperthyroidism is a common condition, more common in women then in men. There is frequently a positive family history for thyroid disease. Hyperthyroidism often presents in the third to sixth decades of life.

DIFFERENTIAL DIAGNOSIS

The initial test is for highly sensitive thyroid-stimulating hormone (TSH). In hyperthyroidism, a low TSH indicates that the pituitary gland is being suppressed by an excessive amount of thyroid hormone. If hyperthyroidism is suspected and the TSH level is low, the next step is to check the T_4 level and the triiodothyronine (T_3) resin uptake. The free thyroxine index (FTI) is calculated using these values. The FTI approximates the level of free T_4 in the serum. If the FTI is normal, measurement of the free T_3 is necessary. Up to 10% of people who are hyperthyroid are hyperthyroid strictly with T_3. This condition is known as T_3 thyrotoxicosis. Once the diagnosis of hyperthyroidism has been confirmed, the next step is to see if the thyroid gland is overproducing thyroid hormone or simply oversecreting stored thyroid hormone. This is accomplished with a radioactive iodine (^{131}I) thyroid scan and uptake.

In some forms of hyperthyroidism, the thyroid gland produces an excessive amount of thyroid hormone. In other conditions the thyroid gland secretes an excessive amount of thyroid hormone that is already stored in the gland. Common conditions of overproduction are Graves' disease, toxic adenoma, and toxic multinodular goiter. A common condition of oversecretion is thyroiditis. The thyroid scan and uptake can differentiate between a single nodule producing excessive thyroid hormone, multinodular goiter, or Graves' disease. The scan and

> Common causes of hyperthyroidism are Graves' disease, toxic adenoma, multinodular goiter, thyroiditis, and iodine-induced hyperthyroidism. Less common causes are iatrogenic hyperthyroidism, factitious hyperthyroidism (particularly people who report taking diet pills or pills for weight loss), and TSH-secreting tumors.

uptake can also differentiate between overproduction of thyroid hormone by the thyroid gland and oversecretion of existing hormone in the gland.

Graves' disease is an autoimmune disease and is the most common form of hyperthyroidism. In Graves' disease, thyroid receptor antibodies stimulate the gland to overproduce thyroid hormone. The pretibial myxedema, dermopathy, and exophthalmos appear to be caused by the autoimmune component of the disease and not the hyperthyroidism. Much less common causes of hyperthyroidism are TSH-producing tumors and excess iodine intake. Factitious hyperthyroidism (taking unneeded thyroid hormones) is seen, particularly in people trying to lose weight.

TREATMENT

In Graves' disease, the production of thyroid hormone needs to be decreased. At the same time, some of the symptoms of hyperthyroidism need to be blunted. Beta-blockers such as propranolol will blunt some of the somatic symptoms of hyperthyroidism such as palpitations and tremor. Thyroid-suppressing drugs such as propylthiouracil (PTU) will decrease the amount of hormone that is produced by the thyroid gland, and prolonged treatment sometimes leads to remission of Graves' disease. Surgery or ^{131}I to ablate the thyroid gland are the definitive treatments, but these may render the patient hypothyroid, in which case thyroid hormone supplementation is necessary. Often thyroid-suppressing drugs are used to get the patient euthyroid prior to definitive treatment.

In severe or "malignant" exophthalmos associated with Graves' disease, treatment is necessary to improve eye comfort and to prevent vision loss. Local treatment to keep the cornea moist is very important. Steroids are often used to decrease the inflammation in the orbit. Diuretics and elevation of the head of the bed may also help with the swelling. Surgical decompression or radiation of the orbit has been used in severe cases. Rendering the person euthyroid may have no effect on the course of the exophthalmos.

In a condition such as thyroiditis the gland does not continue to produce excessive thyroid hormone; it simply secretes the thyroid hormone that it has in reserve. Thus, thyroiditis is typically a self-limiting condition. It is often painful and aspirin or oral steroids are used for pain control. Beta-blockers are used for symptomatic control. Frequently, after an episode of acute thyroiditis, the person will become hypothyroid for the rest of their life, and this needs to be evaluated and treated accordingly.

PROGNOSIS

Severe hyperthyroidism (thyroid storm) can be fatal, particularly in people with other underlying medical conditions. When diagnosed in a timely fashion, most hyperthyroidism can be treated effectively. The exophthalmos of Graves' disease can persist even when normal thyroid function is restored.

SUGGESTED READING

Knudson P: Hyperthyroidism in adults: variable clinical presentations and approaches to diagnosis. *J Am Board Fam Pract* 8:109–113, 1995.

CHAPTER 66
Gout

-- -- -- -- -- -- -- -- -- -- -- -- -- -- -- --

Gaetano P. Monteleone, Jr., M.D.

PATIENT

M. Lockwood, a 53-year-old man, complains of pain in the right great toe. He was awakened from a sound sleep last night by a sharp, burning pain. He denies any recent trauma. He says that he also has a low-grade fever. On further questioning, he admits to increased alcohol consumption yesterday. Pertinent medical history includes a history of high blood pressure, for which he takes a "water pill."

Physical examination reveals a first metatarsophalangeal (MTP) joint that is erythematous, locally edematous, and very tender to palpation. There is warmth to palpation of the first MTP joint and pain with active and passive range of motion.

CLINICAL PRESENTATION

Gout represents a heterogeneous group of disorders resulting in periarticular deposition of uric acid (monosodium urate) crystals.

The principal metabolic abnormality is hyperuricemia, either because of increased production (75%) or underexcretion (25%) of uric acid in the body. Common causes of overproduction of uric acid include aberrant purine metabolism, increased cell turnover (myeloproliferative disorders, multiple myeloma), and certain enzyme deficiencies. Common causes of underexcretion of uric acid include diuretics (thiazide, loop), low-dose aspirin, niacin, and alcohol consumption.

> The term gout is derived from the Latin word "gutta," or drop. The ancient Greeks believed that a drop of poison in the joint caused pain and inflammation.

Over 50% of the time the first joint affected is the MTP. This type of gouty attack is also known as podagra. Other joints can be affected (mid-foot, ankle, knee). If untreated the acute attack will last a few days to weeks. Resolution of the inflammatory process heralds desquammation

> The classic presentation is an abrupt onset of nocturnal pain, usually monoarticular.

and pruritus of the overlying skin. Symptoms generally resolve in a few hours with appropriate treatment. Subsequent attacks may affect the upper extremities, including the elbow, shoulder, wrist, or hands. The arthritis typically progresses to asymmetric, polyarticular distribution.

The classic appearance on physical examination demonstrates localized erythema and edema of the affected joint. Exquisite point tenderness and pain with joint motion also occur. The joint may appear warm to touch. Some patients develop a low-grade fever.

EPIDEMIOLOGY

Gout is more prevalent in middle-aged men and postmenopausal women. Approximately 90% of patients with gout are men.

Asymptomatic hyperuricemia is seen in approximately 5%–8% of adult men. The prevalence of gout in the United States is less than 3%. Hyperuricemia is not required for the diagnosis of gout though the risk of gout increases with the level and duration of hyperuricemia.

DIFFERENTIAL DIAGNOSIS

Gout may mimic trauma, septic joints, rheumatoid arthritis, cellulitis, and other deposition diseases (such as pseudogout or calcium pyrophosphate deposition disease). An accurate history will disclose previous trauma. Rheumatoid arthritis is generally associated with more systemic symptoms (generalized malaise, fever, weight loss), different joint predilection, and a female predominance (3:1). Cellulitis has a more diffuse erythematous reaction and lacks the exquisite, localized pain associated with gout.

DIAGNOSIS

Diagnosis of gout is usually established by thorough history and physical examination. Serum uric acid may or may not be elevated. Aspiration of the affected joint demonstrates negative birefringent crystals under polariscopic examination.

X-ray results are highly variable depending on the duration of disease. In chronic tophaceous gout, x-rays may demonstrate normal mineralization, punched-out erosions with sclerotic borders, and tophi. On completion of the initial acute gouty attack, some physicians suggest obtaining a 24-hour urine uric acid level to differentiate overproduction (high urinary uric acid) from underexcretion (normal or low urinary uric acid), which will guide therapeutic decisions.

TREATMENT

Treatment options are nonpharmacologic and pharmacologic. Pharmacologic intervention depends on the current phase of gout. Nonpharmacologic modifications may contribute to significant symptom reduction. Bed rest may be helpful in the acute phase. In addition, heat will help ameliorate symptoms (cold or ice may actually exacerbate symptoms). Dietary changes should occur. For instance, hyperhydration and avoidance of alcohol are paramount. Decreased purine intake (i.e., red meat, alcohol, beans, lentils, cauliflower, asparagus) may be of some benefit although this is controversial. Weight reduction is also warranted.

- **Acute therapy** consists of nonsteroidal anti-inflammatory drugs (NSAIDs), such as naproxen, ibuprofen, and indomethacin. In the beginning daily doses are high and then tapered with symptom control. Colchicine is effective for acute and prophylactic therapy. Significant side effects, including diarrhea, abdominal cramping, and nausea limit its use. Corticosteroids, taken orally, effectively decrease inflammation and pain. If septic arthritis is a significant possibility, however, corticosteroids should be avoided. Analgesics, including opiates, may be required.

  > NSAIDs and colchicine are commonly used as treatment for acute gouty arthritis. Rapid pain resolution with colchicine verifies the diagnosis.

- **Prophylactic therapy** includes colchicine, allopurinol, and probenecid. Colchicine inhibits the phagocytosis of urate crystals by white blood cells and is helpful for overproduction and underexcretion of uric acid. Allopurinol blocks uric acid synthesis. It helps to mobilize tophi and decrease renal exposure to uric acid. It is more effective in overproducers. Probenecid is a uricosuric agent designed to increase urinary excretion in underexcreters. Prophylactic therapy should commence at least several weeks after the last attack of gout to avoid precipitation of an acute attack. Intermediate goals of prophylactic therapy are to maintain serum uric acid levels lower than 5.0–6.0 mg/dL and to maintain a hyperhydrated state (greater than 2 L/d urine output). This hyperhydrated state decreases the risk of uric acid stone formation within the kidney and deterioration of kidney function.

PROGNOSIS

There are four commonly recognized phases of gout:

- Asymptomatic hyperuricemia
- Acute gouty arthritis
- Interval or intercritical gout
- Chronic tophaceous gout

Asymptomatic hyperuricemia may be present for up to 30 years. This phase ends with the occurrence of the *first gouty attack*. With resolution of the acute attack, a symptom-free period of time will exist (*intercritical gout*). The disease usually progresses with shorter durations of intercritical gout and more frequent attacks. Prophylactic pharmacologic therapy during the intercritical period may decrease uric acid deposition and increase the duration of symptom-free periods between attacks.

After 10 years of acute gouty attacks, tophi begin to form in the periarticular areas. Tophi represent conglomerations of monosodium urate crystals associated with an inflammatory reaction. Tophi can be destructive to the surrounding bone, cartilage, and tissue. Common locations of tophi include synovium, subchondral bone, olecranon bursa, Achilles tendon, helix of the ear, and other subcutaneous tissue. Tophi can be confused with rheumatoid and other subcutaneous nodules. The risk of progressive, destructive arthropathy is greatest in patients whose first attack occurs before the age of 50. Kidney disease from urate crystal deposition can occur. Gout may be associated with hypertension, renal disease, diabetes mellitus, obesity, and atherosclerosis. The mechanism for these associations is not known.

SUGGESTED READING

Emmerson BT: Drug therapy—management of gout. *N Engl J Med* 334(7):445–451, 1996.

Goroll AH: Management of gout. In *Primary Care Medicine—Office Evaluation and Management of the Adult*, 3rd ed. Edited by Goroll AH, May LA, Mulley AG. Philadelphia, PA: J. B. Lippincott, 1995, pp 700–703.

Hellmann DB: Arthritis and musculoskeletal disorders. In *Current Medical Diagnosis and Treatment*, 36th ed. Edited by Tierney LM, McPhee SJ, Papadakis MA. Stanford, CT: Appleton & Lange, 1997, pp 750–799.

CHAPTER 67
Rheumatoid Arthritis

Laure L. Veet, M.D., and Eileen E. Reynolds, M.D.

PATIENT

S. Reynolds, a 39-year-old woman, comes into the office complaining of fatigue, pain, swelling, and occasional redness of both wrists, both knees, and the knuckles of both hands. These symptoms started about 6 months ago and recently have become so intense that she has cut back her hours working as a chef. She says the pain is at its worst throughout the mornings when her joints are particularly stiff. She has been using over-the-counter ibuprofen with some relief.

CLINICAL PRESENTATION

Though the presentation of rheumatoid arthritis (RA) may vary, the "classic" presentation is like that of the patient above with the gradual onset of symptoms of inflammatory arthritis, morning stiffness, and generalized fatigue. Joints in the hands, particularly the proximal interphalangeal (PIP) and metacarpophalangeal (MCP) joints, and joints in the wrists are most commonly affected. RA can also affect the knees, ankles, feet, hips, and neck. Though patients may have a little more redness or swelling on one side or the other, the distribution of joints involved is remarkably symmetric. The morning stiffness that also is characteristic of RA can take hours to get better. If the disease is longstanding, cartilage, bone, and tendons that make up the joint become damaged, causing classic deformities of the hand and wrist, such as ulnar drift at the MCP joints and swan neck deformity of the fingers (PIP hyperextension and distal interphalangeal [DIP] flexion).

> **Classic Joint Findings**
> Redness and swelling
> Hands and wrists
> Multiple joints
> Morning stiffness
> Symmetric involvement

Since RA is a systemic illness, it may involve more than just joint inflammation. Constitutional symptoms and signs such as fever, weight loss, and fatigue often accompany joint symptoms. Other extra-articular manifestations of RA include: vasculitis, rheumatoid nodules (usually on the skin but also pulmonary nodules), pulmonary interstitial fibrosis, mononeuritis multiplex (simultaneous damage to several peripheral nerves), Sjögren's syndrome (dry eyes and dry mouth that may also occur in patients without RA), and Felty's syndrome (splenomegaly, anemia, thrombocytopenia). Some complications, such as vasculitis or pulmonary involvement, can be serious and even life-threatening.

ETIOLOGY

RA is a systemic, autoimmune disease that is commonly seen in primary care practice. Though RA may affect multiple systems of the body, the primary area affected is the synovial lining of the joints. Inflammation from the autoimmune process causes scarring in the joint space and outgrowths of the synovium known as pannus formation. This in turn leads to destruction of the joint cartilage and eventually of the surrounding bones or arthritis.

The cause of this autoimmune attack is unknown. Genetic factors probably predispose some patients. Researchers have postulated an infectious etiology, but none has ever been convincingly identified.

EPIDEMIOLOGY

Rheumatoid arthritis is a fairly common disorder, affecting about 1%–2% of adults. It is two and a half times more likely to occur in women than in men. Rheumatoid arthritis can begin almost anytime during adulthood, but the peak age of onset is between 25 and 55 years of age.

DIFFERENTIAL DIAGNOSIS

At times it is difficult to tell if a patient's symptoms are due to RA or other diseases. Connective tissue disorders (e.g., systemic lupus erythematosus, scleroderma, the spondyloarthropathies, sarcoidosis, vasculitis) and systemic infections (e.g., Lyme disease, subacute bacterial endocarditis, hepatitis B, rheumatic fever, disseminated gonococcal infection) may present with constitutional symptoms and inflammatory arthritis, which may be difficult to distinguish from RA. Gout and pseudogout are other types of inflammatory arthritis that also may be confused with RA, especially if multiple joints are involved. However, constitutional symptoms are not typically present with gout and pseudogout. Osteoarthritis, usually a noninflammatory degenerative disease, may occasionally present with warm, swollen joints, which mimic those of inflammatory arthritis and so may also be mistaken for RA.

DIAGNOSIS

There is no single finding or test that is diagnostic of RA. It is a clinical diagnosis and requires the presence of *several* characteristic signs and symptoms. The American Rheumatism Association has developed a list of seven diagnostic criteria for RA (Table 67-1). To be diagnosed with RA, a patient must meet four of the seven defined criteria. The sensitivity and specificity of having four or more of these criteria are thought to be around 90%.

TABLE 67-1
DIAGNOSTIC CRITERIA FOR RHEUMATOID ARTHRITIS

(should have four or more of the following symptoms)

1. Morning stiffness ($\geq$ 1 hour, for more than 6 weeks)
2. Symptoms in three or more joint areas for more than 6 weeks
3. Arthritis of hand joints or wrists for more than 6 weeks
4. Symmetric joint involvement
5. Rheumatoid nodules
6. Serum rheumatoid factor in elevated titers
7. Typical x-ray changes (osteopenia, erosions, joint-space narrowing)

Source: Adapted with permission from Arnett FI, et al: The American Rheumatism Association 1987 revised criteria for the classification of rheumatoid arthritis. *Arthritis Rheum* 31:315, 1988.

There are two tests included in the list of diagnostic criteria that, in the right clinical setting, may contribute to the diagnosis of RA. These are rheumatoid factor (RF) and plain x-rays. RF is an antibody found in about 75%–80% of patients with RA. A positive RF supports the diagnosis of RA only in the appropriate clinical context since it may also be present in patients with other diseases and even in many normal people with no symptoms who will never develop RA.

X-ray findings, if classic, may contribute to the diagnosis as well. Early in the disease process x-rays may be normal or may show soft tissue swelling around the involved joints. Eventually, more classic x-ray findings may develop. One classic x-ray finding is that of decreased bone density (osteopenia) in the parts of the bones surrounding the joints. A little later, bite-like erosions may be seen, then joint-space narrowing, and eventually joint destruction may become evident on x-ray.

Another test that some physicians use is the erythrocyte sedimentation rate (ESR), which is a marker for inflammation. The ESR may be elevated when the inflammatory disease is active, but it is not specific for RA. It may be elevated in other diseases as well. The

ESR may also be near normal or even in the normal range if the patient with RA is not having an active flare.

TREATMENT

The optimal treatment for RA is under debate. In the past, the goal of initial treatment has been to control symptoms and inflammation using anti-inflammatory medications like nonsteroidal anti-inflammatory drugs (NSAIDs) and salicylates. More aggressive intervention with "disease-modifying" medications with potentially severe side effects (e.g., gold, penicillamine, azathioprine, cyclosporine, methotrexate) were used only when first-line agents did not control the signs and symptoms of disease.

NSAIDs are still used as first-line agents to help control inflammation and pain in most patients. Recently, however, studies have shown that some of the more aggressive medications are able to delay progression of bone destruction seen on x-ray, probably by altering the immune system and actually slowing down the immune-mediated damage to the joints. Many physicians are changing their treatment strategies to include these agents along with NSAIDs *early* in the disease, in hopes of preventing or delaying disabling joint destruction. Because these medications slow down the progression of disease, many believe that they will improve patients' disabilities and improve mortality of patients who take them despite the lack of evidence. Studies trying to answer these clinically relevant questions are currently underway.

"Disease-modifying" agents are listed in Table 67-2. These drugs often have significant side effects. Methotrexate, the most frequently used drug in this group, likely has the most benefit and the fewest side effects. Methotrexate is administered once a week and may be taken orally. Side effects include stomatitis, gastrointestinal toxicity, rash, accelerated nodule formation, cytopenias, and pneumonitis. Methotrexate has also been associated with hepatic toxicity and requires monitoring of liver function tests (baseline levels and then every 4–8 weeks while on therapy).

TABLE 67-2
POTENTIAL DISEASE-MODIFYING AGENTS

Hydroxychloroquine	D-Penicillamine
Methotrexate	Cyclosporine
Auranofin	Azathioprine
Gold	Cyclophosphamide
Sulfasalazine	

Occasionally, there are other medications that may be useful in treating the inflammation of RA. Oral corticosteroids are useful to control severe, acute flares or as a bridge while changing from one disease-modifying agent to another. The long-term use of oral corticosteroids should be limited if possible because of the side effects of long-term use (e.g., cataracts, decreased bone density, adrenal suppression, glucose intolerance). Corticosteroids injected directly into joints also work well to improve joint symptoms without incurring substantial systemic side effects. Relief can be achieved for days to weeks, but injected corticosteroids should not be used in the same joint more than 2–3 times a year.

PROGNOSIS

The clinical course of RA is variable. About 25% of patients will actually have complete resolution of their symptoms. After an initial flare, another 25% of patients will go on to have mild or moderate disease and will be only slightly limited in their activities, if at all. The other half of patients will have a more severe form of the disease, which will significantly limit their activities. Severe joint disease may leave patients wheelchair-bound and unable to perform the activities of daily living, making them prone to complications of prolonged disability, including infections and skin breakdown. Patients with RA, particularly those with more severe disease, are likely to have a shorter life span than people without RA.

SUGGESTED READING

Pope RM: Rheumatoid arthritis: pathogenesis and early recognition. *Am J Med* 100(Suppl 2A):2A–3S–2A–9S, 1996.

Jain R, Lipsky PE: Treatment of rheumatoid arthritis. *Med Clin North Am* 81(1):57–84, 1997.

CHAPTER 68
Degenerative Joint Disease (Osteoarthritis)

Gaetano P. Monteleone, Jr., M.D.

PATIENT

K. Walker, a 60-year-old man, complains of knee pain. The pain has occurred "off and on for years" but has intensified over the last few months. On further questioning, he admits knee stiffness, especially in the morning. This usually subsides when he gets "up and about." There is no significant recent or distant trauma, weakness, fever, weight loss, or malaise.

CLINICAL PRESENTATION

Osteoarthritis (OA) is a slow progressive degeneration of the articular cartilage of the body. During the progression of the disease, hypertrophy of the underlying bone may contribute to irregularities such as subchondral sclerosis and osteophytes. The arthropathy is typically devoid of inflammation, though adjacent synovitis may exist. The term degenerative joint disease (DJD) is more appropriate as the term OA incorrectly implies an inflammatory process.

The most commonly affected joints include the distal interphalangeal (DIP), proximal interphalangeal (PIP), metacarpophalangeal (MCP), and interphalangeal (IP) joints of the thumb, hip, knees, cervical spine, and lumbar spine. The articular changes can progress to nodule formation in the DIP and PIP joints, termed Heberden's and Bouchard's nodes, respectively.

Common symptoms include pain, brief duration of stiffness (especially with disuse), clicking, grinding, and occasional swelling. Physical examination may yield biomechanical changes (genu varum), minimal-to-no effusions, disuse atrophy of surrounding musculature (especially the knee), crepitus, and decreased range of motion. There may also be diffuse tenderness to palpation of the individual joint.

DJD is generally divided into two categories: primary (idiopathic) or secondary. Secondary DJD is caused by previous trauma or internal derangement of the joint, metabolic disorders, or deposition diseases.

EPIDEMIOLOGY

DJD is one of the most common disorders requiring medical attention in a family physician's office. In men, the predominant joint involved is the knee, while the first metatarsophalangeal (MTP) and DIP joints are most commonly involved in women. Radiographic evidence of DJD can be seen in up to 40 million Americans. Approximately 25 million will actually experience symptoms or dysfunction. The prevalence of DJD in patients over the age of 65 years is estimated to be 65%–85%.

Multiple risk factors for DJD have been proposed. The lack of prospective, well-controlled human studies, however, make definitive assessment of risk difficult. Proposed risk factors include:

- Age
- Previous injury, internal derangement, or both
- Obesity
- Gender (women may demonstrate a higher prevalence of DJD)

The question of whether exercise (such as jogging and sports) increases the risk of DJD of the knees, hips, and lumbar spine has not been fully answered. While anecdotal and retrospective studies imply an associated risk, the available prospective, controlled human studies do not support this. There *does* appear to be an increased risk of DJD in joints with internal derangement or biomechanical abnormalities.

DIFFERENTIAL DIAGNOSES

With the dearth of systemic signs and symptoms as well as the classic joint involvement, the diagnosis of DJD of a joint is relatively simple. Rheumatoid arthritis (RA) is usually associated with more redness and swelling of the joints and systemic symptoms (fever, weight changes, dermatologic changes, gastrointestinal symptoms). In addition, RA is associated with a different pattern of joint involvement with a predilection for the second through fifth MCP joints, wrists, elbows, shoulders, and MTP joints. Rheumatologic and collagen vascular disorders typically affect younger populations (ages 25–50). Gout, pseudogout, and Lyme disease should also be considered. Internal joint derangements, ligamentous injuries, and bony fractures can usually be detected by a good physical examination.

Generally, pain with resisted range of motion indicates a more musculotendinous cause of pain, while pain with passive range of motion indicates DJD.

DIAGNOSIS

The typical history and physical examination features assist with the diagnosis. Laboratory testing is only necessary if the diagnosis is unclear. The complete blood count (CBC), chemistry profile, and urinalysis are usually normal. Markers for inflammation (erythrocyte sedimentation rate [ESR], C-reactive protein) are usually normal, although they may be slightly elevated during the acute phase of erosive DJD. Rheumatoid factor (RF) and antinuclear antibody titers are normal. Radiographic evidence of DJD includes:

- Subchondral sclerosis and cysts
- Osteophyte formation
- Narrowing of joint space
- Deformity and malalignment

Occasionally, small intra-articular effusions may be present. If the diagnosis is still in question, a joint aspiration may be considered. Synovial fluid analysis may demonstrate clear-to-yellow color, few white blood cells ($< 300/\mu L$, $< 25\%$ neutrophils), negative culture, and fluid glucose roughly equal to serum.

TREATMENT

Mainstays of treatment include non-pharmacologic and pharmacologic measures.

Nonpharmacologic Management

- Weight-reduction techniques (a loss of just 5 kg may significantly decrease symptoms)
- Aerobic conditioning (low impact)
- Joint-specific physical therapy and rehabilitation (range of motion, stretching, strengthening exercises)
- Thermal and cryotherapy
- Emotional and social support
- Aids for activities of daily living, such as walkers or braces

> Because of the chronicity and risks from co-morbid conditions in this age group, nonpharmacologic measures may be more important than pharmacologic interventions.

Pharmacologic Management

Pharmacologic management includes acetaminophen, nonsteroidal anti-inflammatory drugs (NSAIDs), nonacetylated salicylates, opiates, corticosteroids, over-the-counter capsaicin or salicylate creams, and low-dose antidepressants. **Acetaminophen** should be the drug of choice. It has a good safety profile, and it is frequently effective. NSAIDs are commonly used and sometimes preferred by patients. Because of significant risk for gastric, renal, and hepatic toxicity with long-term use, consider the lowest effective doses, pulse therapy, or drug holidays. Toxicity is higher in the elderly.

Nonacetylated salicylates (e.g., salsalate and choline-magnesium-trisalicylate) are often overlooked but provide good analgesia. These medications do not inhibit prostaglandins that are protective to gastric mucosa. Opiates may be a short-term alternative for more severe pain. Keep in mind that opiates may be sedating, are addictive, and increase the risk of falls. Opiates generally should be avoided because of the long-term nature of the disease. Intra-articular injections of corticosteroids may offer modest benefit and should be used sparingly. Optimal dosing and frequency are not known, but many physicians suggest no more than 2–3 injections a year. Over-the-counter capsaicin or salicylate creams can be helpful for local joint pain, and low-dose antidepressants are sometimes helpful for chronic pain relief. Concurrent treatment of osteoporosis may also be helpful.

Surgery, such as hip or knee replacements, are appropriate for patients with substantial disability and joint abnormality.

PROGNOSIS

DJD is considered a progressive arthropathy. The rapidity of this progression, however, is highly variable. Progression is not guaranteed, and radiographic regression has been demonstrated in some patients.

SUGGESTED READING

Brandt KD: Nonsurgical management of osteoarthritis with an emphasis on nonpharmacologic measures. *Arch Fam Med* 4:1057–1064, 1995.

Griffin MR, Brandt KD, Liang MH, et al: Practical management of osteoarthritis—integration of pharmacologic and nonpharmacologic measures. *Arch Fam Med* 4:1049–1055, 1995.

Hellmann DB: Arthritis and musculoskeletal disorders. In *Current Medical Diagnosis and Treatment*, 36th ed. Edited by Tierney LM, McPhee SJ, Papadakis MA. Stanford, CT: Appleton & Lange, 1997, pp 750–799.

CHAPTER 69
Polymyalgia Rheumatica and Giant Cell Arteritis

David A. Simpson, M.D.

PATIENT 1

H. Maxwell, a 63-year-old women, complains of a 1½-month history of difficulty rising from her bed and chairs. She complains of localized pelvic and shoulder pain and stiffness mostly in the morning. Laboratory studies are significant for an erythrocyte sedimentation rate (ESR) of 75 mm/hr and a mild normochromic normocytic anemia.

CLINICAL PRESENTATION

Polymyalgia rheumatica (PMR) is a debilitating musculoskeletal syndrome of older patients and is characterized by pain and marked morning stiffness in the shoulders and pelvic girdle. Multiple studies suggest that many of the symptoms of PMR are secondary to a chronic low-grade synovitis that primarily affects the proximal joints. Low-grade fever, weight loss, malaise, and anorexia are common.

> Shoulder aches and an elevated ESR in an older person is highly suspicious for PMR.

PMR should be suspected in any elderly patients who have new acute onset of aching and stiffness in their shoulders, neck, and hips with or without systemic signs. The aching and stiffness should last longer than 1 month. There is no significant loss of muscle strength.

EPIDEMIOLOGY

Evidence suggests that the incidence of PMR and giant cell arteritis (GCA) varies with ethnicity, sex, and geography. Women are affected in a 2 to 1 ratio, and 95% of patients with PMR are Caucasian. Prevalence increases with advancing age. The etiology of both PMR and GCA remains unclear.

DIFFERENTIAL DIAGNOSIS

The relationship between PMR and GCA (also known as temporal arteritis [TA]) is now firmly established. Patients with GCA have a symptom complex consistent with PMR in approximately 50% of the cases, and some patients with PMR develop GCA. With this degree of overlap, it is sometimes difficult to make a clinical distinction between these two disease entities.

The variety of different presentations of PMR and GCA make the differential diagnosis extensive. Depression, early dementia, and fibromyalgia are all conditions associated with malaise, weight loss, and muscle aches. However, all are marked by a normal ESR and a lack of significant response to low-dose corticosteroids. Fever, appetite loss, and aching may represent an infectious process, but localizing signs, as well as an elevated white blood cell count, should suggest a specific site of infection. Certain malignancies may present with PMR- and GCA-like symptoms, especially diffuse hematologic malignancies or metastatic disease. Patients with these diseases do not respond to corticosteroids nor do they have a positive temporal artery biopsy.

Thyroid disease should be considered in the differential, as it may be associated with constitutional and musculoskeletal complaints. The ESR will be normal in these settings. Appropriate diagnostic hormonal testing should be pursued.

Rheumatic diseases should also be considered. Systemic lupus erythematosus (SLE) will be marked by a positive ESR, a positive antinuclear antibody (ANA), low complement levels, and some evidence of other organ system involvement. Rheumatoid arthritis (RA) is marked by a positive rheumatic factor (RF) and synovitis with profound stiffness, aching, or both. However, PMR is seronegative, does not involve peripheral joints, and never produces erosive changes in the joints. Polymyositis will cause true weakness on examination and will be accompanied by elevated muscle enzymes such as creatinine kinase.

DIAGNOSIS

An elevated ESR is the laboratory hallmark of PMR. More than 95% of patients present with an ESR of greater than 40 mm/hr at the time of disease activity. A diagnosis of PMR can be made in the face of a normal ESR but only if there is a clear history of the onset of new symptoms that is marked by morning stiffness, the exclusion of other diagnoses, and complete and prompt relief of symptoms with low-dose corticosteroids. Once the diagnosis is made and remission is achieved, the ESR is used as an aid in following PMR patients. C-reactive protein is a useful marker of disease activity. Approximately 60% of patients have a normochromic normocytic anemia, and 20%–55% show elevated liver enzymes especially alkaline phosphatase. These symptoms usually resolve with treatment.

TREATMENT

Prednisone is usually initiated at a single oral dose (10–20 mg/d). This is usually maintained for 2–4 weeks, at which time the dose is tapered by approximately 2.5 mg every 3 weeks until a dose of 10 mg/d is reached. Prednisone is then decreased by 1 mg/d monthly as tolerated by the patient. Mean duration of therapy with PMR is approximately 24 months.

PROGNOSIS

PMR is thought to be a self-limiting condition. Relapses while tapering steroid therapy are common, and more than half of one large panel of patients experienced at least one relapse.

PATIENT 2

B. Caldwell, a 65-year-old woman, complains of persistent bilateral frontal headaches for the past month. Her headaches worsened over the past week, and she notes visual blurring bilaterally, which is greater in her left eye. She has a loss of appetite secondary to pain in her jaws when she chews. Laboratory studies show a normochromic normocytic anemia and an ESR of 120 mm/hr. A temporal artery biopsy was positive for giant cells.

CLINICAL PRESENTATION

Giant cell arteritis (GCA) is a systemic vascular inflammatory disease involving medium- and large-sized arteries. It has a predilection for vessels originating from the aortic arch and the branches supplying the head, neck, and upper extremities. Only two-thirds of biopsies show evidence of giant cells; thus, absence of giant cells does not rule out the diagnosis.

Patients with GCA usually present with symptoms that are either of a nonspecific nature or are secondary to vascular ischemia, including headaches, fever, malaise, chronic depression, confusion, anorexia, weight loss, night sweats, fatigue, blurred vision, and jaw claudication.

> A new-onset headache in an elderly patient should make the physician suspicious of GCA.

Headache is the most common complaint of a patient with GCA. The headache can present in various locations and to variable degrees. The most common location is the temporal area and is described as throbbing. Pain can be either intermittent or continuous, and in most cases is severe and progressive in nature. The temporal artery may be swollen, nodular, pulseless, or indurated. Scalp tenderness in the area of the temporal artery occurs and can be elicited by washing, combing or brushing hair, resting the head on a pillow, or wearing a hat or eyeglasses. Jaw claudication is present in up to 50% of patients. The pain in the jaw is usually relieved after the person stops chewing.

A sore throat can occur secondary to a lesion in the ascending pharyngeal artery, causing pain in the internal pharyngeal muscles. Weight loss partially occurs when the patients only eat small amounts secondary to jaw pain while chewing.

Auricular pain is felt as an earache and occurs with involvement of the temporal or occipital arteries. Vestibular involvement can occur with vertigo, tinnitus, or nystagmus and can disappear spontaneously or with treatment.

Ophthalmologic involvement is the most dreaded presentation of GCA. Unilateral blindness occurs in up to 15%–20% of all cases of GCA and is followed by blindness in the second eye one-third of the time, usually within 7 days of the first eye. It is uncommon to have recovery of visual acuity once it is lost, but rapid (within 12–24 hours) intervention with corticosteroid therapy can at times spare vision. Blindness in GCA is predominantly because of ciliary artery involvement resulting in ischemic optic neuropathy. In some patients, intermittent blurred vision is reported as the initial symptom. Intracranial central nervous system symptoms are uncommon but include transient ischemic attacks (TIAs), hemorrhage, or infarct.

GCA can involve large- and medium-sized arteries outside the head and neck in 10%–15% of cases. Aortic valve insufficiency, aortic aneurysm, and rupture have been reported. Coronary involvement resulting in angina or myocardial infarction can occur, as well as mesenteric ischemia.

The patient's physical examination may be normal depending on the arteries that are involved. The key point is to palpate and auscultate all accessible arteries and to obtain blood pressures in each arm, looking for differences that suggest possible aneurysms.

EPIDEMIOLOGY

GCA is a form of vasculitis of unknown origin, affecting middle-aged and older adults. Although the etiology has not been established, certain environmental predispositions seem to exist. GCA is common in certain populations and certain geographic areas. There is an increased incidence in Northern European populations as well as northern regions of the United States.

GCA occurs up to seven times more frequently in Caucasians than in other races. Female sex predominates by a ratio of 5 to 2. It has been documented in multiple family situations including siblings, identical twins, and parent-child combinations.

DIAGNOSIS

No one laboratory test is diagnostic for GCA. The ESR is the most frequently used test and is greater than 40 mm/hr in more than 90% of patients. C-reactive protein, fibrinogens, and hapto-globin also act as acute phase reactants and frequently are elevated with disease activity and fall with disease quiescence. Anemia that is normochromic and normocytic can be present in 50% of patients. Other tests may be suggested by the patient's clinical presentation.

The test for a definitive diagnosis is a temporal artery biopsy. If GCA is clinically suspected, an ESR should be obtained. If there are any suspicions of GCA and no other cause of the patient's symptoms can be found, a temporal artery biopsy should be performed. It is best to obtain at least a 4-cm specimen of the artery because of the presence of skip areas. The overall sensitivity varies from 65%–97%. If the initial biopsy is negative and there remains a high index of suspicion for GCA, the second side should undergo biopsy. Bilateral biopsy increases the yield by 5%–10%. In a patient suspected of having GCA, particularly with any visual symptoms, corticosteroid treatment should not be withheld while awaiting biopsy results. The temporal artery biopsy can be obtained 1–5 days after starting corticosteroids.

TREATMENT

Steroids are the primary treatment. Prednisone is started at 60–90 mg once a day. Most patients experience a quick if not dramatic response. In the face of an abrupt loss of vision or progressive visual loss, patients have been given pulse intravenous doses of methyl-prednisolone in doses of 1000 mg over 1 hour daily, or 250 mg intravenously every 6 hours for 3–5 days. Once the patient's symptoms have resolved on the intravenous methylprednisolone, the patient may then be placed on oral prednisone at 90 mg/d, which can be reduced by 10 mg/d every 2–3 weeks until a dose of 30–40 mg/d is achieved. The dose can then be decreased by 5 mg/d every 2–3 weeks until a dose of 15–20 mg/d is reached.

Once a full remission is obtained, the ESR generally reverts to less than 50 mm/hr. ESR can be used to follow patients; however, more importantly, symptomatology should be followed, and prednisone should be increased for any suggestion of increased disease activity.

PROGNOSIS

GCA, in general, is self-limited, and most patients will be off treatment in 2 years.

SUGGESTED READING

Kelly WN, Harris ED: *Textbook of Rheumatology*, 4th ed. Philadelphia, PA: W. B. Saunders, 1993, pp 1103–1112.

Nordborg E: Giant cell arteritis. *Rheum Dis Clin North Am* 21(4): 1013–1025, 1995.

Silver RM: *Rheumatology Pearls*. Philadelphia, PA: Hanley and Belfus, 1997, pp 53–55.

CHAPTER 70
Fibromyalgia

Valerie P. Pendley, M.D.

PATIENT

G. Conway, a 27-year-old woman, comes to the office with the complaint of "feeling like an old lady" for the last 3 months. She feels achy all over, especially in the neck and shoulders, and her sleep is restless. Other symptoms include fatigue and morning stiffness lasting over 15 minutes. Her complaint seemed to coincide with starting a new aerobics class, which she subsequently stopped. She has returned to her usual sedentary life style. Anxiety and stress worsen her pain. A massage and a warm bath improve it. On physical examination, she has widespread tender areas on muscles without joint involvement. The rest of the examination is normal, including a normal complete blood count (CBC), erythrocyte sedimentation rate (ESR), and thyroid studies.

CLINICAL PRESENTATION

Fibromyalgia is primarily a syndrome without a well-defined pathophysiologic basis. It includes widespread pain of at least 3-months duration, tenderness on palpation of greater than 10 of 18 designated tender points, fatigue, and sleep disturbance. Other symptoms include morning stiffness, stiffness after a prolonged posture, headache, and paresthesia. Often anxiety or depression accompany this diagnosis. Stressful circumstances seem to worsen symptoms. Other aggravating factors include cold or humid weather, excessive physical activity, and conversely, lack of physical activity. A warm bath, warm and dry weather, restful sleep, and moderate physical activity relieve symptoms.

> **Symptoms of Fibromyalgia**
> Widespread pain
> Fatigue
> Morning stiffness lasting more than 15 minutes
> Sleep disturbance
> Paresthesias
> Headache
> Anxiety

EPIDEMIOLOGY

Fibromyalgia is more common in women, especially women between the ages of 20 and 50, although it can be found in adolescents and elderly women. At any given point in time, 3%–6% of the population meet the criteria for a diagnosis of fibromyalgia.

DIFFERENTIAL DIAGNOSIS

Fibromyalgia has many symptoms that overlap with numerous rheumatologic disorders. This overlap can lead to expensive and unnecessary testing. Recognizing a symptom complex and a careful history and physical examination will help to differentiate fibromyalgia from the following illnesses:

- **Myofascial pain syndrome**—a nonchronic, more localized disorder. This also has painful, tender areas in the involved muscles associated with a muscle twitch and a zone of referred pain.
- **Chronic fatigue syndrome (CFS)**—a chronic, persistent, disabling fatigue, often following a virus-like illness. Chronic fatigue syndrome can last months to years but is usually worse in its first year.
- **Multiple areas of bursitis** or **tendonitis, connective tissue disease** (rheumatoid arthritis, systemic lupus, polymyalgia rheumatica), **endocrine myopathy, drug-related myopathy,** and an **occult malignancy.**

DIAGNOSIS

A few simple tests are useful to exclude other diagnoses, mainly other rheumatologic, endocrine, or malignant disorders. Commonly used tests are CBC with differential, chemistry profile, thyroid-stimulating hormone (TSH) level, and ESR.

TREATMENT

Treatment of fibromyalgia includes pharmacologic as well as nonpharmacologic approaches. Treatment includes extensive patient education and change in behavior patterns. Education begins with acknowledgment of all symptoms. Patients should be told that death or serious damage will not occur despite the pain they are experiencing. Although no cure is available, the course of fibromyalgia is likely to be chronic and fluctuating, and treatment requires an active role by the patient. Behavior modification should emphasize improvement of sleep by encouraging sleep hygiene techniques, biofeedback, and stress reduction. Moderate exercise, especially low-impact aerobics and stretching exercises, beginning at a very low level and increasing slowly, works best. Pharmacologic treatment includes low-dose tricyclic antidepressants such as amitriptyline (25 mg) taken 2–3 hours before bedtime.

PROGNOSIS

Often fibromyalgia resolves after several months only to return 1 or 2 years later, initiated by stress, trauma, or an overzealous initial attempt at an exercise program.

SUGGESTED READING

American College of Rheumatology: 1990 criteria for the classification of fibromyalgia, report of the Multicenter Criteria Committee. *Arthritis Rheum* 33:160–172, 1990.

CHAPTER 71
Chronic Fatigue Syndrome

Judith A. Long M.D., and Eileen E. Reynolds, M.D.

PATIENT

C. Lang, a 36-year-old woman, was in good health until she suffered an acute viral illness 3 years ago. Since then she has never felt well. Her main symptoms are postexertional fatigue, difficulty concentrating, myalgias, weakness, and forgetfulness. She sleeps 10–12 hours a night but wakes up unrested. During the first year of her illness she felt tired all the time. Since then she has had a waxing and waning course, although she is far from her baseline. She lost her job, lost her apartment, and has moved back in with her parents. At the end of her first year of illness, she experienced an episode of major depression.

CLINICAL PRESENTATION

There are no physical findings or laboratory tests that define chronic fatigue syndrome (CFS), thus it is a diagnosis of exclusion. In 1988 the Centers for Disease Control and Prevention (CDC) developed a working case definition, which was updated in 1994. The definition requires a complaint of chronic (> 6 months), disabling fatigue that is not explained by a medical or psychiatric diagnosis. In addition, the patient must complain of four out of eight possible minor symptoms: impaired memory or concentration, sore throat, painful nodes, muscle pain,

> Only think chronic fatigue syndrome if fatigue has been present for at least 6 months.

arthralgias, new headaches, unrefreshing sleep, or postexertional malaise. Although the fatigue must not be explained by a medical or psychiatric illness, there are certain conditions that do not exclude the diagnosis of CFS. These are well-treated diseases or disorders defined solely by symptoms (anxiety disorders, fibromyalgia, somatoform disorders, uncomplicated major depression, multiple chemical sensitivity disorder). Thus, one can be diagnosed with both depression and CFS.

The main symptom of CFS is profound fatigue. The patient in the case has had disabling fatigue for 3 years and has five of eight symptoms; thus she meets the CDC's definition of CFS. In addition her social functioning has been greatly diminished, and she has experienced depression during her illness. All of these findings are typical of CFS.

ETIOLOGY

No known cause of CFS exists, although speculations abound. At this time, there are four main theories postulating that CSF is:

- An infectious disease
- The result of immune dysfunction
- A neuroendocrine disease
- A psychiatric entity

Each theory has some evidence to support it, but a direct link to the disease has not been made. The cause of CFS remains unclear.

CFS patients have a higher prevalence of psychiatric diseases than the general population. One-fourth to one-half of patients are estimated to have evidence of a preexisting psychiatric disorder (dysthymia, major depression, generalized anxiety disorder, panic disorder, somatoform disorder). One-half of CFS patients experience depression, anxiety disorder, or both during their lifetime. CFS is a depressing illness. Not only is it debilitating, but there is no known cause, and treatment is poor. All patients with chronic medical disorders have higher rates of depression than their healthy counterparts, and these rates increase when findings or symptoms are unexplained. Providers must remember that psychiatric disease often presents with fatigue, and they must evaluate and treat any psychiatric disorders before making the diagnosis of CFS.

EPIDEMIOLOGY

Fatigue is common; it is reported by up to one-fourth of patients seeking medical care. On the other hand, CFS, as defined by the CDC, is rare. In a large population-based study, the point prevalence of CFS was one person in a thousand.

The workup for CFS is straightforward: a good history, a physical examination, and basic screening laboratory tests. Further evaluation is dictated by clinical suspicion.

DIAGNOSIS

Since there is no known etiology of CFS, a diagnostic evaluation should be simple and should focus on excluding other treatable illnesses. The physician should perform a thorough history and physical examination and pay special attention to medical and psychosocial circumstances. Depression or other psychiatric disorders, episodes of medically unexplained symptoms, or substance abuse should be determined. The physician should also ask about the use of prescription or over-the-counter medications or food supplements that may contribute to symptoms. A mental status examination to identify abnormalities in mood, intellectual function, and personality should also be completed. The CDC recommends a minimum battery of screening tests to rule out other medical illness: complete blood count (CBC), erythrocyte sedimentation rate (ESR), liver function tests (LFTs), albumin, total protein, calcium, phosphorus, glucose, electrolytes, blood urea nitrogen (BUN), creatinine, thyroid-stimulating hormone (TSH), and urinalysis. Additional tests should be ordered only as indicated to confirm or exclude another suspected diagnosis. Since there is not enough evidence to implicate CFS as an infectious disease or as a result of immune dysfunction, viral markers (e.g., cytomegalovirus [CMV] or Epstein-Barr virus [EBV]) or immune cell levels (e.g., CD_4 or CD_8) should not be ordered. They are expensive and can neither confirm nor exclude the diagnosis.

TREATMENT

At present there is no treatment specifically for CFS. Many treatments have been studied and reported, but the results are inconclusive. Often initial studies have shown promising responses to therapies, but when followed by placebo-controlled trials, results have been disappointing. One promising therapy undergoing study is treating patients as though they have neurocardiogenic syncope. Patients are treated with fludrocortisone, a diet high in salt, and beta-blockers or disopyramide (either alone or in combination). Initial results have been promising but further, more rigorous studies are required.

Currently, most care is directed towards reducing symptoms. Although antidepressants have not been formally studied in CFS patients, they are the mainstay of treatment because they help ameliorate symptoms of fatigue in depressed patients, they have been proven effective in treating fibromyalgia (a disorder with many symptoms similar to CFS), and they alleviate depression (which may be a concomitant, exacerbating disorder in CFS patients). The most frequently used antidepressants for CFS are doxepin and amitriptyline. For many CFS patients normal doses can be intolerable; providers should start patients at the lowest dose possible and increase slowly.

Other symptomatic treatments include anti-inflammatory agents for generalized aches and pains, anxiolytics for anxiety, muscle relaxants for muscle spasms, and graded exercise regimens to improve exercise tolerance. Behavioral therapy aimed at modifying disease perception may also benefit the patient. Many patients who have found no relief through Western medicine have turned to other medical approaches such as acupuncture and Chinese herbs. Support groups and information services abound, and they often provide information for patients and practitioners regarding alternative methods.

Finally, forging an alliance with patients and showing a willingness to search for the most efficacious treatment for them is paramount. Both physician and patient must come to accept that treatment responses to known therapies are variable and that although, over time, many patients improve, return to premorbid functioning is uncommon.

PROGNOSIS

CFS waxes and wanes and is a disabling disease with a poor chance for complete recovery. Psychiatric disease is common in CFS patients, but in general, its presence does not predict who will improve and who will remain debilitated. Although return to premorbid function is rare, over time most patients improve.

SUGGESTED READING

Epstein KR: The chronically fatigued patient. *Med Clin North Am* 79(2):315–327, 1995.

McKenzie R, Straus SE: Chronic fatigue syndrome. *Adv Intern Med* 40:119–153, 1995.

CHAPTER 72
Acute and Chronic Renal Failure

Peter DeLong, M.D., and Lisa M. Bellini, M.D.

PATIENT 1

S. Wells, a 70-year-old woman with congestive heart failure (CHF), presents to the office with a 1-week history of dizziness when she stands up. She has been in her apartment for 6 days without air conditioning. She says she has been taking extra doses of her "water pills" because she thought they would help her feel better. She notes that she has been urinating less than normal and that her shoes fit better than usual. Her laboratory tests reveal a blood urea nitrogen level (BUN) of 50 mg/dL and a creatine level of 4.5 mg/dL.

CLINICAL PRESENTATION

Acute renal failure (ARF) is defined as a sudden decrease in glomerular filtration and renal function that causes an increase in creatinine and nitrogenous waste. It is often reversible. Many clinical situations can cause ARF, and symptoms and therapy vary with each cause. Thus, there is no classic clinical presentation specific for ARF.

The most common symptom is a decreased urine output, which occurs in about 70% of cases. While this is not a specific finding for diagnosis, it is useful to quantitate the urine output and classify it as oliguric (< 400 mL/d) or nonoliguric (> 400 mL/d). Patients with nonoliguric failure have a better prognosis than those with oliguric failure. About 40% of patients with ARF require dialysis, but only about 25% of these patients require long-term dialysis. Common late manifestations of renal failure include uremia, hyperkalemia, acidosis, and complications of volume overload.

> ARF is classified as prerenal, intrinsic, or postrenal.

ETIOLOGY

ARF is classified according to the three major steps of urine production.

1. Blood is delivered to the kidney to be filtered by the glomerulus. ARF resulting from clinical causes of decreased blood flow is classified as *prerenal*.

2. Blood is filtered, and the ultrafiltrate is processed by the tubules in the kidney. ARF resulting from factors adversely affecting the glomerulus and tubules is classified as *intrinsic*.

3. Urine is excreted through the ureters, bladder, and urethra. ARF resulting from problems with these structures is classified as *postrenal*.

Prerenal ARF

The most common form of ARF is prerenal. It accounts for approximately 50% of all ARF cases and approximately 70% of community-acquired cases. The elderly are at increased risk for prerenal ARF because of their tendency to become hypovolemic; their increased incidence of renal artery atherosclerotic disease; and the gradual, functional decline in renal function that occurs as a natural consequence of aging. The causes of prerenal failure can be further classified based on the mechanisms of decreased renal artery perfusion.

- *Inadequate circulating blood volume* is due to hypovolemia. Symptoms and signs include nausea, vomiting, diarrhea, fever, dizziness, palpitations, dry mucous membranes, tachycardia, decreased blood pressure, and cool extremities.

- *Cardiovascular problems* such as inadequate cardiac output, renal vascular disease, and drug effects also cause prerenal failure. Symptoms and signs of CHF include shortness of breath, dyspnea on exertion, angina, elevated neck veins, a third heart sound (S_3), abdominojugular reflux, and lower extremity edema. The most important renal vascular diseases are renal artery stenosis, seen in younger women, and atherosclerotic disease, seen in older men. Drug effects are a very important cause. Angiotensin-converting enzyme inhibitors (ACEIs) dilate the efferent blood supply to the glomerulus, making the kidney more preload dependent. Nonsteroidal anti-inflammatory drugs (NSAIDs) can have a similar effect.

Intrinsic ARF

The major categories of intrinsic ARF are ATN, interstitial diseases, and glomerular diseases.

This is the least common form of ARF in the ambulatory setting. This type can be subdivided into acute tubular necrosis (ATN), interstitial diseases, and glomerular diseases.

- *Acute tubular necrosis (ATN)* is the most common cause of intrinsic ARF. It can be further classified as *ischemic* (related to low circulating blood volumes), *toxic* (related to the use of antimicrobial agents, contrast dyes, chemotherapeutic agents, 3-hydroxy-3-methylglutaryl coenzyme A [HMG-CoA] reductase inhibitors, cocaine), and as myoglobinuria resulting from rhabdomyolysis. ATN typically occurs in three stages: (1) urine output diminishes within 24–48 hours of the injury, and the patient remains oliguric for about a week (the timing is variable); (2) urine output gradually returns to normal; and (3) there is a polyuric phase, which indicates some degree of persistent tubular damage.
- *Interstitial disease* can result from the use of certain drugs, systemic vasculitis, or infections such as pyelonephritis. Drugs are a primary cause and include NSAIDs, loop diuretics, and antimicrobial agents (e.g., penicillins, cephalosporins, sulfonamides).
- *Glomerular diseases* are the least common cause of intrinsic ARF and include post-streptococcal glomerulonephritis, rapidly progressive glomerulonephritis, nephrotic syndrome, Wegener's granulomatosis, and Goodpasture's syndrome.

Postrenal ARF

ARF resulting from postrenal causes frequently presents in an ambulatory setting and is directly related to the anatomy of the urinary collecting system. Symptoms are secondary to urinary obstruction or to an underlying disorder. Postrenal ARF can be further classified as intrarenal or extrarenal.

- *Intrarenal causes* include renal calculi, papillary necrosis, and crystal accumulation. The latter is seen as a complication of acyclovir, sulfonamides, or ethylene glycol intoxication.
- *Extrarenal causes* include benign prostatic hypertrophy, tumors of the urinary tract, and extrinsic compression of the ureter resulting from tumor or retroperitoneal fibrosis.

DIFFERENTIAL DIAGNOSIS

The diagnosis of ARF is based on a thorough history and physical examination. Risk factors for acute renal failure, particularly prerenal ARF, include age, a history of diabetes, prior renal insufficiency, and dehydration. Concurrent hemoptysis suggests Wegener's granulomatosis or Goodpasture's syndrome. Bone pain, symptoms of anemia, and frequent infections should suggest multiple myeloma. Recent hot weather in the setting of diuretic use should suggest dehydration. A recent contrast dye exposure should suggest dye-induced ATN. A careful medication history must be obtained and should include questions on over-the-counter medications. The presence of a rash may suggest allergic interstitial nephritis. An elevated blood pressure may suggest malignant hypertension.

DIAGNOSIS

In the absence of an obvious cause, the initial workup should proceed systematically. Volume status should be evaluated first, followed by elimination of obstruction as a cause. Urine flow should be documented, and the patient should be catheterized if necessary. Finally, intrinsic disease should be considered (Table 72-1).

The evaluation of a patient with suspected ARF should begin with a urinalysis, an inexpensive screening tool. Urine indexes, including urine osmolarity, sodium concentration (Na^+), and fractional excretion of Na^+ ($FeNa^+$), differentiate between prerenal and intrinsic ARF. $FeNa^+$ is the fraction of filtered Na^+ in the urine. Values less than 1 imply a prerenal cause; values greater than 1 imply a renal cause.

$$FeNa^+ = \frac{urine\ Na^+}{plasma\ Na^+} \div \frac{urine\ creatinine}{plasma\ creatinine} \times 100$$

TABLE 72-1
ACUTE RENAL FAILURE

Site of Process	Urinalysis Findings	Osmolarity (osmoles/L)	FeNa$^+$
Prerenal	Normal, possibly some hyaline casts	>500	<1
Intrinsic			
Tubular (ischemia or toxin)	Pigmented "muddy brown" granular casts	<350	>1
Interstitial	White blood cell (WBC) casts, eosinophils, and red blood cells (RBCs)	<350	>1
Glomerulonephritis	RBC casts and protein	>500	<1
Postrenal	Crystals, WBCs, and RBCs	<350	>1

Following the urinalysis, an assessment of serum chemistry, including creatinine, BUN, Na^+, potassium (K^+), and bicarbonate (HCO_3^-), should be performed. Later, antinuclear antibody, calcium (Ca^{2+}), uric acid, and creatine kinase can be obtained according to clinical suspicion. Imaging studies such as renal ultrasound or a renal computed tomography (CT) scan can identify obstruction, stones, or suggest acute presentations of a chronic problem. For example, the small kidneys in a diabetic patient suggest medical renal disease from longstanding diabetes. Renal biopsy is useful in determining the etiology of an intrinsic renal disease that remains unclear after other diagnostic tests are performed. Most patients undergo biopsy prior to the use of immunosuppressive medications.

TREATMENT

ARF can often be prevented by adequate hydration of patients at risk (the elderly, patients with a history of diabetes or renal insufficiency), especially before surgical procedures and studies using radiocontrast dye. It is also important to avoid or discontinue drugs that reduce renal function.

Management of ARF centers on reversing the cause of renal failure and correcting any fluid and electrolyte abnormalities. This requires hospitalization. A daily assessment of creatinine, BUN, K^+, and HCO_3^- is performed until renal function stabilizes or improves. Urine output and fluid intake should be monitored. Daily weights can assist in the determination of fluid status. Fluid should be restricted to a volume equal to urine output plus approximately 500 mL/d. If the patient is oliguric, addition of diuretics will not change the prognosis but may make the management of volume status easier. Volume as normal saline should be given to patients who are hypovolemic. All nonessential medications with a potential for decreasing renal function should be discontinued. Hyperkalemia should be treated promptly, as many patients with ARF are elderly and less able to tolerate the cardiac arrhythmias associated with hyperkalemia. If phosphate (PO_4^-) is elevated, PO_4^- binders can be started to keep $PO_4^- < 5.5$ mg/dL. Specific conditions may respond to steroids or immunosuppressive therapy.

Dialysis may be considered as an emergent therapy in selected patients. The list of conditions for which emergent dialysis is appropriate is short and includes acidosis, electrolyte abnormality (hyperkalemia), ingestion of toxic substances, volume overload in patients with poor cardiovascular reserve, and symptomatic uremia (e.g., mental status changes, pericardial rub).

PATIENT 2

J. Barker, a 67-year-old man with a 17-year history of diabetes mellitus type 1 (type 1 DM), presents to the office with weight gain, hypertension, and fatigue. He has not seen his physician for a year. He was told during his last visit that his kidneys were not working well. His wife says that he is "not on top of things" anymore and that he is eating poorly. She also says that he seems to itch all over. His laboratory tests reveal a BUN of 85 mg/dL and a creatine of 6.7 mg/dL.

CLINICAL PRESENTATION

Chronic renal failure (CRF) involves the progressive loss of all renal functions, but its development is usually staged by the degree of uremia present. It can be broken down functionally into three stages: diminished renal reserve, renal insufficiency, and uremia.

1. *Diminished renal reserve* is identified by a chronically decreased glomerular filtration rate (GFR) and is usually asymptomatic.
2. *Renal insufficiency* is marked by elevated BUN and serum creatinine.
3. *Uremia* occurs when renal insufficiency has progressed to the point where symptoms develop.

The clinical syndrome of uremia resulting from an elevated BUN affects the neurologic system, the gastrointestinal (GI) tract, the cardiovascular system, the hematologic system, and the skin. Neurologically, patients develop muscle twitches, cramps, and a metabolic encephalopathy. GI manifestations include nausea, vomiting, anorexia, and an unpleasant taste in the mouth. Patients often develop malnutrition. Cardiovascular effects include hypertension, lower extremity edema, and occasionally CHF secondary to hypervolemia. Pericarditis is often seen in chronic (and sometimes acute) uremia. Hematologic abnormalities include poor platelet function and GI bleeding. Finally, the skin may become a yellow-brown color and itch. Sweat from patients with uremia may crystallize into what is called "uremic frost."

> ESRD refers to chronic renal failure resulting in acid–base and electrolyte derangements, endocrine deficiencies, volume overload, and the syndrome of uremia.

End-stage renal disease (ESRD) refers to CRF that has resulted in acid–base and electrolyte derangements, endocrine deficiencies, and volume overload in addition to the syndrome of uremia. Serum chemistry abnormalities other than increased BUN and creatinine levels include a metabolic acidosis, hyperkalemia, hyperphosphatemia, hyperuricemia, and hypermagnesemia. Hypertriglyceridemia is also a common finding. Endocrine abnormalities include a failure to convert vitamin D to its active form $(1,25[OH]_2D_3)$, secondary hyperparathyroidism, and decreased erythropoietin secretion. Lack of erythropoietin causes a normocytic anemia. The increased parathyroid hormone (PTH) causes osteitis fibrosa cystica, a syndrome involving subperiosteal erosions and bone cysts. Lack of vitamin D causes osteomalacia, known as "renal rickets."

EPIDEMIOLOGY

There are approximately 200,000 dialysis patients in the United States. Incidence increases with age and is four times greater in African Americans and Hispanics. The major causes of CRF are diabetes (30%), hypertension (25%), and chronic glomerulonephritis (approximately 15%). It occurs in approximately 40% of all insulin-dependent diabetic patients after a mean of 10 years.

DIAGNOSIS

CRF is suspected in patients with an underlying disorder (e.g., diabetes, hypertension) that can affect the kidneys with the symptoms described above. The diagnosis is confirmed by the laboratory findings of nitrogen retention, elevated creatinine level, acidosis, hyperkalemia, hyperphosphatemia, and hypocalcemia.

TREATMENT

Initially, CRF may be controlled by managing its complications. It is necessary to monitor physical signs and symptoms of volume overload, mental status, and anemia. Intake of Na^+ and water must be limited. Antihypertensives may be required to control blood pressure. Serum chemistry and blood counts should be obtained on presentation and followed regularly. If anemia is severe, blood transfusions may be required. K^+ levels must be monitored and lowered with binding resins if high. HCO_3^- may be necessary to control the metabolic acidosis. Uremia can be partially controlled by adherence to a low-protein diet, which should be instituted in all patients with ESRD. Restriction of protein can reduce nausea and vomiting, lethargy, and encephalopathy. PO_4^- can be limited in the diet also, but a PO_4^- binder is usually employed because a PO_4^--free diet is unpalatable. Supplements are used to replace calcium, vitamin D, and erythropoietin. Diabetic patients usually need to have their dose of insulin reduced to avoid hypoglycemia. All renally cleared medications need dose adjustments to prevent toxicity, mostly in patients with mild renal insufficiency.

> All renally cleared medications need dose adjustments to prevent toxicity, mostly in patients with mild renal insufficiency.

When these measures fail to control the manifestations of uremia, acidosis, and electrolyte imbalance, dialysis is necessary. (It is important to note that dialysis does not treat the endocrine deficits of renal failure.) Dialysis is the process of separating soluble elements by diffusion across a semipermeable membrane. Thus, nitrogenous wastes, K^+, hydrogen (H^+), and other accumulated substances can be removed from the blood when the kidneys do not function. There are two types of dialysis: hemodialysis and peritoneal dialysis.

> The two types of dialysis are hemodialysis and peritoneal dialysis.

In *hemodialysis*, blood is removed from the body, pumped through a membrane unit that allows diffusion of the above-mentioned substances, and then returned to the body. This must be performed at a dialysis center. Access is obtained through surgically placed arteriovenous fistulas. Heparin is required to prevent clotting of blood in the lines. A treatment usually lasts about 3–5 hours. Advantages of hemodialysis include a three times per week schedule; rapid and efficient removal of accumulated toxins; correction of hypervolemia, acidosis, and hyperkalemia; and improvement of uremic symptoms. Disadvantages include complications such as infection at the site of access, hypotension and chest pain from excessive fluid removal, bleeding from the heparin load, hypokalemia and hyponatremia, restlessness, muscle cramps, pruritus, and seizures. The only contraindication is active bleeding.

Peritoneal dialysis relies on the peritoneum to act as a semipermeable membrane. Fluid is instilled into the peritoneum through a permanent catheter, allowed to "dwell" for a period of time, and then is removed. Instillation and removal can be performed manually (continuous ambulatory peritoneal dialysis [CAPD]) or by automated cycler. CAPD uses long "dwell" times, so fluid is exchanged three or four times a day. Automated cyclers can be set to cycle at night, leaving the patient free during the day. Peritoneal dialysis has the advantages of being administered by the patient at home and being mobile (patients can travel for several days with their own dialysis setup). Disadvantages include complications such as peritonitis, cellulitis at the site of the catheter, abscess in the catheter tract, inadequate glucose control, leakage of dialysate around the catheter, poor catheter flow resulting from clots, hypotension, hypoalbuminemia, pulmonary edema, peritoneal sclerosis, small bowel obstruction, and inguinal hernias.

SUGGESTED READING

Andreoli TE: Acute and chronic renal failure. In *Cecil's Essentials of Medicine*, 3rd ed. Philadelphia, PA: W. B. Saunders, 1993, pp 238–252.

Editor: *Merck Manual*, 16th ed. Rahway, NJ: Merck, 1992, pp 1661–1677.

Humes HD, Messana JM: Approach to the patient with oliguria and acute renal failure. In *Textbook of Internal Medicine*. Edited by Kelley WN. Philadelphia, PA: Lippincott-Raven, 1997, pp 929–936.

CHAPTER 73
Peripheral Neuropathy

Marjorie A. Bowman, M.D., M.P.A.

PATIENT

J. Sever, a 45-year-old man, fell from his bike 4 days ago. He injured his right arm with diffuse bruises, contusions, and swelling around the elbow. There were no fractures, and his treatment was ice, wound measures, and rest. He complains of numbness and tingling in the fourth and fifth fingers of the right hand with intact muscle strength.

CLINICAL PRESENTATION

There are several types of neuropathies, such as cranial, sympathetic, autonomic, or peripheral neuropathies with many causes. Peripheral neuropathy refers to sensory problems, motor problems, or both in the peripheral nervous system.

EPIDEMIOLOGY

The most common peripheral neuropathies in primary care practice are probably disk compression syndromes, carpal tunnel syndrome, and diabetic neuropathy. It is estimated that over half of diabetic patients have neuropathy. Table 73-1 lists common types of peripheral neuropathy seen in primary care practice.

TABLE 73-1
COMMON PERIPHERAL NEUROPATHIES IN PRIMARY CARE PRACTICE

Pressure, entrapment, and trauma neuropathies
  Carpal tunnel syndrome (associated with overuse, hypothyroidism, autoimmune disease, pregnancy)
  Ulnar palsy (cubital tunnel syndrome)
  Meralgia paresthetica (lateral femoral cutaneous nerve, upper outer thigh)
  Tarsal tunnel syndrome
  Cervical or lumbar disk
  Common peroneal nerve palsy
  Morton's neuroma (plantar nerve between third and fourth toes)
  Thoracic outlet syndrome
Diabetic neuropathy
Postherpetic neuralgia
Vitamin B_{12} deficiency (alcoholism, diet, pernicious anemia)

TABLE 73-1 (CONTINUED)

Neuropathy associated with alcoholism (direct toxic effects; thiamine, folate, or vitamin B_{12} deficiencies; and pressure palsies resulting from prolonged compression of a nerve during blackouts)
Human immunodeficiency virus (frequency depends on risk factors of the practice's patient population)
Chemotherapy-induced
Uremic polyneuropathy

DIAGNOSIS

The patient usually complains of numbness, tingling, burning pain, or other descriptions of dysesthesias and may have concurrent motor weakness. It is common for diabetic patients to have detectable neuropathy (loss of vibration sense, loss of ankle reflexes) without complaints. Less complete compression is associated with milder sensory complaints, such as partial numbness, with more complete compression associated with more complete numbness and accompanying motor complaints.

For local compression or traumatic neuropathies, the sensory and motor problems are in the anatomic territory of the compressed nerve or nerves. For many toxic or metabolic causes of peripheral neuropathy, the complaints are more diffuse, less anatomically specific, and worse distally. For example, the feet are primarily affected in diabetic neuropathy, and a stocking–glove distribution is often found with vitamin B_{12} deficiency.

The physical examination can be normal in early or mild neuropathies; the sensory complaints appear before the damage is severe enough to be readily detected on examination. Thus, if the patient complains of numbness in a specific distribution, but this distribution cannot be verified on examination, it still can truly be present and represent an organic problem. Similarly, some motor weakness can be detected by a patient before it is detectable on examination. Complete sensory loss or marked motor deficiencies can be detected through light touch testing and muscle resistance testing. Visual inspection can detect muscle wasting.

The diagnosis is frequently made on clinical history and physical examination alone, such as for diabetic neuropathy and mild carpal tunnel syndrome. However, the presence of neuropathy can be confirmed through peripheral nerve conduction studies and electromyelograms. The cause of the neuropathy may need to be determined more specifically with laboratory tests, including: thyroid-stimulating hormone (TSH), serum vitamin B_{12}, red blood cell folate, serum or urine methylmalonic acid, heavy metal screening, human immunodeficiency virus (HIV) testing, complete blood count, erythrocyte sedimentation rate, serum protein electrophoresis, electrolytes, blood urea nitrogen (BUN), creatinine, liver function tests, rheumatoid factor, antinuclear antibody, blood glucose, glycosylated hemoglobin, or chest x-ray (Table 73-2). The exact testing will depend on what disorders are suggested by a complete history and physical examination.

TABLE 73-2
CAUSES OF PERIPHERAL NEUROPATHIES

Toxic	**Inflammatory**
Heavy metals: lead, arsenic, thallium, and mercury	Rheumatoid arthritis Polyarteritis nodosa Sarcoidosis
Drugs: phenytoin, vincristine, high-dose pyridoxine, cisplatin, nitrofurantoin, and alcohol	**Vitamin deficiencies** Vitamin B_{12} Folate
Chemicals: organophosphates, methyl alcohol, and benzenes	Thiamine
Metabolic	**Ischemia**
Diabetes	**Cancer associated**
Uremia	Multiple myeloma
Hypothyroidism	Paraproteinemias
Infectious	Cancer of the lung
Human immunodeficiency virus	**Genetic**
Lyme disease	Charcot-Marie-Tooth disease
Leprosy (important international cause)	Friedreich's ataxia Porphyria
Diphtheria	**Mixed or other**
Postherpetic	Amyloidosis
Local compression, entrapment, or trauma	Idiopathic

TREATMENT

Treatment specific to the cause of the peripheral neuropathy should be the first priority. Diabetic patients should tightly control their blood glucose. Vitamin B_{12} deficiency should be treated with vitamin B_{12} replacement (oral or intramuscular). With alcoholism, alcohol treatment should be initiated. For other toxic neuropathies, exposure to the inciting agent should be stopped. There are many treatments for the more ongoing, symptomatic neuropathies such as diabetic neuropathy. Common treatments include:

- Capsaicin, an over-the-counter cream made of an extract of hot peppers
- Amitriptyline in low doses (10–75 mg) or other antidepressants
- Phenytoin, carbamazepine, or clonazepam (for shooting or lightning pain)

Simple analgesics, antiarrhythmic drugs, and opioids are also used.

For patients with anesthesia of the extremities, care should be taken to prevent injury. For example, shoes should fit well, and patients should be cautious of objects or footwear that might injure a foot. Water temperatures for baths should be checked before entry. Physical therapy can be useful for muscular weakness, and splints are sometimes indicated.

PREVENTION AND SCREENING

There is no routine screening for peripheral neuropathies in the general population. However, it is useful to ask questions and examine the lower extremities of diabetic patients to look for early signs and symptoms of peripheral neuropathy. Monofilaments are useful for testing sensory loss in diabetic patients. For prevention, many industries have designed programs to prevent toxic exposure or to help prevent carpal tunnel syndrome, such as by providing ergonomically correct work stations.

SUGGESTED READING

Emanuele NV: Diabetic neuropathy: therapies for peripheral and autonomic symptoms. *Geriatrics* 52:40–49, 1997.

Lipnick JA, Lee TH: Diabetic neuropathy. *Am Fam Phys* 54:2478–2484, 1996.

Venna N: Peripheral neuropathies. In *Primary Care Medicine*, 2nd ed. Edited by Noble J. Philadelphia, PA: Mosby, 1996, pp 1408–1431.

CHAPTER 74
Epilepsy

Sarah A. Stahmer M.D.

PATIENT

A. Mitchell, a 45-year-old woman, is referred for evaluation after being treated in a local emergency department for her first seizure. Her medical history reveals that she has had a number of episodes of focal arm twitching associated with brief lapses in memory over the past few years, which have never been formally evaluated. Two days ago she experienced similar symptoms, which progressed to generalized tonic-clonic activity. She was taken to the emergency department and was evaluated by laboratory tests, toxin screen, and head computed tomography (CT) scan—all of which were normal. Her physical examination at that time was also "nonfocal." She was discharged with instructions not to drive and to follow up with her family physician within a week. At the present time she feels well with no interim seizure activity. The patient denies a history of alcohol dependence, recent or past head injury, or significant co-morbidities.

CLINICAL PRESENTATION

The classification of epilepsy is based on whether the seizure activity is *focal* (localized to a particular brain region or focus) or *generalized*. Focal seizure activity, also referred to as partial seizures, can be either simple or complex depending on whether the patient has an associated alteration in level of consciousness. Many patients describe an aura prior to the onset of seizure activity. This aura represents the spread of a partial seizure from simple to complex. The aura varies from patient to patient and has been described as a "sinking feeling," flashing lights, disagreeable taste or odor, lip or finger numbness, tingling, involuntary movements, or twitching. Partial seizures may clinically manifest as involuntary movements or sensations, which may be associated with a period of unresponsiveness, staring, or eye deviation.

Generalized seizures can either be primarily generalized or begin as partial seizures and subsequently spread to both cortical hemispheres. The clinical manifestations of generalized seizures can vary from periods of inattention or unresponsiveness, as in absence seizures, to full-blown, tonic-clonic movements associated with grand-mal seizures. These relatively broad categories are broken down into subcategories (Table 74-1). Accurately classifying an individual patient's seizure disorder helps to guide the choice and timing of anticonvulsant therapy.

TABLE 74-1
SEIZURE CLASSIFICATION

Partial seizures
  Simple partial seizures
    With motor symptoms
    With sensory symptoms
    With psychic or autonomic symptoms
  Complex partial seizures
    Beginning as simple partial seizures
    Beginning with impairment of consciousness
    With secondary generalization
Generalized seizures
  Absence
  Atonic
  Tonic
  Clonic
  Tonic-clonic
  Myoclonic
Unclassified seizures

EPIDEMIOLOGY

Epilepsy is a condition of recurrent seizures, which have no apparent cause. This is distinctly different from seizures that occur in the setting of acute head injury, toxin ingestion, hemodynamic instability, or metabolic derangement. Seizures occurring under such conditions usually resolve with treatment of the underlying process, are unlikely to recur, and rarely require chronic treatment. Approximately 0.5%–1% of the United States population has epilepsy.

DIAGNOSIS

Patients usually appear well between seizures. The role of the physician is to search for an underlying cause, which can be found in up to 50% of patients, and to initiate and monitor anticonvulsant therapy. A neurologist can help determine if the patient truly has epilepsy, classify the type of epilepsy, and guide initial and "breakthrough" drug therapy. Subsequent management of patients with epilepsy is usually performed by the primary care physician. The initial evaluation should include:

- A detailed history of the seizure:

    Prodrome. Symptoms (such as headache or nausea) experienced in the days prior to the seizure

Aura. Symptoms that immediately precede the seizure

Behavior. Behavior exhibited during the seizure

Postictal State. Duration, focal symptoms (headache), and signs (paralysis)

Triggers. Recent stressors, diet changes, menstrual history, loud noises, and flashing lights

- A complete medical history including head trauma, family history of seizures, toxin exposures, and co-morbid conditions, particularly in the elderly
- A complete physical examination with vital signs
- A complete neurologic examination
- Head CT scan, magnetic resonance imaging (MRI), or both to exclude structural causes of seizures
- Electroencephalogram (EEG) preferably when the patient is awake and sleeping (Photostimulation and sphenoidal and anterior temporal electrodes may increase diagnostic yield.)

TREATMENT

Most patients with true epilepsy (i.e., multiple seizures) require chronic drug therapy. Patients for whom the evaluation reveals a "treatable" cause, such as an arteriovenous malformation or tumor, can be managed as outlined below but may need reassessment after the underlying condition is treated. The choice of treatment is based on whether the patient has partial or generalized epilepsy, age and life style of the patient, tolerance of drug side effects, and co-morbidities (e.g., pregnancy, liver disease, extremes of age).

Partial Seizures

The initial drug of choice is *carbamazepine*. Potential side effects include ataxia, nausea, sedation, and diplopia. Most of these are usually transient or experienced at higher doses. Patients must be closely monitored for hepatic and bone marrow toxicity in the first 3 months of treatment and less frequently after this period. For patients who are intolerant of the drug side effects or who experience breakthrough seizures, the second drug of choice is *phenytoin*. Common dose-related side effects of phenytoin include nystagmus, ataxia, lethargy, and cognitive problems. Non–life-threatening but potentially troubling side effects associated with long-term use include gingival hyperplasia, osteopenia, hirsutism, coarsening of features, and acne.

Other agents that have demonstrated clinical efficacy for the treatment of partial seizures refractory to either carbamazepine or phenytoin include valproic acid, felbamate, gabapentine, or lamotrigine. These agents can be used as monotherapy, although the newer agents are most often used as second-line or "add-on" therapy. The side effects and toxicities of valproic acid are discussed below. *Gabapentine* is a newer anticonvulsant medication that is relatively easy to use and well tolerated. It is usually administered as adjunctive therapy for partial and secondary generalized seizures. *Lamotrigine* is also indicated as adjunctive therapy for partial seizures. It is more difficult to use than gabapentine because its hepatic metabolism is easily affected by other medications. The most frequently reported side effect of lamotrigine is skin rash, which has been reported in 10% of patients. The rash can be serious, requiring hospitalization, withdrawal of the drug, or both. *Felbamate* is used as monotherapy and adjunctive therapy for partial and secondary generalized seizures. Serious potential side effects include aplastic anemia and hepatic failure; therefore, it is recommended only for patients with severe symptoms refractory to alternative regimens (Table 74-2).

TABLE 74-2
TREATMENT GUIDELINES FOR ANTICONVULSANT MEDICATIONS

	First Choice	Second Choice
Partial seizure		
All types	Carbamazepine	Phenobarbital
	Phenytoin	Gabapentine
	Valproic acid	Lamotrigine
	Divalproex sodium	Felbamate
Generalized seizure		
Tonic-clonic	Valproic acid	Carbamazepine
	Divalproex sodium	Phenobarbital
	Phenytoin	Primidone
Tonic, clonic, and atonic	Valproic acid	Phenobarbital
	Divalproex sodium	
Absence	Ethosuximide	Trimethadione
	Valproic acid	
	Divalproex sodium	
Myoclonic	Valproic acid	Benzodiazepine
	Divalproex sodium	

Generalized Seizures

Patients in this category may have more than one seizure type and often require more than one agent to control their seizures. *Valproic acid* is generally considered the first drug of choice because it is broad spectrum and generally well tolerated. Common side effects include tremor, hair thinning and color change (red to brown), fluctuations in weight (up and down), and nausea. Because valproic acid can impair platelet function, and at higher doses cause thrombocytopenia, patients should be advised to watch for abnormal mucosal bleeding. For absence seizures, *ethosuximide* can be used as either monotherapy or in combination with valproic acid. Myoclonic seizures, which may be difficult to control with valproic acid alone, often respond to the addition of benzodiazepines.

Second-line therapy for refractory seizures include phenytoin and the newer agents gabapentine, lamotrigine, and felbamate, which are usually used in combination with either valproic acid or phenytoin. Also, phenobarbital and primidone are useful agents to consider as second-line therapy, either alone or in combination with valproic acid. A major limitation in the use of either of these sedating agents is that, if the agent does *not* work, withdrawal can precipitate worsening symptoms (Table 74-3).

Table 74-3
Monitoring of Drug Treatment

Medication	Starting Dose	Serum Monitoring	Serum Levels (mg/L)	Side Effects
Carbamazepine	100 mg tid × 3 d 100 mg qid × 3 d 200 mg tid × 1 wk; check level and adjust dose	CBC with differentials, LFTs, electrolytes; repeat at 3, 6, and 12 mos	4–12	Diplopia, ataxia, lethargy, liver and marrow toxicity, SIADH, pancreatitis, and hepatitis
Valpoic acid Divalproex sodium	125 mg bid × 3 d 250 mg bid × 3 d 250 mg qid × 1 wk; check level and adjust dose	CBC with differentials, LFTs, amylase, electrolytes; repeat 3, 6, and 12 mos	50–120	Nausea, thrombocytopenia, hepatitis, pancreatitis, hair loss, tremor, weight gain or loss, and polyuria
Phenytoin	100 mg tid × 1 wk check level at 1 wk; 1, 3, 6, and 12 mos	CBC with differentials, LFTs	10–20	Ataxia, nystagmus, peripheral neuropathy, gingival hyperplasia, and hepatitis

Table 74-3 (Continued)

Medication	Starting Dose	Serum Monitoring	Serum Levels (mg/L)	Side Effects
Ethosuximide	500 mg qd	CBC with differentials; repeat at 1, 3, 6, and 12 mos	40–100	Abdominal discomfort, leukopenia, rash, and dizziness
Gabapentine	300 mg qd × 1 d 300 mg bid × 1 d 300 mg tid × 1 d	CBC with differentials; repeat at 1, 3, 6, and 12 mos	5–7	Lethargy, ataxia, and nystagmus
Lamotrigine	50 mg qd × 2 wk 50 mg bid × 2 wk; reduce dose if pt is on valproic acid	CBC with differentials, LFTs; repeat at 1, 3, 6, and 12 mos	2–5	Rash, dizziness, and lethargy
Felbamate	400 mg tid	CBC with differentials, LFTs; repeat at 1, 3, 6, and 12 mos	32–137	Anorexia, insomnia, abdominal discomfort, aplastic anemia, and hepatic failure
Phenobarbital	30–120 mg/d		10–40	Ataxia, cognitive slowing, lethargy, rash, and Stevens-Johnson syndrome

Note. qd = everyday; qid = four times a day; tid = three times a day; bid = two times a day; d = day; wk = week; mos = months; pt = patient; CBC = complete blood count; LFTs = liver function tests; SIADH = syndrome of inappropriate antidiuretic hormone.

Refractory Seizures

Reasons to change medications include patient intolerance of side effects or inadequate seizure control. Side effects are often seen with the introduction of new medication, and most dissipate over time. Once a patient has failed initial treatment, it is less likely that a second-choice medication will be effective. Thus, it is important for the physician to ensure that the maximum tolerated dose is used before switching to second-line therapy. It is also critically important that antiepileptic medications are not abruptly discontinued; medications should be slowly tapered only after therapeutic levels of the new medication have been achieved.

Refractory epilepsy has been defined as either seizures that are unable to be controlled with antiepileptic drugs or as epilepsy in patients who are experiencing intolerable side effects from the medications. Such patients should be referred to a neurologist for evaluation. The neurologist may suggest alternative treatment strategies or surgical intervention. For selected patients, surgical resection of the seizure focus or commissurotomy can significantly reduce seizure frequency and drug therapy.

Special Circumstances

ELDERLY

Epilepsy in the elderly is often a symptom of an underlying medical condition. Common causes of their seizures include cerebrovascular accidents, brain tumors, toxic or metabolic syndromes, trauma, medication effects, and degenerative disorders such as Alzheimer's disease. The presentation of seizures can be atypical or easily confused with other disorders such as syncope, transient ischemic attacks, tremor, dementia, or sleep disorders. In addition, many elderly patients live alone, are unable to describe their seizure, or have other disorders that may mask seizure symptoms (e.g., preexisting paralysis resulting from a cerebrovascular accident). For patients with recurrent "events" that defy characterization, EEG or video monitoring may be useful to confirm the diagnosis.

Anticonvulsant therapy is often complicated by age-related changes in pharmacokinetics and potential for interactions with other medications. In addition, the elderly are highly susceptible to side effects, particularly those that affect cognition. Benzodiazepines and barbiturates tend to be the most problematic. Fortunately, most anticonvulsant medications are well tolerated by the elderly, as long as one follows the philosophy of "starting low and going slow" with dosing changes.

WOMEN

Many commonly used anticonvulsant agents reduce the effectiveness of oral contraceptive agents. This is due to enhancement of the activity of the liver microsomal enzyme cytochrome P-450 by the medications, which increases steroid metabolism. Women of childbearing age should be counseled appropriately and barrier protection should be used until the physician is sure that ovulation is being suppressed consistently.

Many of the anticonvulsant agents also have significant cosmetic side effects: weight gain, gum hyperplasia, coarsening of facial features, and abnormal hair growth are some of the most common ones. Although not life-threatening, these may be important to the patient (particularly younger patients) and can result in poor medication compliance. Physicians should carefully weigh the potential for side effects against clinical efficacy and counsel patients accordingly.

Pregnancy poses a special set of problems to the epileptic patient. There is a potential for teratogenic effects, which are higher in women with epilepsy. Use of valproic acid has been associated with higher rates of fetal malformations, specifically neural tube defects. There is a risk of subtherapeutic levels of medications with pregnancy-related changes in volume of distribution and drug elimination kinetics, and poorly controlled seizures are a risk to the fetus. In spite of this, most women with epilepsy are able to have a normal healthy pregnancy as long as they are carefully monitored by their physician. Anticonvulsant drug levels need to be closely followed, and folate supplementation reduces the risk of neural tube defects. Patients on valproic acid should be offered prenatal screening (ultrasound, chorionic villus sampling, alpha-feto-protein) for neural cord defects. The risk of major birth defects with the use of newer anticonvulsant drugs remains to be defined.

COMPLIANCE

Patients should be counseled about the importance of compliance with medications, potential side effects, and the need for periodic monitoring of serum levels. They should be encouraged to maintain a life style that includes regular eating habits, adequate sleep, and avoidance of excessive alcohol and known seizure-inducing stimuli. Patients should be encouraged to wear a medical alert bracelet and carry a medical information card. Women considering pregnancy should consult with their primary care physician before conceiving to minimize fetal exposure to medications. All driving must be suspended until seizures are controlled: the required duration of a seizure-free interval varies from state to state, but in general is at least 6 months. Physicians are often required to report seizures to the state.

SUGGESTED READING

Brodie MJ, Dichter MA: Antiepileptic drugs. *New Engl J Med* 334(3):168–175, 1996.

Gilliam F, Wyllie E: Diagnostic testing of seizure disorders. *Neurol Clin* 14(1):61–84, 1996.

Kerrigan JF, Fisher RS: Recurrent generalized and partial seizures. In *Current Therapy in Neurologic Disease*, 5th ed. Edited by Johnson RT, Griffen JW. Philadelphia, PA: Mosby-Year Book, 1997, pp 47–55.

Schachter SC, Yerby MS: Management of epilepsy: pharmacologic therapy and quality-of-life issues. *Postgrad Med* 101(2):133–138, 141–144, 150–153, 1997.

Schwartz BE: Complex partial seizures. In *Current Therapy in Neurologic Disease*, 5th ed. Edited by Johnson RT, Griffen JW. Philadelphia, PA: Mosby-Year Book, 1997, pp 55–60.

Shuster EA: Epilepsy in women. *Mayo Clin Proc* 71(10):991–999, 1996.

Thomas RJ: Seizures and epilepsy in the elderly. *Arch Intern Med* 157(6):605–617, 1997.

Wilder BJ: The treatment of epilepsy: an overview of clinical practices. *Neurology* 45(3)[Suppl 2]:S7–S11, 1995.

CHAPTER 75

Stroke

Peter DeLong, M.D., and Lisa M. Bellini, M.D.

PATIENT

J. Willus, a 72-year-old woman with a history of poorly controlled hypertension and coronary artery disease, is brought in by her daughter because she suddenly became confused and impossible to understand during lunch. The daughter noticed that her mother drooled from the left side of her mouth and that her right arm and leg seemed very weak as she was helped from her chair to the car. She says her mother appears to understand what is being said to her but garbles her words. Her mother seems frustrated.

CLINICAL PRESENTATION

Stroke is the acute onset of a neurologic deficit. Its symptoms are focal and referable to a vascular distribution. Brain tissue can tolerate ischemia for 4–5 minutes before undergoing necrosis. Many events can result in ischemia and therefore some degree of long-term neurologic deficit.

> Stroke is the acute onset of a neurologic deficit with symptoms that are focal and referable to a vascular distribution.

Strokes are broadly classified according to whether they result from a lack of perfusion (ischemic) or from bleeding (hemorrhagic). In addition, there are fleeting neurologic deficits that result from vascular events, which resolve completely within minutes. These are called reversible ischemic neurologic events.

ETIOLOGY

Ischemic Strokes

These are classified as focal or global with most being focal.

FOCAL STROKES

Focal strokes are further classified as either *embolic* or *thrombotic*. The deficit produced by focal strokes is partially determined by the ischemia-modifying effect of collateral circulation. Acute obstruction allows no chance for the development of collateral circulation, while gradual loss of flow may increase collaterals and minimize damage. Anatomic variation also contributes to focal strokes.

TABLE 75-1
CLASSIFICATION OF STROKES

Classification	Mechanism	Etiology
Ischemic strokes		
Embolic	Artery to artery	Atherosclerosis from carotid artery or aortic arch post-MI, and mural thrombus
	Cardiogenic	Atrial fibrillation, valvular-endocarditis, rheumatic atherosclerosis, mitral valve prolapse, and atrial septal defect secondary to venous thrombosis
	Hematologic	Cell dyscrasia, hematocrit > 55, white blood cells > 500,000, platelets > 600,000, coagulation disorders, sickle cell disease, factor V Leiden, lupus anticoagulant, and cardiolipin antibody
Thrombotic	Atherosclerosis	Any cerebral vasculature
	Arteritis	Polyarteritis nodosa, granulomatous arteritis, and neoplastic invasion
	Cocaine	Arterial spasm
	Other	Carotid dissection, trauma to carotid artery, complicated migraine, postpartum state, postoperative state, and hypertension
Hemorrhagic strokes		
	Vascular catastrophes	Aneurysm, arteriovenous malformation, and rupture
	Malignancy	Tissue and vascular necrosis
	Bleeding diatheses	Hemophilia and anticoagulation

Note. MI = myocardial infarction.

- **Embolic strokes** are the most common type of stroke (ischemic or hemorrhagic), making up approximately 30% of the total. They are characterized by the sudden onset of a focal neurologic deficit that improves slowly over time. They can occur at any time and without warning. Approximately 40% of emboli are from the heart with the majority of the others originating from artery-to-artery emboli secondary to atherosclerosis in the aortic arch and carotid arteries.
- **Thrombotic strokes** are less common than embolic strokes. They may have the same abrupt onset and commonly occur at night. The classic presentation involves a patient awaken-

ing with weakness and falling to the floor unaware of the event. Many have a protracted evolution over minutes or hours. Often this occurs in a stepwise (saltatory) fashion with new deficits appearing suddenly after a period of brief stability. Strokes that develop over time are called "strokes in evolution." This temporal progression usually represents the extension of the thrombus. Thrombotic strokes that occur in this stuttering fashion are commonly preceded by transient ischemic attacks (TIAs).

- **Miscellaneous strokes** include stroke caused by internal carotid artery dissection, spinal stroke, and cerebral venous sinus thrombosis. *Internal carotid artery dissection* can cause decreased blood flow and cerebral ischemia. The resulting stroke is usually preceded by facial pain and headache behind the eye on the same side. There is often an associated Horner's syndrome (ptosis, miosis, anhydrosis). *Spinal stroke* is ischemic infarction of the spinal cord. This occurs most commonly after episodes of severe hypotension or shock or from compression of the blood supply by an intraspinal mass, usually a tumor. *Cerebral venous sinus thrombosis* can decrease cerebral blood flow and cause infarction; this occurs most often in postpartum women.

GLOBAL STROKES

Global strokes result from hypoperfusion of the entire brain. This can result from systemic hypotension and shock, from severely or acutely elevated blood pressure, or most commonly from carotid dissection. Cardiac arrhythmias account for the overwhelming majority of hypotensive ischemic events, often in the context of cardiopulmonary resuscitation. Elevated blood pressure can produce multifocal cerebral ischemia and hypertensive encephalopathy. Patients may have a headache; become confused or stuporous; and develop cortical blindness, hemiparesis, and hemisensory deficits. Severe hypertension and severe hypotension can cause focal or global deficits that tend to be more severe than isolated focal strokes.

COMPLICATIONS OF ISCHEMIC STROKES

Complications of ischemic strokes include cerebral edema, hemorrhage, and occasionally seizures. Cerebral edema occurs in large strokes and is particularly dangerous when it occurs in the poste-

> Complications of ischemic strokes include cerebral edema, hemorrhage, and occasionally seizures.

rior fossa because it can compress the brainstem. The risk period for significant cerebral edema is 12–72 hours poststroke. Hemorrhage is another complication of large strokes. When the hematoma from a bleed extends to the cortex, seizures can occur.

Hemorrhagic Strokes

This is the third most common cause of stroke after embolic and thrombotic events. Hypertension and aneurysmal rupture account for most hemorrhagic strokes. Bleeding disorders also contribute and clinically resemble hypertensive hemorrhages.

HYPERTENSIVE STROKES

Hypertensive intraparenchymal strokes are more common in African Americans than in Caucasians. Clinically, these strokes often cause vomiting, and headache is seen in 50% of these patients. Loss of consciousness, delirium, and seizures are also common. Large intraparenchymal strokes are fatal in more than 50% of cases. Hypertensive hemorrhage occurs in several well-known locations in the brain. They are (in order of frequency in which they occur): (1) the putamen and internal capsule—50% of all hypertensive strokes; (2) temporal, parietal, or frontal white matter (lobar hemorrhages); (3) thalamus; (4) cerebellar hemispheres; and (5) pons.

ANEURYSMAL STROKES

The rupture of an aneurysm causes a subarachnoid hemorrhage that typically presents as vomiting in association with "the worst headache of my life." These occur most often at arterial bifurcations at the base of the brain. Rapid loss of consciousness occurs in half of these patients. There is often dizziness, headache, and vomiting. A stiff neck, not present at the onset, can develop over the following 24 hours from irritation of the meninges by blood. The mortality rate is 35%.

Complications of hemorrhagic strokes include ischemia, infarction, communicating hydrocephalus, and recurrent hemorrhage.

COMPLICATIONS OF HEMORRHAGIC STROKES

Complications of hemorrhagic strokes include ischemia and infarction from vasospasm, communicating hydrocephalus, and recurrent hemorrhage. Between 10%–30% of patients will rebleed within 2–3 weeks, often with progression of neurologic deficits. The mortality rate of rebleeding is 60%.

Stroke Syndromes

The symptoms of a stroke result from the cause and, more importantly, from the location and size of the vascular territory involved. Each syndrome has general characteristics that are helpful in evaluating a patient with suspected stroke. Several of the most common stroke syndromes are listed in Table 75-2. These are listed by vascular territory, not by cause, because the neurologic deficit results from the location and the size of the event.

TABLE 75-2
STROKE SYNDROMES

Anatomic Distribution	Vascular Distribution	Symptoms
Hemispheric	Anterior cerebral artery (ischemic lesions of this artery are uncommon)	Contralateral hemiparesis, leg greater than arm or face, with gait disturbance Contralateral grasping and sucking reflexes (frontal release) Apathy and loss of will (abulia) Perseveration Urinary incontinence Expressive (Broca's) aphasia
	Middle cerebral artery (most common lesion)	Contralateral hemiparesis, face and arm greater than leg Contralateral sensory loss Horizontal gaze palsy, gaze preference to side of lesion Homonymous hemianopsia Expressive or receptive aphasia in dominant hemisphere Neglect, apraxia in nondominant hemisphere
	Posterior cerebral artery	Contralateral homonymous hemianopsia or quadrantanopsia Frank cortical blindness if both hemispheres involved Possible memory loss Sensory loss Painful dysesthesias Choreoathetosis

Brainstem	Vertebrobasilar system	Weber's syndrome
		  Ipsilateral third nerve palsy
		  Contralateral hemiparesis
		Lateral medullary syndrome (Wallenberg's syndrome)
		  Vertigo
		  Vomiting
		  Nystagmus

TABLE 75-2 (CONTINUED)

Anatomic Distribution	Vascular Distribution	Symptoms
Brainstem	Vertebrobasilar system	Ipsilateral decreased pain and temperature sensation in face
		Horner's syndrome (ptosis, miosis, anhydrosis)
		Ataxia (falling toward lesion)
		Contralateral loss of pain and temperature sensation
Cerebellar		Dizziness
		Nausea and vomiting
		Nystagmus
		Ataxia

Transient Ischemic Attacks and Reversible Ischemic Neurologic Events

These are brief episodes of focal neurologic deficit that resolve completely. A TIA is the common term that has been used for many years to describe neurologic events that last minutes to hours then resolve. The newer term, reversible ischemic neurologic events (RINE), is more often used for other longer lasting yet completely reversible events. Some people use the term RINE for both events. These reversible ischemic events are most often due to atherosclerotic disease. They may occur in isolation, or they may herald the coming of a more severe stroke. Up to 30% of those patients with untreated TIAs or RINEs will have a significant stroke in 5 years. They may occur in any distribution but are most common in the carotid and vertebrobasilar distributions.

- **Carotid TIAs or RINEs** commonly cause ipsilateral blindness ("amaurosis fugax," classically described as a shade being lowered), contralateral hemiparesis and paresthesias, and dysarthria.
- **Vertebrobasilar TIAs or RINEs** cause vestibular symptoms, vertigo, drowsiness, diplopia, dysarthria, and ataxia.

It is important to discover whether TIAs or RINEs cause the same or different symptoms. Recurrent deficits imply atherosclerosis and thrombosis from the same source and are most often seen in the distribution of the carotid artery. Different symptoms imply either embolization or involvement of the vertebrobasilar arteries. TIAs or RINEs are also markers for patients at high risk for MI, probably because both of these diseases result from atherosclerotic processes.

RINEs can present a diagnostic dilemma because of the varied symptoms they produce. Conditions often mistaken for stroke include focal seizures, glaucoma diagnosed as retinal artery occlusion, positional vertigo or Meniere's disease attributed to vertebrobasilar RINEs, and cardiac syncope. Complicated migraine headaches may also be diagnosed as a stroke.

EPIDEMIOLOGY

Stroke is the third leading cause of death in the United States behind heart disease and cancer. Stroke causes approximately 85,000 deaths per year. The morbidity of stroke is tremendous with

> Stroke is the third leading cause of death in the United States.

approximately 1 million stroke survivors living with a severe disability. There has been a reduction in the rate of stroke over the last 30–35 years probably attributable to improved control of blood pressure and increasingly frequent anticoagulation of patients at risk.

Risk factors for stroke include *hypertension, atrial fibrillation, alcohol abuse, carotid stenosis* (> 70%), *oral contraceptive use, valvular heart disease* (mitral valve prolapse is six times more common in people over the age of 45 with stroke), *intracardiac shunts* (atrial septic defect, patent foramen ovale), *smoking, hyperlipidemia, diabetes, MI* (people with MIs are at an increased risk of stroke; conversely, people with stroke are far more likely to have MIs than those without stroke), and RINEs (up to 30% of untreated RINE patients suffer a stroke within 5 years).

DIAGNOSIS

Though the diagnosis of stroke is largely clinical, it is very important to determine whether the cause is ischemic or hemorrhagic. A patient with a hemorrhagic stroke should not be anticoagulated. After this distinction is made, the search for a cause is tailored to each patient. A typical evaluation includes a noncontrast computed tomography (CT) scan, an electrocardiogram (ECG), and blood work consisting of a complete blood count and coagulation times. Further studies are obtained based on the clinical presentation. For instance, a patient with a severe headache and a normal CT should have a lumbar puncture to rule out a subarachnoid hemorrhage. Although stroke is usually a catastrophe of old age, it is not uncommon in young people, and its occurrence in this population should prompt a more aggressive workup for the cause, particularly embolic causes. Commonly used tests in the evaluation of stroke include:

- **CT Scan without Contrast.** This is used to rule out hemorrhage and signs of increased intracranial pressure. It misses approximately 10%–15% of subarachnoid hemorrhages, however, and is a poor method of imaging the posterior fossa. In addition, it does not reliably detect infarcts that are less than 48 hours old.

- **Lumbar Puncture.** This is used when a high clinical suspicion exists for subarachnoid hemorrhage and the CT scan is negative. Essentially, the only way for blood to get into the cerebrospinal fluid (CSF) is by rupture of an aneurysm into the subarachnoid space. Thus, xanthochromia in the CSF is virtually diagnostic of a subarachnoid bleed.

- **Prothrombin Time and Partial Thromboplastin Time.** This combination of tests may uncover a bleeding disorder and is used for monitoring patients receiving anticoagulation therapy. Other blood tests for specific coagulopathies can also be done if there is a high clinical suspicion or a family history.

- **ECG, Cardiac Monitoring, and Echocardiography.** These procedures can detect abnormal cardiac rhythms, mural thrombi, atrial septal defects, and valvular irregularities that would predispose a patient to an embolic stroke.

- **Carotid Ultrasound and Transcranial Doppler Studies.** These studies assess the degree of vascular stenosis in the large vessels of the head. Such disease, if significant, predisposes a patient to an ischemic stroke.

- **Magnetic Resonance Imaging (MRI).** MRI provides better resolution and enables earlier detection of cerebral infarction than CT. It also visualizes the posterior fossa, improving the detection of cerebellar lesions.

- **MRI Angiography.** This procedure can image blood flow in the carotid and vertebrobasilar arteries and detect many carotid dissections.

- **Cerebral Angiography.** This can detect aortic dissection, mural thrombi, emboli, and collateral circulation. It is the best method for visualization of the basilar artery. The procedure entails substantial risk as it can precipitate strokes.

TREATMENT

> Because of the high morbidity, prevention in the form of risk-factor modification is the best strategy.

Because stroke involves neurologic deficits that resolve incompletely, prevention in the form of risk-factor modification is the best strategy. Hypertension is the most important risk factor and should be aggressively controlled. Smokers should be encouraged to stop. Those patients with atrial fibrillation, severe carotid stenosis, valvular disease, or previous MI should be maintained on antiplatelet therapy and possibly anticoagulated. Diabetes and hyperlipidemia should be treated. Women over the age of 35 who smoke should be educated not to use oral contraceptives. For selected patients with asymptomatic carotid stenosis greater than 70%, endarterectomy has been shown to reduce the risk of stroke compared to medical therapy. Once a stroke has occurred and been identified as ischemic or hemorrhagic, care is guided by several principles, which are discussed below.

Ischemic Stroke

- **Support the Acute Deficits.** Patients should be intubated if control of the airway is compromised, and blood pressure must be controlled. Blood pressure is often allowed to run higher immediately poststroke than would otherwise be tolerated to ensure cerebral perfusion. This is done with normal saline to avoid cerebral edema, which could result from free water. Nutrition is also important and often requires consideration of a feeding tube after 48 hours.

- **Restoration of Blood Flow.** Patients must be anticoagulated with heparin to prevent extension of thrombus or recurrent emboli if thrombolytics are not to be used. The use of thrombolytics must be considered as they are being increasingly used for acute strokes. If thrombolytics are indicated, patients must be referred (within 3 hours of the onset of symptoms) to a tertiary care center with the capability to give thrombolytics and manage the complications of bleeding.

- **Prevention of Recurrent Thrombosis.** This is done with antithrombotic therapy and risk-factor modification as described above.

- **Rehabilitation.** Occupational and physical therapy are the mainstays of long-term recovery. Speech therapy will also play a role for those who have dysarthria or aphasia. Depression following a stroke is common and should be treated. Early involvement of social services is also important to identify community resources. More debilitated patients require institutional care and monitoring of skin breakdown, nutrition, airway control, and infection.

Hemorrhagic stroke

There are three principles guiding the treatment of an intracerebral hemorrhage.

- **Neurosurgical evaluation** should be scheduled to evaluate for the possibility of surgical evacuation of the hematoma.

- **Coagulopathies** should immediately and aggressively be reversed.
- **Anticonvulsants** should be used, especially when the bleed extends to the cortical surface.

A subarachnoid hemorrhage is treated similarly to an intra-parenchymal bleed except that surgical intervention may be even more urgent if hydrocephalus develops. Aneurysms and arte-riovenous malformations that bleed are treated surgically. Often surgeons wait 10–14 days before operating, but in emergencies they will intervene more quickly. Patients should be put at bed rest, and factors that increase intracranial pressure should be limited: cough should be suppressed, constipation treated with stool softeners, and benzodiazepines given for restlessness. In addition, vasospasm is often treated with calcium channel blockers to prevent cerebral infarction.

SUGGESTED READING

Adams RD, Victor M: *Principles of Neurology*, 4th ed. New York, NY: McGraw-Hill, 1994, pp 617–692.

Pulsinelli WA, Levy DE: Cerebrovascular disease. In *Cecil's Textbook of Medicine*. Edited by Wyngaarden JB, et al. Philadelphia, PA: W. B. Saunders, 1992, pp 2145–2169.

CHAPTER 76
Dementia of the Alzheimer's Type

Mark D. Andrews, M.D.

PATIENT

D. Cates, a 65-year-old woman, is brought into the office by family members. She is feeling well and is without complaints. The family reports that she has had gradually progressive difficulty with memory over the past 6–12 months, including difficulty locating familiar objects in the house, forgetting well-known recipes, occasionally repeating words or actions, and more frequently becoming lost when driving in the local neighborhood. She denies depressive feelings or crying and has not had any weight loss, change in her skin, or constipation. She has experienced increasing difficulty handling her financial affairs and occasionally has left a burner operating on the stove. In casual conversation she remains alert, sociable, and appropriate. More recently she has become withdrawn, somewhat apathetic, and disinterested in her usual hobbies. In the last few months she has been unusually suspicious of family members trying to help her with household chores.

CLINICAL PRESENTATION

Dementia of the Alzheimer's type (DAT) is an insidious disease. The early symptoms tend to be so mild and gradually progressive that they may easily go unrecognized. A social facade or a capacity to look and behave well in brief social encounters is often maintained in the early stages of the illness. Once the evolving loss of intellectual functioning and memory is of sufficient severity to cause dysfunction in daily living, the clinical syndrome can usually be identified. DAT is not always evident to families until the later stages of the illness. Contributing to this delay in recognition is the unfortunate acceptance by families of cognitive change as an expected part of normal aging. Shadowing or following a family member into the bathroom or around the house is not uncommon. New demands, irritability, or obsessive-compulsive traits with low frustration tolerance are frequently encountered as the disease progresses. Hiding and losing things and accusations of theft are common behavioral changes, as well as constantly packing, pacing, rummaging, searching, or moving things around.

The rate and pattern of progression of symptoms is particularly important in classifying the type of dementia. Cognitive impairment that occurs suddenly over days, rather than over months or years, particularly when associated with fluctuating symptoms and altered levels of consciousness, should suggest a potentially reversible state of delirium. Multi-infarct dementia, DAT, and dementia associated with other neurologic disorders (e.g., Parkinson's disease, Huntington's disease) tend to progress more slowly over months to years. A gradual, but irregular or stepwise deterioration in cognitive function over time suggests a pattern of multi-infarct dementia.

> DAT is insidious, progressive, and often unrecognized.

The key features of DAT include:

- Impairment in short- and long-term memory (short-term deficits are usually more prominent)
- Deficits in two or more areas of cognitive function
    - Abstract thinking
    - Judgment (often early manifestation)
    - Language (aphasia)
    - Motor skills (apraxia)
    - Perception (agnosia)
- Progressive worsening of memory and other cognitive functions
- No disturbance of consciousness
- Onset between ages 40 and 90 but usually after age 65
- Absence of systemic disorders or other brain diseases that might explain symptoms
- Impaired activities of daily living and altered patterns of behavior (may become unusually withdrawn, hostile, or aggressive)
- Normal laboratory studies, including lumbar puncture, electroencephalogram (EEG), computed tomography (CT), and magnetic resonance imaging (MRI) [except for possible non-specific slowing on EEG or atrophy on the imaging study]

DIFFERENTIAL DIAGNOSIS

> When evaluating cognitive changes in the elderly, exclude reversible causes, especially medication.

Whenever evaluating cognitive changes in the elderly, it is important to rule out reversible causes. The leading cause of a reversible dementia syndrome in the elderly is drug therapy. Other causes of reversible cognitive deficits include emotional disturbances, endocrine disorders, nutritional problems, tumors, trauma, infections, and alcohol abuse.

EPIDEMIOLOGY

Dementia in the elderly can be grouped into five broad categories listed below (Table 76-1):

Table 76-1
Categories of Dementia

Type of Dementia	Percent of Dementia
Primary degenerative dementia (mainly DAT)	50%–60%
Multi-infarct or vascular dementia	20%–30%
Mixed dementia	10%
Reversible or partially reversible dementia	5%–10%
Other disorders (mainly neurologic)	5%

DAT usually starts in older adults over 65 years of age but can be seen in younger adults who are in their late 40s or 50s. It is an all too common disease with increasing prevalence as our population ages and life expectancy increases. The prevalence of DAT is 5% at age 65, 20% at age 80, and approximately 40%–50% at age 85.

DIFFERENTIAL DIAGNOSIS

DAT is not a part of normal aging, and the diagnosis is one of exclusion. Amnestic syndromes and benign senescent forgetfulness are related disorders that need to be differentiated. The predominate feature in these syndromes is memory impairment with sparing of other intellectual functions. Amnestic syndromes may be associated with thiamine deficiency, trauma, or transient global ischemia. Benign senescent forgetfulness involves minor degrees of memory loss that are not observed to be progressive, associated with dysfunction in daily living, or associated with deterioration of intellectual function in other areas. The key alternative diagnoses to consider in evaluating DAT include multi-infarct dementia, reversible drug-induced syndromes, and pseudodementia of depression. A chronic dementing illness with periods of rapid "stepwise" decline in function, often associated with focal neurologic findings and chronic essential hypertension, suggests a multi-infarct etiology. Drug-induced dementias are often subacute in onset but usually are associated with the introduction of the offending pharmacologic agent. A trial off the medication is diagnostic.

The interrelationship between depression and dementia is very complex. Many patients with early demential illness can be depressed, and likewise many patients with more severe major depressive illnesses may present with cognitive impairment, which may resemble DAT. This condition has been labeled "pseudodementia." These patients usually have significant reversal of cognitive impairment with treatment of their depression. When in doubt, a trial of antidepressant therapy and subsequent reassessment of cognitive function are always appropriate.

DIAGNOSIS

There is no specific test for DAT. Factors that place people at increased risk include age, family history, early head trauma, and low linguistic ability early in life. The diagnosis of "definite" DAT can only be made by brain biopsy, which for obvious reasons is infrequently pursued. The diagnosis of "probable" or "possible" DAT is made on clinical grounds. Greater insight has been gained recently into some of the genetic issues of DAT—particularly those involving familial cases, which account for 2%–10% of all DAT cases. However, current genetic knowledge cannot account for 15%–20% of familial DAT cases. The presence of measurable APOE$_4$, a cholesterol-carrying protein manufactured in the liver and brain, increases the risk of DAT but is neither necessary nor sufficient for the development of DAT. Therefore, APOE$_4$ cannot be used as a predictive test. It may, however, be useful in some clinical situations to help clarify the diagnosis.

Laboratory testing can play a role in diagnosing potentially reversible causes of dementia. Thyroid function tests (particularly thyroid-stimulating hormone [TSH]) are helpful in identifying hypothyroidism. Serologic tests for syphilis and human immunodeficiency virus (HIV) are important, as well as serum vitamin B$_{12}$ and folate levels to identify deficiency states. Serum creatinine, sodium (Na$^+$), calcium (Ca^{2+}), magnesium (Mg^{2+}), and glucose levels are valuable to identify reversible metabolic abnormalities. The Westergren sedimentation rate may be obtained to screen for collagen vascular diseases, which may create mental status changes resembling dementia. A CT scan of the head may be useful but is not always required in the patient with a "classic" presentation. A CT scan may identify mass lesions, a subdural hematoma, or a meningioma, or it may suggest changes of normal pressure hydrocephalus that may produce dementia-like symptoms.

TREATMENT

There is no current cure for DAT. Two drugs are presently approved by the Food and Drug Administration (FDA) for the early treatment of DAT, tacrine and the newer agent donepezil. Both agents are cholinesterase inhibitors and have the potential to improve or stabilize function in 25%–50% of patients treated, but the disease will continue to progress. The ease of once daily dosing, fewer adverse side effects, and a reduced need for laboratory monitoring makes donepezil the likely choice to dominate the market place. Second-generation drug therapies are rapidly being developed, and vitamin E is under investigation. Preliminary studies have indicated that there is a decreased incidence of DAT in individuals taking vitamin E (400 IU a day). Studies with aspirin and other nonsteroidal anti-inflammatory drugs (NSAIDs) have also suggested a trend toward a decreased incidence of DAT compared with a placebo group. Recent reports on estrogen and hormonal replacement therapy in women, although involving limited patient numbers, have suggested a significant impact on reducing the risk of DAT. The cognitive performances of the women mentioned in those reports were improved at least temporarily.

Sleep disorders are common in patients with DAT and should be treated by avoiding daytime naps and alcohol and sedative use when possible. Chloral hydrate titrated to need or short-acting benzodiazepines can be used for short-term insomnia. In patients exhibiting aggressive, delusional, psychotic, or paranoid behavior, small doses of haloperidol (0.5–1 mg, twice a day) may be effective.

The use of restraints remains a controversial issue in the treatment of demented elderly patients, and it is important to maintain options for monitored wandering in institutional settings. Daily routines need to be maintained and activity reminders provided. Support, counseling, and education of family members are critical in the treatment process, so that they can better cope with this devastating illness.

Behavioral problems are common in demented persons, and the most frequently encountered include memory disturbance, restlessness, catastrophic reactions, nonspecific agitation, day-and-night disturbance, and delusions. It is important to modify the home environment to avoid over- and understimulation and to reduce injury potential. A number of stressors can increase agitation in the cognitively impaired, including fatigue, change of routine, excess demands, overwhelming stimuli, and physical stressors. Principles that may help families manage agitation are:

- Correct sensory impairments (eyeglasses, hearing aide, dentures).
- Approach patients in a nonconfrontational manner.
- Find an optimal level of patient autonomy.
- Simplify and structure daily routine and living environment.
- Provide multiple cues (repeated and varying instructions).
- Guide and demonstrate.
- Repeat information and instructions.
- Provide positive and negative reinforcement.
- Reduce choices.
- Optimize stimulation.

- Avoid excessive new learning.
- Determine and use overlearned skills.
- Couple learning with emotional arousal.
- Minimize anxiety and situational stressors.
- Distract the patient.

It is important to direct families to help with behavioral symptoms in DAT. Support groups are a valuable resource and can provide creative solutions from experienced family caregivers who have survived similar behavioral disruptions. The national Alzheimer's Association can provide referrals. The Alzheimer's Association chapters have telephone help lines with experienced peer counselors to answer questions or just talk to family members experiencing difficulty with behavioral symptoms. There are also e-mail discussion groups for family and professional caregivers, as well as disease-specific chat groups, bulletin boards, and web sites, all of which offer immediate real-time help with behavioral symptoms.

PROGNOSIS

DAT is an insidious and progressive disease that eventually results in total loss of independence and the need for round-the-clock supervision and nursing care. With more advanced disease, individuals may demonstrate motor signs such as increased muscle tone, myoclonus, or gait disorders. Associated symptoms are incontinence, delusions, hallucinations, depression, emotional outbursts, weight loss, and, in more advanced stages, seizures. As function declines there is an increased risk for common infections such as urinary tract infections and pneumonia. There is also a gradual loss of interest in food and worsening nutritional status. In the most advanced stages, patients become bedridden, minimally interactive, and totally dependent on caretakers.

SUGGESTED READING

American Psychiatric Association: *Diagnostic and Statistical Manual of Mental Disorders*, 4th ed. Washington, DC: American Psychiatric Association, 1994.

Beck JC, Benson DF, Schiebel AB, et al: Dementia in the elderly: the silent epidemic. *Ann Intern Med* 97:231–241, 1982.

Kane RL, Ouslander J, Abras I: Confusion. In *Essentials of Clinical Geriatrics*, 3rd ed. New York, NY: McGraw-Hill, 1994, pp 83–114.

Katzman R: Alzheimer's disease. *N Engl J Med* 314:964–973, 1986.

CHAPTER 77
Alcohol and Drug Abuse

Robin M. Clemons, M.D., M.P.H.

PATIENT

P. Stack, a 41-year-old schoolteacher, comes into the office for a routine annual examination. The patient complains of having a great deal of difficulty falling asleep. To help her get to sleep, she has been drinking four or more glasses of wine or other alcohol-containing beverages each evening. The patient wonders if she may be drinking too much. On further questioning, the physician finds that she has several family members who are alcoholics. Her father and her uncle have continuing drinking problems.

CLINICAL PRESENTATION

Alcoholism and drug abuse are elusive diseases. Because taking illicit drugs is not a socially acceptable behavior in many cultures, patients hide the degree of their illness and ask for help at the same time. Drug abuse and alcoholism are illnesses that many physicians do not feel comfortable diagnosing or treating. Some physicians fear opening Pandora's box and do not know what to do about the problem, whereas other physicians fear that they are labeling patients and could cause future problems with the patient's insurance and occupational status.

Abuse of alcohol or drugs is actually one disease process. In alcoholism, the drug of choice is a legal one, whereas with drug abuse the choice of drug can be legal (e.g., prescription drugs) or illegal (e.g., heroin, cocaine). In either case there is misuse, overuse, and abuse of a substance. Alcoholism and drug abuse are illnesses that will not be discovered unless the physician is sensitive to these issues. Often people come for care after being pushed to treatment by other family members, friends, co-workers, or the judicial system (Table 77-1).

> Alcoholism and drug abuse are illnesses that will not be discovered unless they are considered. Patients both minimize symptoms and under-report alcohol and drug intake.

TABLE 77-1
CHARACTERISTICS THAT CAN HELP DIAGNOSE SUBSTANCE ABUSE

Feature	Description
Increased tolerance	It takes more of the substance to provide the desired effect.
Withdrawal symptoms	Eliminating the substance produces unwanted symptoms in the patient.
Impairment of social or occupational functioning	As people spend more and more time on acquiring the substance, they stop performing other important tasks (e.g., spending time with family members, doing treasured hobbies, performing well at work).
Continued use	Despite the intellectual knowledge that the substance is creating problems for them, they continue using it.
Complications	The long-term complications of alcohol and drug abuse go far beyond the health of a single individual. It leads to physical illness in the patient but can also destroy the patient's ability to earn a living. It can lead to social isolation or dissolution of the family. It affects the community in general when patients have legal problems such as driving while intoxicated, receiving illegal drugs, engaging in prostitution or commiting theft to support a drug habit. In pregnancy, alcohol and drug use can lead to complications for mother and infant. Alcohol ingestion during pregnancy can lead to fetal alcohol syndrome, which is characterized by mental retardation, small birth weight, and dysmorphic features in the infant. Cocaine and other drug use can lead to premature or small-for-gestational-age infants.

Physical signs of this disease depend on whether the patient is withdrawing from the drug or under its direct effects (intoxication or overdose) when he or she comes to medical attention. Physical signs also depend on the stage of the disease process (Table 77-2). In the early stages of the disease, patients are indistinguishable from other people by their physical appearance. As they progress in their dependence, patients can appear older than their stated age, disheveled, and thin and gaunt from lack of nutrition (cachectic). Vital signs taken during acute alcohol withdrawal can show a patient to be hypertensive and tachycardic with an elevated temperature. In cases of central nervous system depressant overdose with narcotics, patients can be bradycardic, hypotensive, and have a decreased respiratory rate.

TABLE 77-2
PHYSICAL SIGNS OF DRUG ABUSE

Drug of Abuse	Physical Sign
Cocaine sniffing	Irritated nasal mucosa, chronic sniffing, and perforation of nasal septum
Narcotics	Pinpoint pupils and nonreactive pupils
Intravenous drugs of abuse	Needle marks, tracks, or both; bruises on forearms and legs; skin abscesses, cellulitis, or both; and multiple excoriations
Alcohol	Enlarged, tender, or shrunken liver; dilated peripheral veins; (telangiectasia); dilated capillary beds (spider angioma); palmer erythema; and rosacea

EPIDEMIOLOGY

Alcoholism and drug abuse are nondiscriminating diseases. They can affect any gender, any cultural group, and any racial or ethnic group. There does appear to be a genetic predisposition to the development of alcoholism and drug dependence. The prevalence of alcohol and drug abuse in the United States population is 15%–20%. It is a very common problem seen in the primary care setting.

SCREENING

Initial screening involves obtaining a good history. A supportive and nonjudgmental environment encourages honesty about substance use. Questions should include what drugs are currently taken, how often, in what amounts, and, if appropriate, what route is being used (e.g., oral, nasal, intradermal, or intravenous)?

There are several screening questionnaires that family physicians use routinely in their practices. CAGE is a brief screening test for alcoholism that can be given in a few minutes during an interview and consists of four questions. The name is an acronym, which is reminiscent of the questions themselves. Two or more positive responses indicate a drinking problem.

1. Have you ever felt you should *cut down* on your drinking?
2. Have people *annoyed* you by criticizing your drinking?
3. Have you ever felt bad or *guilty* about your drinking?
4. Have you ever taken a drink first thing in the morning (*eye opener*) to steady your nerves or get rid of a hangover?

The Michigan Alcoholism Screening Test (MAST) is a longer questionnaire also routinely used in practice to screen patients.

Other questions are asked to determine how alcohol or drugs affect the patient's daily life, job, and family. Have there been hospitalizations, arrests, or previous attempts to stop use? How is drug use supported financially?

Drug screening in office practice can be very useful in diagnosing and managing these patients. Individuals often abuse more than one drug and often minimize their illness. Other drugs that patients may be taking (often called secondary drugs of abuse) can be important, because in a patient's quest to change these behaviors, it is not only necessary to abstain from the main drug of abuse but all drugs of abuse that potentiate the addictive behavior. If a patient has a problem with cocaine but also drinks alcohol, both drugs need to be eliminated. If the patient continues to drink alcohol, it may lead to behaviors that can promote a return to cocaine abuse in the future.

To follow patients who are undergoing maintenance therapy, obtaining random drug screens can be very useful in verifying the information the patients give. When things are not going well with treatment, drug screening may confirm drug use. Voluntary drug screening with the patient's approval is highly recommended. The patient can be told that the drug screen is an important tool that is used routinely in practice. Involuntary drug screening is very controversial. It places the physician in an adversarial role with the patient, and for that reason it is not recommended.

In the case of alcohol abuse, because alcohol has a characteristic odor and causes familiar behaviors, drug screening for alcoholism in the office is less common. It is possible to obtain an accurate serum level for alcohol from most laboratories.

DIAGNOSIS

Diagnostic tests are used in this disease mainly to assess end-organ damage and to confirm which drugs are being used by the patient (Table 77-3).

TABLE 77-3
DIAGNOSTIC TESTS TO ASSESS END-ORGAN DAMAGE

Test	Reason For Testing
Complete blood count with differential platelet count	Anemia and bone marrow suppression
Vitamin B_{12} and folate levels	Vitamin B_{12} or folate deficiency
Creatinine, blood urea nitrogen, and urinalysis	Kidney function
Electrolytes	Fluid and electrolyte status
Creatine phosphokinase	Rhabdomyolysis

TABLE 77-3 (CONTINUED)

Test	Reason For Testing
LDH, GOT, alkaline phosphatase, bilirubin, and GGT	Liver function
Amylase and lipase	Pancreatic function
Ammonia level	Hepatic encephalopathy
Toxicology screen	Test for other drugs of abuse
VDRL, HIV, pregnancy screen, hepatitis panel, gonorrhea, *Chlamydia* cultures	Tests for other sexually transmitted diseases and diseases transmitted by blood products

Note. LDH = lactate dehydrogenase; GOT = glutamine-oxaloacetic transaminase; GGT = γ-glutamyltransferase; VDRL = Venereal Disease Research Laboratory; HIV = human immunodeficiency virus.

TREATMENT

Treatment of alcoholism or a drug abuse problem is accomplished in two phases. The first is getting rid of the substance from the body and treating the related symptoms of withdrawal (detoxification). The second phase is usually more problematic. This involves psychologic and behavioral therapies to continue abstaining from the drug or drugs of abuse.

Detoxification usually involves careful management of a patient in an inpatient setting or an intensive outpatient setting. Patients must be monitored for signs of withdrawal and given medical therapy to modify acute symptoms. It should be noted that withdrawal symptoms can be mild or severe in nature.

In the case of alcohol withdrawal, patients can have nervous system hyperexcitability, which can lead to uncontrollable shaking (tremors) or severe seizures. Symptoms can occur within 6–12 hours after ingestion of their last drink. These symptoms are usually controlled with benzodiazepines and fluid and electrolyte management. Severe symptoms such as headache; disorientation; autonomic hyperactivity; agitation; and tactile, visual, and auditory hallucinations indicate that the patient is developing delirium tremors. This occurs usually 2–4 days after cessation of alcohol ingestion. Patients may need intravenous benzodiazepines on fixed dosage schedules to prevent them from doing harm to themselves or others. Thiamine, magnesium, folate, and pyridoxine are useful in preventing Wernicke's syndrome, an acute nervous system disorder caused by nutritional deficiency, which produces symptoms of confusion, unsteady gait (ataxia), and rapid eye movements (nystagmus).

During opioid detoxification patients may demonstrate mild symptoms, which consist of anxiety, insomnia, tearing, increased perspiration, mydriasis, loss of appetite, tremors, hot and cold flashes, and generalized aching. More severe symptoms include these features plus changes in vital signs with increased blood pressure, increased temperature, increased pulse, increased respirations, vomiting, diarrhea, and hemoconcentration. Clonidine is helpful in controlling the cardiovascular symptoms but not the insomnia, anxiety, or generalized aching.

Methadone can also be used for narcotic withdrawal, but since methadone is a narcotic itself, there is controversy as to whether to replace the harmful effects of one form of a narcotic with another. Also since it is very difficult to withdraw most patients from methadone completely, the usual treatment is to wean them down to a minimum dose and have them placed in a methadone treatment program for ongoing maintenance.

There is no specific treatment for cocaine withdrawal. Withdrawal can produce insomnia, anxiety, increased appetite, and severe depression. Cocaine withdrawal is usually not life-threatening. Drugs used to help resolve these symptoms are bromocriptine, carbamazepine, and desipramine.

The second phase of treatment involves getting the patient the social, psychologic, and behavioral support they need to remain drug free for a lifetime. This support usually involves a team approach so that patients can obtain the occupational training, drug counseling, family therapy, and group and individual therapy that they may need. Twelve-step programs such as Alcoholics Anonymous and Narcotics Anonymous have been extremely useful in helping some patients remain in recovery.

PROGNOSIS

Alcoholism and drug abuse are lifelong chronic disease processes. They can have periods of exacerbation and remission. Patients that drop out of therapy are more likely to go back to their previous drug-seeking behaviors. It is a struggle that continues throughout the patient's life.

SUGGESTED READING

Goodwin DW: *Alcoholism: The Facts*. Oxford, UK: Oxford University Press, 1994.

Johnson VE: *Intervention. How to Help Someone Who Does Not Want Help*. Minneapolis, MN: Johnson Institute, 1986.

Winger G, Hoffman FG, Woods JH: *A Handbook on Drug and Alcohol Abuse*, 3rd ed. New York, NY: Oxford University Press, 1992.

CHAPTER 78
Anxiety Disorders

Kevin S. Ferentz, M.D.

INTRODUCTION

Anxiety is a symptom, not a disease. Just as patients with chest pain are given a specific diagnosis (e.g., angina), patients with anxiety should also be given a specific diagnosis. This means becoming familiar with the different forms anxiety can take and recognizing that there may be considerable overlap in patients. Most patients with anxiety disorders are treated with various anxiolytic or antidepressant medications along with psychotherapy and self-help materials. In general, anxiety disorders begin in early adulthood.

PATIENT 1

S. Harding, a 23-year-old physical therapy student, is brought in by her friend because of several "attacks" she has had over the past few weeks. The episodes occurred in school and at home. During the attacks the patient reported feeling her heart racing, shortness of breath, tingling in her hands, nausea, and "feeling like something terrible was going to happen." She feels well between attacks, although she is increasingly concerned that she will have another attack while she is in class.

CLINICAL PRESENTATION

Panic disorder is characterized by recurrent, unexpected panic attacks, which cause the patient concern. A panic attack is the sudden onset of intense fear in which at least four of the following fourteen symptoms develop:

- Palpitations
- Trembling or shaking
- Choking
- Nausea
- Fear of losing control or going crazy
- Numbness or tingling
- Derealization (feelings of unreality)
- Depersonalization (feeling detached from oneself)
- Sweating
- Shortness of breath or smothering
- Chest pain
- Feeling dizzy or lightheaded
- Fear of dying
- Chills or hot flushes

Panic attacks reach peak intensity within 10 minutes and typically last for about 30 minutes.

EPIDEMIOLOGY

The lifetime prevalence of panic disorder is 1.5%–3.5%. One-year prevalence rates are between 1%–2%. Panic disorder occurs twice as often in women as in men. While many patients with panic disorder can be cured, as many as 25% of patients with panic disorder have a chronic course.

> Patients with panic disorder often present to the emergency room and are worked-up for medical complaints such as chest pain. The average patient with panic disorder sees more than 10 physicians before a diagnosis is made.

TREATMENT

Panic disorder must always be treated initially with education. Patients should be offered a self-help book (see Suggested Reading), which may be all they need. While benzodiazepines are often used to treat panic disorder, the issues of dependence and sedation make alternative drug choices desirable. Both tricyclic antidepressants and selective serotonin-reuptake inhibitors (SSRIs) have been found to be effective in reducing panic.

PATIENT 2

T. Holmes, a 27-year-old man, has been experiencing panic attacks for the past several months. He now reports that he is afraid to take the bus to work since he has had several attacks while on the bus. On further questioning, he also admits to avoiding restaurants and theaters since he is afraid he might have a panic attack while in those public places.

CLINICAL PRESENTATION

Agoraphobia commonly occurs in patients with panic disorder but can occur in the absence of panic. It is defined as anxiety about being in places from which escape might be difficult in the event of a panic attack. If a patient has an attack in a certain location he may begin to avoid that location. As more situations are avoided, the patient's life becomes more affected and constricted.

EPIDEMIOLOGY

In clinical settings, most patients with agoraphobia have a diagnosis of panic disorder. Agoraphobia occurs three times more often in women than in men.

TREATMENT

As with panic disorder, patients with agoraphobia must learn to expose themselves to the situations they fear. Patients begin to see that panic is uncomfortable but not life-threatening. A number of excellent self-help books are available along with programs that use "exposure therapy." Antidepressants are often helpful.

PATIENT 3

G. Stevens, a 25-year-old woman, comes to see the physician for help dealing with her extreme fear of flying in an airplane. Her mother has become ill and is a great distance away, necessitating her to fly home to see her. The patient reports that she has only flown once, as a child, and she now has intense fear of getting on an airplane.

CLINICAL PRESENTATION

Patients with a *specific phobia* develop a significant and persistent fear of a specific object or situation. Exposure to this stimulus causes the patient to experience anxiety, often in the form of a panic attack. The phobic stimulus is generally avoided. The diagnosis is made when the avoidance or fear of the stimulus interferes with the person's daily living.

EPIDEMIOLOGY

Women are affected by specific phobia more often than men. The lifetime prevalence is approximately 10%.

TREATMENT

Patients with specific phobias are often treated with gradual exposure to the phobic stimulus; this is called desensitization. Patients with specific phobia who must infrequently face the inciting experience can also be treated with short-acting benzodiazepines.

PATIENT 4

J. Harrison, a 45-year-old man, has just gotten a job as a salesman and, as part of his job, he must make presentations to his fellow salesmen. However, he reports an intense fear of getting up to speak in front of a group of people. He is afraid he is going to have to change jobs.

CLINICAL PRESENTATION

Social phobia is a marked and persistent fear of social or performance situations. The fear may take the form of a panic attack. The fear or avoidance must significantly affect the person's life in order to make the diagnosis.

EPIDEMIOLOGY

The lifetime prevalence of social phobia ranges from 3% to 13%, and men appear to be affected as often as women.

TREATMENT

Social phobia can be treated with psychotherapy, although many patients are now effectively treated with SSRIs. Small doses of beta-blockers can also be used to treat acute performance anxiety, which shares some of the symptoms of social phobia.

PATIENT 5

K. Lang, a 32-year-old woman, presents with raw, red skin on her hands. Although embarrassed, she admits that she has a great fear of "germs," and she washes her hands as often as 100 times each day. While she realizes her hand washing is excessive, she tells the physician that she gets extremely anxious if she tries to stop.

CLINICAL PRESENTATION

Obsessive-compulsive disorder (OCD) is characterized by recurrent obsessions (thoughts, ideas, images) or compulsions (repetitive behaviors or mental acts). To meet criteria for OCD, the obsessions or compulsions must be time-consuming (at least 1 hour a day) or cause distress or impairment. Common obsessions are thoughts of contamination, doubts (having left a door unlocked or an iron left on), or a need to have things in a particular order (need for symmetry). Compulsions are usually performed in response to an obsession. Common compulsions are hand washing, counting, and "checking" (testing many times to see if a door is locked).

EPIDEMIOLOGY

Once thought relatively rare, OCD is now thought to have a lifetime prevalence of 2.5%. It occurs equally in men and women.

TREATMENT

OCD is usually treated with SSRIs (usually at higher doses than required to treat depression) or clomipramine, a tricyclic anti-depressant.

PATIENT 6

B. Simms, a 49-year-old Vietnam War veteran, is brought in by his wife because of problems he has been having for years, which have recently worsened. He has trouble falling asleep and is plagued by dreams of his war experience. He recently attended a reunion of his combat unit, and since then he has been having frequent "flash-backs" to his days in Vietnam.

CLINICAL PRESENTATION

Post-traumatic stress disorder (PTSD) can occur after a person is exposed to an extremely traumatic event that often involves actual or threatened death or serious bodily harm. Common stressors include military combat, violent personal assault (rape, mugging), and disasters. Affected persons relive the event through recurrent thoughts or dreams. Patients with PTSD try to avoid stimuli that they might associate with the traumatic event. In addition, they experience ongoing symptoms of anxiety. PTSD can occur from days to years after the traumatic event and lasts longer than 1 month.

EPIDEMIOLOGY

Any age group can be affected by PTSD, including children. The lifetime prevalence in the community ranges from 1% to 14%, although studies of at-risk individuals (e.g., combat veterans) indicate a prevalence of 3%–58%.

TREATMENT

Treatment of PTSD often requires long-term psychotherapy. Several studies of SSRIs have shown some promise as an adjunct to psycho-therapy.

> Victims of child-hood physical abuse, sexual abuse, or both can present in adulthood with PTSD.

PATIENT 7

R. Adams, a 35-year-old man, was held-up at gunpoint 2 weeks ago. He comes in stating that since the robbery he feels like he is "in a daze." The patient cannot stop thinking about the robbery, and he finds that he is always looking over his shoulder, worried that he is being followed. The patient is having trouble concentrating at work.

CLINICAL PRESENTATION

Acute stress disorder (ASD) is similar to PTSD, in that it occurs after experiencing a potentially life-threatening event. Unlike PTSD, ASD always occurs within 4 weeks of the traumatic event and lasts for up to 4 weeks.

EPIDEMIOLOGY

The prevalence of ASD depends on the severity and persistence of the traumatic event.

TREATMENT

Acute stress disorder is treated with supportive psychotherapy along with anxiolytic medications, as needed.

PATIENT 8

N. Miche, a 32-year-old man, complains of feeling nervous. He states that he has felt this way "all my life." He states that he is concerned about his job, although his evaluations are excellent. He also complains about decreased energy and muscle aches, although these have been present for some time.

CLINICAL PRESENTATION

Generalized anxiety disorder (GAD) is characterized by excessive worry for at least 6 months, although most patients report these feelings for many years. Patients with GAD worry excessively about routine life circumstances and are unable to keep the anxious thoughts from interfering with their lives. In addition to their anxiety, patients with GAD must also have at least three other symptoms from the following list:

- Restlessness
- Easily fatigued
- Difficulty concentrating
- Irritability
- Muscle tension
- Sleep disturbance

EPIDEMIOLOGY

As with most anxiety disorders, GAD often begins in adolescence. The lifetime prevalence rate is believed to be 5%. GAD is diagnosed somewhat more frequently in women. The course of the illness tends to be chronic, but it fluctuates in intensity.

TREATMENT

Patients with GAD may benefit from psychotherapy as well as general stress-reduction techniques such as exercise and meditation. Buspirone, a unique anxiolytic medication, is primarily indicated for the treatment of GAD. Benzodiazepines can also be used to treat this disorder.

SUGGESTED READING

American Psychiatric Association: *Diagnostic and Statistical Manual of Mental Disorders*, 4th ed. Washington, DC: American Psychiatric Association, 1994.

Marks IM: *Living With Fear*. New York, NY: McGraw-Hill, 1980.

Weeks C: *Hope and Help For Your Nerves*. New York, NY: Hawthorne Books, 1968.

CHAPTER 79
Depressive Disorders

Marcia B. Szewczyk, M.D.

PATIENT

M. Werson, a 35-year-old woman, complains of not feeling well and having no energy. As she talks to the physician, she begins to cry, stating that she feels so bad that she is unable to concentrate at work or take care of her children at home. On further questioning she reports that she felt like this once before after her divorce when she was treated by her physician for depression.

CLINICAL PRESENTATION

Most patients who are depressed initially seek treatment through their primary care physician. However, depression is frequently not recognized as the patient often does not complain of depression but rather reports vague somatic symptoms such as fatigue. Frequent office visits for unexplained physical symptoms or complaints of marital discord, job-related difficulties, or problems with children may also reflect depression. The physician needs to have a high index of suspicion, enquiring about symptoms of depression when this occurs. There are no laboratory tests to confirm the presence of depression. It is a clinical diagnosis based on the presence of classic symptoms.

> Depression can seriously impair patients' ability to function in any sphere of their lives. The worst case scenario is suicide.

To meet the *Diagnosis and Statistical Manual of Mental Disorders*, 4th ed. (*DSM-IV*) criteria for *major depressive disorder*, the patient must have either anhedonia or depressed mood accompanied by at least four of the following symptoms:

- Appetite disturbance
- Fatigue
- Loss of motivation
- Low self-esteem
- Poor concentration or indecisiveness
- Psychomotor agitation or retardation
- Sadness
- Sleep disturbance

> Major depression is an acute and severe episode of depression, which has been present for at least 2 weeks.

- Somatic complaints
- Suicidal ideation

Signs of depression may include significant weight changes (most often decreased), poor eye contact, anxious behavior (such as pacing or hand wringing), tearfulness, and psychomotor retardation.

EPIDEMIOLOGY

Depression is a common disorder that affects women more often than men. It most frequently occurs between ages 18 and 44 with the average age of onset in the mid-twenties. Often a chronic disease, depression is characterized by repeat episodes. Relapse, which is defined as recurrence of symptoms within 6 months after treatment, occurs often because of inadequate length of treatment. An initial diagnosis of depression in the elderly is often associated with medical illness, especially myocardial infarction, cancer, and stroke.

Depression is thought to occur secondary to changes in the levels of central nervous system (CNS) neurotransmitters and is probably also influenced by hormonal factors. It can occur as a result of diseases such as hypothyroidism and multiple sclerosis. Medications may also cause depression. Other psychiatric illnesses in which depression is a predominant finding include:

Dysthymia—depression that is milder than that characterized as major depression but still interferes with optimal functioning. Symptoms must be present for at least 2 years and may lead to major depression.

Premenstrual syndrome—depression that occurs only during the luteal phase of the menstrual cycle

Seasonal affective disorder—depression that recurs seasonally, most often in the winter

Abnormal grief reaction—depression that occurs in relation to grieving but is particularly severe or persistent

Adjustment reaction with depressed mood—depression that occurs in response to a significant stressor or stressors

Postpartum depression—depression that occurs in a woman during the first year after childbirth

Bipolar disorder—depression that alternates with episodes of mania

Risk factors for depression include the following:

- Family history of depression (except for late onset depression after age 45)

- Previous depression
- Prior suicide attempts
- Postpartum state
- Presence of other psychiatric disease (particularly anxiety)
- Serious medical illness
- Chronic pain syndrome
- Substance abuse
- Social stressors such as sexual abuse and domestic violence
- Lack of social support
- Major losses such as death of a loved one, divorce, or a job loss

> The presence of risk factors for depression should alert the physician to the possibility of depression.

DIAGNOSIS

A thorough history and physical examination are necessary to identify risk factors, drug or medication use, concurrent medical or psychiatric illness, and to evaluate depressive symptoms. Depressive symptoms and alcohol dependence frequently occur together and both are risk factors

> To make a diagnosis of depression one has to suspect it.

for each other. Suicide risk and intent should be ascertained by asking if patients have considered death or suicide, if they have thoughts of how they would commit suicide, and whether or not they have the means to do so. The need for laboratory work depends on the degree of suspicion of other medical disorders. Screening questionnaires such as the Beck, Zung, or Hamilton Depression Scales can help uncover depression and are useful but are not a replacement for sound clinical judgment.

> Optimal treatment of depression often combines drug therapy with counseling.

TREATMENT

Early treatment increases the likelihood of a successful response. Counseling may be given by the primary care physician or involve the use of support groups or a mental health professional. If possible, involvement of the patient's family during treatment is advised. Counseling is especially useful when psychosocial stressors are present, and it is often adequate treatment alone for adjustment or grief reactions. Patients with wintertime seasonal affective disorder (SAD) frequently respond to light therapy, which may also be

> Patients with depression need to have close follow-up for multiple reasons: to assess safety issues; provide support, therapy, or both; and monitor medication side effects and response.

used prophylactically. However, most patients with major depression require antidepressant medications. Response to medication may take anywhere from 2 to 6 weeks. The goal of treatment should be *complete* relief from symptoms. Medications should be continued for at least 1 year to prevent relapse and recurrence. In patients who have experienced more than one episode of depression, longer treatment is recommended. Medication should be tapered slowly when discontinued. If there is a high risk of suicide, the patient needs hospital admission.

More than 20 drugs are marketed for depression in the United States. No one antidepressant has been shown to have a therapeutic advantage if used in the proper dosage and for the recommended length of time. Medication choices should be based on an attempt to target the patient's symptoms, side effect profiles, concurrent medication use, prior response to antidepressant treatment, age, and cost.

Referral to a psychiatrist is recommended when the diagnosis is not clear, when there is a high risk of suicide, when the patient has bipolar disorder, when there is an inadequate response to treatment, or when there is another psychiatric illness present that complicates treatment.

There are four major groups of antidepressant medication: the tricyclic antidepressants (TCAs), the selective serotonin-reuptake inhibitors (SSRIs), the monoamine oxidase inhibitors (MAOIs), and several more drugs that are not easily classified, including bupropion, nefazodone, trazodone, and venlafaxine. The TCAs and the SSRIs are usually used initially for treatment with the other medications being reserved as second-line agents. The SSRIs are used most frequently as they have less adverse effects and are better tolerated, particularly by the elderly. The SSRIs also have quicker onset of action and are markedly safer than TCAs in the event of an overdose.

TABLE 79-1
CHARACTERISTICS OF ANTIDEPRESSANT MEDICATIONS

TCAs
- Inexpensive (generic only)
- Sedation, dry mouth, dizziness, weight gain, constipation, and urinary retention
- Arrhythmias
- Overdoses may be fatal

SSRIs
- Expensive
- Nausea, diarrhea, anorexia, and headache
- Sexual dysfunction
- Insomnia and agitation
- Many drug interactions

Trazodone
- Sedation and dizziness
- Priapism
- Expensive

Nefazodone
- Sedation and dizziness
- Sexual dysfunction
- Many drug interactions

Venlafaxine
- Expensive
- Nausea, headache, and dry mouth
- Sexual dysfunction
- Sleep disturbance and anxiety
- Many drug interactions

Bupropion
- Expensive
- Headache, nausea, dry mouth, and constipation
- Agitation, insomnia, and tremor
- Many drug reactions
- Seizures

MAOIs
- Dizziness
- Sleep disturbance
- Strict diet necessary

SUGGESTED READING

American Psychiatric Association: *Diagnosis and Statistical Manual of Mental Disorders*, 4th ed. Washington, DC: American Psychiatric Association, 1994.

Depression Guideline Panel: *Depression in Primary Care*, vol 1. *Detection and Diagnosis. Clinical Practice Guideline*, no 5. AHCPR Publication No. 93-0550, Rockville, MD: Agency for Health Care Policy and Research, Public Health Service, U.S. Department of Health and Human Services, 1993.

Depression Guideline Panel: *Depression in Primary Care*, vol 2. *Detection and Diagnosis. Clinical Practice Guideline*, no 5. AHCPR Publication No. 93-0551, Rockville, MD: Agency for Health Care Policy and Research, Public Health Service, U.S. Department of Health and Human Services, 1993.

Hales RE, Rakel RE, Rothschild S: Depression: practical tips for detection and treatment. *Patient Care Special Report* 100:16–46, 1996.

Sundberg JE: Optimizing treatment of depression. *Postgrad Med* 99:45–56, 1995.

CHAPTER 80
Domestic Violence

Judith A. Fisher, M.D.

PATIENT

C. Golding, a 24-year-old woman, comes to the physician's office to apply for a secretarial position. When asked why she is changing jobs, she replies that it may help her home situation if she works for a woman boss. On further questioning, the physician discovers that her husband accuses her of having an affair with her present boss, often waits outside of her office window, and punches her in the evenings if she smiled while taking dictation. In further discussion, it is discovered that her husband takes her paycheck and demands that she ask him for money when grocery shopping, buying clothing, and paying for household expenses.

CLINICAL PRESENTATION

Domestic violence is thought to be a hidden epidemic. However, those who work with domestic violence contend that it is not hidden, and indeed, the signs and symptoms are obvious. Furthermore, both victims and perpetrators say that they would discuss domestic violence with their physicians if asked.

Domestic violence can take the form of physical, verbal, psychologic, economic, or sexual abuse. Domestic violence is defined as any act of coercion or threat of coercion carried out by an intimate. The term domestic violence is most often used for spousal abuse and, in particular, the abuse of women. It must be remembered that men and same-sex partners may also be victims. Domestic violence reflects uneven power in a relationship. The more powerful partner abuses the less powerful partner. The greater the discrepancy in power, the more severe is the abuse. The perpetrator of the abuse disenfranchises the victim as in the case above where the husband took the patient's pay and demanded that she ask him for small aliquots.

The abuse may be unwittingly revealed by either the perpetrator

> Most victims and perpetrators say that they would discuss their domestic violence if asked by a physician. Victims and perpetrators need to feel safe to answer questions of abuse honestly.

or the victim. Commonly, the victim presents to the emergency room with signs of physical trauma or after a suicide attempt. The primary care physician may see the abused patient with multiple unrelated complaints, such as fatigue, depression, anxiety, panic disorder, insomnia, or substance abuse. Any treating physician must consider domestic violence in the differential diagnosis of chronic fatigue syndrome, fibromyalgia, hypoglycemia, irritable bowel syndrome, chronic headaches, chronic abdominal pain, and post-traumatic stress disorder (PTSD), all of which have vague symptoms and no definitive diagnostic tools. Perpetrators of domestic violence themselves may suffer from substance abuse, personality disorders, PTSD, anxiety, or depression. It is not uncommon for perpetrators to ponder or attempt suicide. Thus, questions concerning domestic violence should be asked in many circumstances.

EPIDEMIOLOGY

Domestic violence strikes one in four families. One-third of women who are murdered in the United States are killed by their husbands or boyfriends. Along with the human cost, the National Crime Survey estimated the cost of domestic violence at 40,000 patient visits, 30,000 emergency room visits, and 100,000 days of hospitalization a year. As many as 35% of women visiting the emergency room are there for symptoms of abuse. Only 4% of these women are diagnosed appropriately. Domestic violence cuts across all socioeconomic groups. For many women, spousal abuse first begins during a pregnancy. Although domestic violence cuts across all socioeconomic classes, the poor and underprivileged are affected in greater proportions.

> Physical safety is a huge issue for the victims of domestic violence. Statistics show that one-third of women who are murdered are killed by a domestic partner.

Unfortunately, the act of leaving a relationship can place women at a 75% greater risk of injury or death. Many women are finally pushed to leave their home or seek help when they discover that the violence is affecting their children.

The violence does affect children. In a home where there is spousal abuse, it is likely that the children are also being abused. With or without direct physical abuse of the children, the children show a greater tendency towards anger, acting out, depression, chronic headaches, chronic abdominal pain, and behavioral problems. Victims and perpetrators are likely to have lived in a home where domestic violence occurred. Thus, abuse spans generations.

SCREENING

Many questions and questionnaires have been developed as screening tools for domestic violence. Domestic violence advocates feel that every patient should be asked about abuse. One should keep in mind that victims must feel secure and safe or they will not answer the questions honestly. Many victims have been threatened with death or death of their children if they seek help for the abuse. When questioning a suspected victim, it is important for the physician to build trust and to have a plan in mind to insure the victim's safety. Any questions could be prefaced with a statement such as "Many people live in fear of being harmed." Good initial questions would be "Is there anywhere in your life that you feel threatened or unsafe?" "Has anyone ever threatened to harm you or your children?" This can be followed with "Do you feel safe at home?" These questions could be followed by a statement such as "Everyone has the right to feel safe; if you ever feel unsafe in any way, I hope that you will be able to contact me as I have helped others and I could help you, too."

> The most important factor in the diagnosis of domestic violence is a high index of suspicion by the health care provider.

Conversely, questions can be asked to screen a perpetrator. These questions could be prefaced with, "Many people have experienced physical, verbal, or psychologic abuse in their lives. Have you ever been abused or been abusive to someone?" Further screening questions would be: "Have you ever harmed anyone?" "Have you ever been so angry or distraught that you felt as if you might harm someone?" "Have you ever felt sorry about something that you have done to someone else?" A statement such as: "Many people do things to others that they regret later. I hope that you would be able to turn to me if these feelings ever occur. I have helped others to stop the pain, and I would help you, too."

DIAGNOSIS

A thorough skin examination may reveal bruises of various ages. For legal reasons skin bruising should be photographed. A radiographic bone survey may reveal multiple fracture sites (old and new).

TREATMENT

It is important for the physician to validate the victim's or perpetrator's feelings, acknowledge that they might have a sense of shame about the abuse, and acknowledge that they may at times feel that they deserve to receive or continue the abuse. It is important to state that no one deserves abuse of any type and that, in fact, we all have a right to personal freedom, safety, and respect. If an individual's safety is threatened, the victim along with children should be sent to a safe place. If the victim refuses or is not in immediate danger, the victim and the perpetrator should be given the name of a local support group, told of the criminal nature of abuse, offered legal aid, sent for counseling, and given a follow-up appointment with the physician. Any suspected victim should be given the National Domestic Violence hot line, 800-333-SAFE, which is a 24-hour resource for victims. Most states have local domestic violence programs. Treating physicians should be aware of these local resources and provide written information to a suspected victim. Treating physicians should also be aware that many people will feel anger toward the perpetrator. It is important to keep in touch with these individuals and offer them empathy and facts while empowering them to seek the help that they need to stop the abuse. It is important that the physician keep meticulous notes and photographs as these will be crucial in any legal proceedings.

SUGGESTED READING

American Medical Association: Diagnostic and treatment guidelines on domestic violence. *Arch Fam Med* 1:39–47, 1992.

American Medical Association: *What You Can Do about Family Violence*. Chicago, IL: American Medical Association, 1992.

Sugg N, Inui T: Primary care physicians' response to domestic violence. *JAMA* 267:3157–3160, 1992.

SECTION III
Pharmacologic Treatment of Ambulatory Care Patients

CHAPTER 81
Frequently Encountered Drugs and Their Clinical Uses

Julienne K. Kirk, Pharm.D.

The following is a list of commonly used drugs and unlabeled uses in clinical practice. An unlabeled use of a drug is also known as off-label prescribing. The American Medical Association estimates that 40%–60% of all United States prescriptions are for off-label use. The labeled indication, which is the Food and Drug Administration approved use of the drug, is also listed. This list is in no way totally comprehensive, but it includes frequently encountered drugs. Some insurance companies will not cover payment of certain medications unless the drug is being used for a labeled indication. In many cases, there are multiple brand names of the product on the market.

Generic Name	Trade Name	Labeled Approved Use	Unlabeled Use
Amitriptyline	Elavil	Depression	Chronic pain[a] CFS IBS Insomnia Fibromyalgia Idiopathic pruritus Pathologic laughing and weeping
Clomipramine	Anafranil	OCD	Chronic pain[a] Eating disorders Panic disorder
Desipramine	Norpramin	Depression	Cocaine withdrawal Eating disorders
Doxepin	Sinequan	Depression	ADHD Chronic pain[a] Dermatologic disorders[b] PUD

Generic Name	Trade Name	Labeled Approved Use	Unlabeled Use
Imipramine	Tofranil	Depression	Chronic pain[a] Enuresis IBS Panic disorder
Nortriptyline	Pamelor	Depression	Dermatologic disorders[b] IBS PMS
Protriptyline	Vivactil	Depression	Obstructive sleep apnea
Trimipramine	Surmontil	Depression	Dermatologic disorders[b] PUD
Bupropion	Wellbutrin	Depression Smoking cessation	Chronic pain[a]
Fluoxetine	Prozac	Bulimia nervosa Depression OCD	Alcoholism Anorexia nervosa ADHD Bipolar disorder Borderline personality disorder Cataplexy and narcolepsy CFS Kleptomania L-Dopa-induced dyskinesia Migraine and tension headaches Obesity PTSD PMS Recurrent syncope Social phobia Tourette's syndrome Trichotillomania
Fluvoxamine	Luvox	OCD	Depression
Paroxetine	Paxil	Depression OCD Panic disorder	Diabetic neuropathy Headaches Premature ejaculation
Phenelzine	Nardil	Depression	Bulimia Cocaine addiction Migraine headache Night terrors Panic disorder PTSD

Generic Name	Trade Name	Labeled Approved Use	Unlabeled Use
Tranylcypro-mine	Parnate	Depression	Bulimia Binswanger's encephalopathy Multiple sclerosis Panic disorder
Methylpheni-date	Ritalin	ADHD Narcolepsy	Depression (elderly) Hiccups (anesthesia-related)
Pemoline	Cylert	ADHD	Narcolepsy
Buspirone	BuSpar	Anxiety	PMS ADHD
Lithium	Eskalith	Manic-depression	Improve neutrophil counts Cluster headache PMS Bulimia Alcoholism SIADH Tardive dyskinesia Hyperthyroidism Postpartum affective disorder Corticosteroid-induced psychosis Topically for dermatitis and genital herpes
Chlorproma-zine	Thorazine	Intractable hiccups Psychotic disorders Nausea and vomiting Severe behavioral problems in children	Agitation in the elderly Acute migraine headaches
Haloperidol	Haldol	Psychotic disorders Tourette's syndrome Severe behavioral problems in children ADHD	Antiemetic Agitation in the elderly
Carbamaze-pine	Tegretol	Seizures Trigeminal neuralgia	Psychiatric disorders[c] Alcohol, cocaine, and benzodiazepine withdrawal Chorea

Generic Name	Trade Name	Labeled Approved Use	Unlabeled Use
Gabapentine	Neurontin	Seizures	Migraine headache Pain Postherpetic neuralgia
Phenytoin	Dilantin	Seizures	Antiarrhythmic Trigeminal neuralgia Preeclampsia
Primidone	Mysoline	Seizures	Benign familial tremor
Clonazepam	Klonopin	Seizures	Periodic leg movement Parkinsonian dysarthria Bipolar disorder Multifocal tic disorders Schizophrenia Neuralgias
Baclofen	Lioresal	Muscle spasms	Trigeminal neuralgia Intractable hiccups Tardive dyskinesia
Dantrolene	Dantrium	Spasticity Malignant hyperthermia	Exercise-induced muscle pain Stroke Neuroleptic malignant syndrome
Levodopa	Larodopa	Parkinsonism	Herpes zoster pain Restless legs syndrome
Nitroglycerin	Various	Acute angina Angina prophylaxis	Impotence Peripheral vascular disease Hypertensive crisis
Clonidine	Catapres	Hypertension	ADHD Alcohol withdrawal Allergen-induced asthma Diabetic diarrhea Growth delay in children Menopausal flushing Methadone/opiate detoxification Postherpetic neuralgia Smoking cessation Tourette's syndrome Ulcerative colitis

Generic Name	Trade Name	Labeled Approved Use	Unlabeled Use
Guanfacine	Tenex	Hypertension	Heroin withdrawal Migraine headache ADHD
Prazosin	Minipress	Hypertension	Refractory CHF Raynaud's vasospasm BPH
Doxazosin	Cardura	Hypertension BPH	CHF
Terazosin	Hytrin	Hypertension BPH	CHF
Hydralazine	Apresoline	Hypertension	Afterload reduction in CHF Severe aortic insufficiency and after valve replacement
Atenolol	Tenormin	Hypertension Angina MI	Ventricular arrhythmias Migraine prophylaxis Anxiety (stage fright)
Metoprolol	Lopressor	Hypertension Angina Acute MI	Aggressive behavior Akathisia Essential tremor Ventricular arrhythmias Enhancement of cognitive performance in elderly CHF Atrial ectopy in COPD Migraine prophylaxis
Nadolol	Corgard	Hypertension Angina	Aggressive behavior Essential tremor Ventricular arrhythmias Anxiety (stage fright) Rebleeding from esophageal varices Migraine prophylaxis Akathisia
Timolol	Blocadren	Hypertension Migraine prophylaxis MI	Anxiety (stage fright) Essential tremor Ventricular arrhythmias

Generic Name	Trade Name	Labeled Approved Use	Unlabeled Use
Propranolol	Inderal	Hypertension Angina Hypertrophic subaortic stenosis Cardiac arrhythmias MI Pheochromocytoma Migraine headache Essential tremor	Anxiety (stage fright) Thyrotoxicosis symptoms Alcohol withdrawal Aggressive behavior Akathisia Essential tremor Migraine prophylaxis Rebleeding from esophageal varices Vaginal contraceptive Schizophrenia Acute panic symptoms Explosive disorder Anxiety
Captopril	Capoten	Hypertension Heart failure MI Left ventricular dysfunction	Hypertensive crisis Rheumatoid arthritis Primary aldosteronism Raynaud's syndrome Bartter's syndrome Renal artery stenosis
Enalapril	Vasotec	Hypertension CHF MI Left ventricular dysfunction	Diabetic nephropathy
Losartan	Cozaar	Hypertension	CHF
Valsartan	Diovan	Hypertension	CHF
Nifedipine	Adalat Procardia	Hypertension Angina	Migraine headache Raynaud's syndrome CHF Cardiomyopathy Esophageal disorders Biliary and renal colic
Diltiazem	Cardizem Dilacor	Hypertension Angina	Migraine headache Non–Q wave MI Raynaud's syndrome Tardive dyskinesia
Verapamil	Verelan Isoptin Calan	Hypertension Angina Arrhythmias	Migraine and cluster headache Cardiomyopathy Asthma Manic depression Nocturnal leg cramps

Generic Name	Trade Name	Labeled Approved Use	Unlabeled Use
Felodipine	Plendil	Hypertension	CHF Raynaud's syndrome
Amlodipine	Norvasc	Hypertension Angina	CHF
Nimodipine	Nimotop	Subarachnoid hemorrhage	Migraine and cluster headache
Hydrocholoro-thiazide	Esidrix Hydrodiuril Oretic	Hypertension Edema	Calcium nephrolithiasis Osteoporosis Diabetes insipidus
Ethacrynic acid	Edecrin	Ascites Nephrotic syndrome	Glaucoma
Amiloride	Midamor	Edema associated with hypertension or CHF	Lithium-induced polyuria Cystic fibrosis (aerosolized)
Spironolac-tone	Aldactone	Hypertension Edema Hypokalemia Hyperaldos-teronism	PMS Precocious puberty Acne vulgaris Hirsutism
Cholestyra-mine	Questran	Hypercholester-olemia Biliary obstruction	*Clostridium difficile* infection Chronic nonspecific diarrhea Chlordecone pesticide poisoning Digitalis toxicity Thyroid overdose
Finasteride	Proscar	BPH	Prostate cancer Male pattern baldness Acne Hirsutism in women
Cimetidine	Tagamet	Ulcer Hypersecretion Gastrointestinal bleeding	Hyperparathyroidism *Helicobacter pylori* Aspiration pneumonia Chronic viral warts Crohn's disease Urticaria Acetaminophen overdose Herpes zoster

Generic Name	Trade Name	Labeled Approved Use	Unlabeled Use
Metoclopramide	Reglan	Diabetic gastroparesis GERD	Migraine headache Improve lactation Postoperative bezoars Atonic bladder Esophageal variceal bleeding Gastric ulcer Nausea and vomiting Anorexia nervosa
Cisapride	Propulsid	Heartburn GERD	Diabetic gastroparesis Idiopathic constipation IBS
Erythromycin	Various	Infection	Diabetic gastroparesis
Minocycline	Minocin	Infection Acne	Malaria Rheumatoid arthritis
Tetracycline	Various	Infection	Pleural sclerosing agent
Demeclocycline	Declomycin	Infection	Chronic hyponatremia
Metronidazole	Flagyl	Infection Rosacea	Crohn's disease Pseudomembranous colitis *H. pylori*
Sulfonamide	Various	Infection	Ankylosing spondylitis Colitis Crohn's disease Rheumatoid arthritis
Ketoconazole	Nizoral	Fungal infection Cutaneous dermatophyte	Onychomycosis Prostate cancer Cushing's syndrome
Amantadine	Symmetrel	Parkinson's disease Drug-induced EPS Influenza A virus	Fatigue of multiple sclerosis
Ethinyl estradiol Norgestrel	Various Birth Control	Contraception	Uterine bleeding Postcoital contraception Turner's syndrome
Misoprostol	Cytotec	Prevention of NSAID-induced gastric ulcers in high-risk patients	Acute graft rejection Abortifacient agent Induction of labor

Generic Name	Trade Name	Labeled Approved Use	Unlabeled Use
Vitamin E		Vitamin E deficiency	Retinopathy of prematurity Hemolytic anemia Heart disease PMS Aging Sexual dysfunction Athletic performance Cancer Skin conditions Nocturnal leg cramps
Tretinoin	Retin-A	Acne vulgaris	Melasma Fine wrinkles Prevention of basal cell carcinoma Sebaceous hyperplasia
Nicotine (transdermal)	Habitrol Nicoderm Prostep	Smoking cessation	Ulcerative colitis
Minoxidil (topical)	Rogaine	Androgenetic alopecia	Impotence
Terbutaline	Brethine	Asthma	Premature labor
Cromolyn	Intal Nasalcrom Gastrocrom	Asthma Allergic rhinitis Mastocytosis	Food allergies Eczema Dermatitis Ulcerations Urticaria Abdominal pain Hay fever
Warfarin	Coumadin	Anticoagulant	Recurrent TIAs Small cell lung carcinoma Recurrent MI
Ticlopidine	Ticlid	Stroke	Intermittent claudication Chronic arterial occlusion Subarachnoid hemorrhage Open heart surgery Coronary artery bypass graft Primary glomerulonephritis Sickle cell disease AV shunts or fistulas

Generic Name	Trade Name	Labeled Approved Use	Unlabeled Use
Cyclosporine	Sandimmune Neoral	Immunosuppression	Alopecia areata Aplastic anemia Atopic dermatitis Behçet's/JEV disease Biliary cirrhosis Corneal transplantation Crohn's disease Dermatomyositis Graves' ophthalmopathy Diabetes mellitus type I Lichen planus (topically) Lupus nephritis Multiple sclerosis Myasthenia gravis Nephrotic syndrome Pemphigus Polymyositis Psoriatic arthritis Pulmonary sarcoidosis Pyoderma gangrenosum Rheumatoid arthritis Severe psoriasis Steroid-dependent asthma Ulcerative colitis Uveitis
Methotrexate	Various	Antineoplastic chemotherapy Psoriasis Rheumatoid arthritis	Crohn's disease Steroid-dependent asthma
Allopurinol	Zyloprim	Gout Malignancies Calcium oxalate calculi	Mouthwash Arrhythmias *H. pylori* Hematemesis Pancreatic pain Prevent tissue damage

Generic Name	Trade Name	Labeled Approved Use	Unlabeled Use
Colchicine	Colchicine	Gout	Multiple sclerosis Familial Mediterranean fever Cirrhosis Amyloidosis Behçet's/JEV disease Idiopathic thrombocytopenia Scleroderma Dermatologic disorders
Prednisolone	Deltasone Various others	Anti-inflammatory and immunosuppressant	Acute mountain sickness Antiemetic Baterical meningitis Contact dermatitis COPD Depression Eczema Muscular dystrophy Graves' ophthalmopathy Alcoholic hepatitis Hirsutism Respiratory distress syndrome Reactive airways disease Septic shock Acute spinal cord injury Tuberculosis pleurisy
NSAIDS	Various	Inflammation	Alzheimer's disease
Pentoxifylline	Trental	Intermittent claudication	Diabetic neuropathy Diabetic angiopathy TIAs Leg ulcers Sickle cell thalassemia Strokes High altitude sickness Asthenospermia Hearing disorders Aphthous stomatitis Raynaud's syndrome Reduction of tumor necrosis factor levels in HIV and AIDs patients

Note. CFS = chronic fatigue syndrome; IBS = irritable bowel syndrome; OCD = obsessive-compulsive disorder; ADHD = attention-deficit hyperactivity disorder; PUD = peptic ulcer disease; PMS = premenstrual syndrome; PTSD = post-traumatic stress disorder; SIADH = syndrome of inappropriate and diuretic hormone; CHF = congestive heart failure; BPH = benign prostatic hyperplasia; MI = myocardial infarction; COPD = chronic obstructive pulmonary disease; GERD = gastroesophageal reflux disease; EPS = extrapyramidal reactions; NSAIDs = nonsteroidal anti-inflammatory drugs; TIAs = transient ischemic attacks; AV = arteriovenous; HIV = human immunodeficiency virus; AIDS = acquired immunodeficiency syndrome.

[a] Chronic pain includes migraine, chronic tension headache, diabetic neuropathy, tic douloureux, cancer pain, postherpetic neuralgia, and arthritic pain.
[b] Dermatologic disorder includes chronic urticaria and angioedema and nocturnal pruritus in atopic eczema.
[c] Psychiatric disorders include bipolar disorder, unipolar depression, schizoaffective illness, resistant schizophrenia, dyscontrol syndrome associated with limbic system dysfunction, intermittent explosive disorder, PTSD, and atypical psychosis.

Index

Note: Page numbers followed by t refer to tables; page numbers in italics refer to figures.